Real Food
for
Healthy Kids

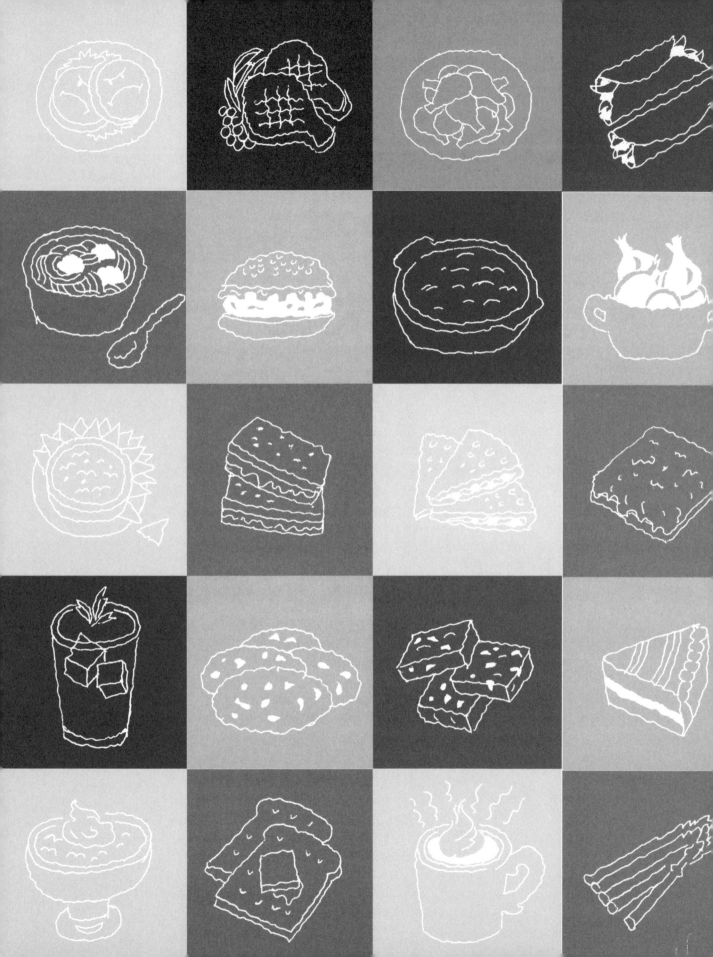

Real Food *for* Healthy Kids

200+ easy, wholesome recipes

Tracey Seaman
and Tanya Wenman Steel

WILLIAM MORROW
An Imprint of HarperCollins*Publishers*

HarperCollins books may be purchased for educational, business, or sales promotional use. For information please write: Special Markets Department, HarperCollins Publishers, 10 East 53rd Street, New York, NY 10022.

Designed by Jaime Putorti
Line art provided and drawn by David Wenman
Pyramid cartoon provided and drawn by Tom Fishburne

Library of Congress Cataloging-in-Publication Data

Seaman, Tracy.
    Real food for healthy kids : 200+ easy, wholesome recipes / by Tracey Seaman and Tanya Wenman Steel.
        p. cm.
    Includes index.
    ISBN 978-0-06-085791-2
1. Cookery, American.   2. Children—Nutrition.   3. Quick and easy cookery.   I. Steel, Tanya Wenman.   II. Title.   III. Title: Real food for healthy kids, 200 plus easy, wholesome recipes.
    TX715.S145718 2008
    641.5973—dc22   200703005

08   09   10   11   12   WBC/QB   10   9   8   7   6   5   4   3   2

The authors will be donating a portion of their proceeds to several children's and hunger-relief charities, including HALO, Helping Autism Through Learning and Outreach, and America's Second Harvest, the nation's largest food bank, which feeds 9 million children annually.

contents

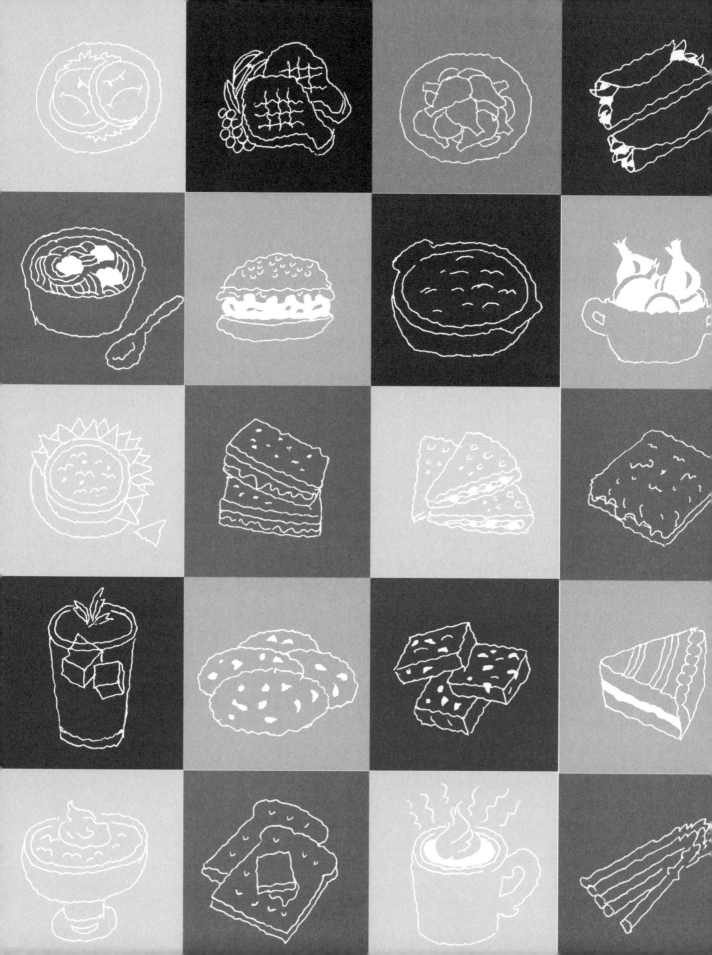

acknowledgments

We would like to thank our agent, David Black, for being such a brilliant mentor and advocate; our hardworking and talented editor, Lyssa Keusch, and her trusty right hand, May Chen; Harriet Bell and Susan Friedland, who both added their vision and expertise in the beginning of the project; and to the staff at Harper-Collins, especially David Sweeney. Our thanks also to Registered Dietician Dana Lilienthal, who analyzed every recipe, as well as to Luanne Petrie, MSRD, CBE, who also gave us invaluable input; Dr. Frank Greer, professor of pediatrics at the University of Wisconsin and chairman of the Committee on Nutrition of the American Academy of Pediatrics; Tom Fishburne, who created the hilarious and quite accurate pyramid cartoon; and David Wenman, Tanya's dad, who drew all the other sweet and funny illustrations.

~ TANYA STEEL'S ACKNOWLEDGMENT ~

I would like to begin by thanking my book partner, Tracey Seaman, for her continual creativity, hard work, and good nature. I'd like to thank all of the thousands of people I've worked with in the past two decades, especially my mentors, who include Felicia Milewicz, Catherine Bigwood, Ila Stanger, Trish Hall, Bill Garry, Barbara Fairchild, and Jamie Pallot. I'd also like to thank my close friends for their support, love, and good humor. I'd like to praise my parents, Carol and David Wenman, for all of their constant love and support, and my sister and brother-in-law, Nicola Wenman and Kevin Hart, for the same daily affection and kindness. A universe-sized thanks to my wonderful husband and partner in life, Bob Steel, who has grown up along with me; together we have carved out a beautiful life. Most of all, I'd like to thank my children, William and Sanger, who not only patiently and willingly tasted every single recipe in this book plus dozens that didn't make it in, but also provided quotes, insight, and inspiration. I dedicate this book—and my heart—to them.

~ TRACEY SEAMAN'S ACKNOWLEDGMENT ~

First and foremost I thank my friend and partner, Tanya, the driving force behind our business, without whom this book would not be a reality; and my parents, from whom I learned my first lessons in cooking.

Love and thanks to my kids, Margot and Darren, who had a less than stellar summer while I typed on my laptop at the beach under an umbrella, and to my longtime love, Jeff—sorry for sometimes paying more attention to food than to you. Thanks for eating everything, repeatedly.

Sincere appreciation to my friends, especially Karen Antone and Lena Pfeffer, who inspired various gluten-free and vegetarian recipes; Anna Coco, Dorothy Stack, and Mike and Alison Betz, who tested lots of recipes; and my chums in the magazine industry, especially Lorilynn Longbotham, Pamela Mitchell, and Jim Standard, who feel like family.

To Diana Sturgis, my friend and mentor, thanks for teaching me how to write a good recipe, and to Silvana Nardone, Dana Cowin, Tina Ujlaki, Kempy Minifie, Susan Spungen, Ellen Jacob, and Carol Guthrie-Dovell—thanks for giving me work when it really counted.

foreword

As a pediatrician and as a result of my recent service on the Committee on Nutrition of the American Academy of Pediatrics, I have become very concerned about the rising obesity epidemic among children and adolescents in the United States. In the last several decades, declining physical activity both at home and in school, and the mass marketing of foodstuffs to the pediatric age group, has led to the alarming statistic that almost 35 percent of American children are now considered to be clinically obese or at risk for becoming clinically obese.

We can't ascribe this obesity epidemic to any single factor such as vending machines in our schools, the large quantities of food eaten outside of the home in fast-food restaurants, or the increasing time spent in front of the television screen. In any event, certainly a significant factor in the etiology of this epidemic is the large amount of calorie-dense but nutrient-poor food eaten by our children, both in and out of the home. Surveys show that the average family sits down at the table together for a meal only a few times a week, and even these dinners are often accompanied by tune-ins to the mass media. To overcome the many factors associated with this obesity epidemic, many small, incremental steps have to be taken by both individuals and families toward changing a lifestyle. *Real Food for Healthy Kids* will allow parents to take control of the kinds of foods their children eat.

This cookbook is a guide to healthier, more wholesome eating for the entire family; it will enable parents to instill in their children an appetite and an appreciation for quality homemade, nutritious food. By preparing meals from this book, families will look forward to sitting down together at the table, particularly if parents empower their kids by making the food together. If parents and children follow just a few of the recommendations in this cookbook, they will be well on their way to preventing obesity and its related disorders, including diabetes and heart disease, in their own families.

Please note that my endorsement of this cookbook does not imply that this book has the endorsement of the American Academy of Pediatrics. After reviewing the recipes and the sage nutritional advice contained within, however, I will pass along a copy of *Real Food for Healthy Kids* to the parents of my grandchildren—and my patients!

—*Frank R. Greer, M.D.*
Professor of Pediatrics,
University of Wisconsin,
Chairman, Committee on Nutrition,
American Academy of Pediatrics

Real Food
for
Healthy Kids

introduction

From the moment your child is born, you promise your little angel your undivided attention and love. You also probably make a promise to yourself to keep him or her away from violent and salacious television shows and video games, ensure that he or she gets the best education possible, and vow that fast food and frozen and highly processed products will never pass your cutie pie's lips. How sweet! How noble! How naïve!

Sadly, for most of us, these best intentions fall faster than our energy level at 3:00 P.M., and we feel pretty proud of ourselves if we've limited our toddler to ninety minutes a day of television and convinced Junior to eat three mini-carrots with his chicken nuggets. It's never been harder to incorporate homemade wholesome food into our daily lives, yet fighting this good fight is important, day by day and bite by bite. The foods your child eats will not only influence his well-being in crucial growing years (to say nothing of setting up a preference for certain flavors and textures) but form a pattern of healthy eating for adulthood. Plus, eating together as much as possible has proved more important than we ever knew. Recent studies show that families who eat together more often than the norm of a few times a week eat a healthier diet than those who don't eat as a family much. Also, when those kids become teenagers, studies show they are less likely to get involved with drugs and alcohol, especially if there is consistent conversation before, during, and after the meal as well.

The main problem for most of us, of course, is time. Factor in finicky eating, high food costs, and cooking skills (or a lack thereof) and you have a generation of kids brought up on microwaved hot dogs and frozen pizza. But it doesn't have to be this way. In fact, you shouldn't allow it to be this way. We believe so strongly in the importance of feeding children well that we have spent the last four years developing and testing recipes to find ones that your kids will actually like, while ensuring that each dish is easy to make and as nutritious and wholesome as possible. We hope *Real Food for Healthy Kids* will become your indispensable guide to feeding your progeny, whether they are toddlers or teenagers.

We've struggled with the same issues you have. When Tanya's identical twin boys were born, she faced the daily problem of creating healthy meals that her boys would like, and that, with a full-time job and a daily commute, she could whip up in less time than it took to watch an episode of Pokemon. Tracey, who also works full-time, is a single mom who wrestled daily with what to give her two children, a daughter who is a very picky eater and a son with special needs who is on a strict gluten-free and casein-free diet. So, we turned to each other for ideas and support, and together we came up with a veritable encyclopedia of simple recipes that have now been table-tested by more than a hundred discriminating kids and their parents. What we discovered is that it is easy to make tasty food; what's challenging is to make a variety of delicious dishes that are nutritious and don't take hours to prepare. To that end, we reduced the amounts of sugar, fat, and white flour as much as possible where we could. We then had a noted nutritionist, Dana Lillenthal, R.D., create nutritional analysis for each recipe so that you can decide which best meet your needs and whether your child should watch his caloric intake or should up it.

We are moms with more than a combined forty years in the food business and have spent the last several years devising these wholesome recipes that not just our own children but kids—from six months to into their twenties—from across the country have tasted. Only those that got a sticky thumbs-up or an enthusiastic "awesome" have made it into the book. These recipes, appropriate for breakfast, lunch, dinner, snacks, and parties, can successfully be made by just about anyone. In fact, some can be made with or by kids (those with the junior chef's hat symbol 🎩 are appropriate for school-aged kids to help make) and will satisfy the entire family, not just its smallest—and pickiest—members. This is important, because one of our strongest beliefs is that just as you don't talk down to a child, you don't cater to an inexperienced palate by constantly making a child his or her own dumbed-down, bland food. Nor are you in the business of being a short-order cook; making a different meal for everyone is highly impractical and often necessitates supplementing of processed foods.

We know that you lack a sous-chef (on weeknights, you usually can't count on your kids), and that time can be more precious than money. The same is true with us, so we have focused on the use of fresh, seasonal items and wholesome premium convenience products so that cooking and prep times are as stripped down as possible. And, we've given you plenty of quick dinners—some take only twenty minutes to make, start to finish. Those that are more involved are written to minimize your time in the kitchen. To help you decide which dishes you have time for, we have given ones under an hour a Speed Limit sign 🚸 with an MPR 🚸 rating (or minutes per recipe), which accounts for preparation and cooking time. For more recipe ideas, new information on kids' health and nutrition, and other parents' ideas on what to feed kids, go to our website, www.realfoodforhealthykids.com.

One last thing: We both believe strongly in teaching children that food is one of life's great pleasures, but as with all pleasures, moderation is the key. After all, as the United Nations noted in a report, "One billion of us eat too much while every year, six million children die quietly of hunger." It is for this reason that the two of us, busy moms, want to help feed other people's children, both with the recipes in this book and with some of the money we earn from its sales. A portion of our profits will go to a national hunger relief organization, America's Second Harvest food bank network. We also will be contributing some funds to several autism organizations, including HALO, due to our personal connection with the condition.

Because we care so deeply about our children, your children, and the world's children, it is our hope that *Real Food for Healthy Kids* will become your daily resource for years to come—a food-splattered treasure that is passed down through the generations.

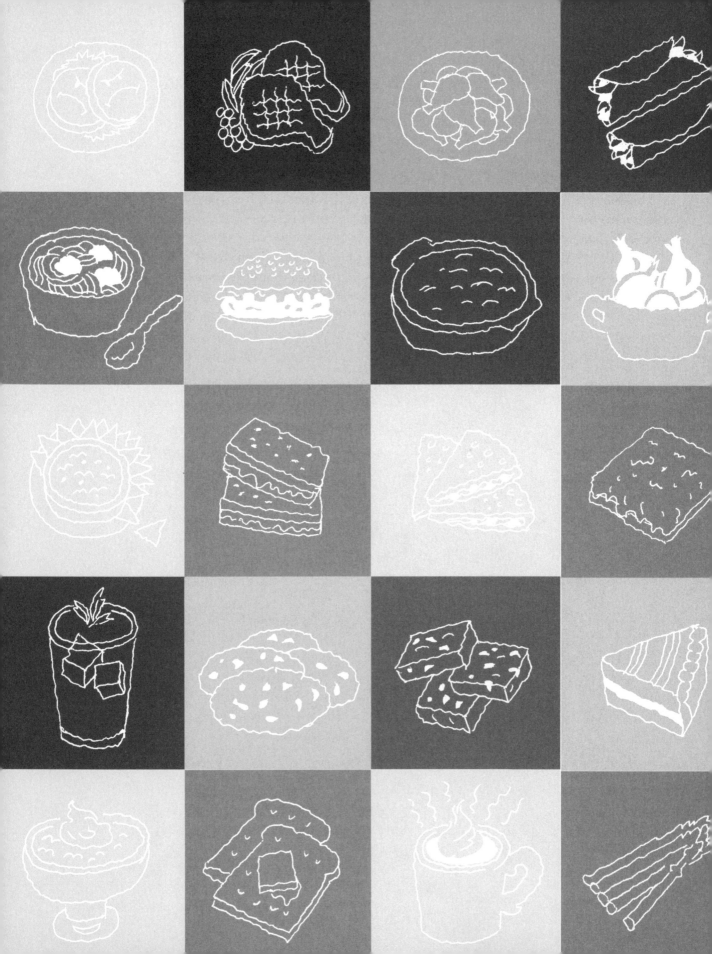

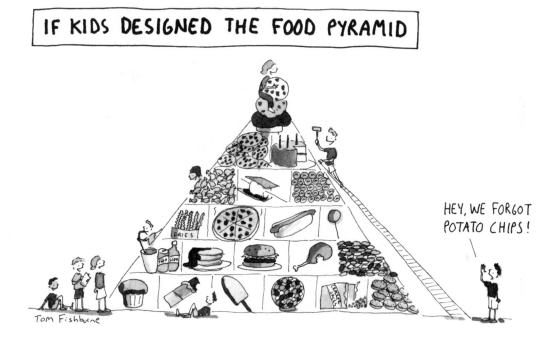

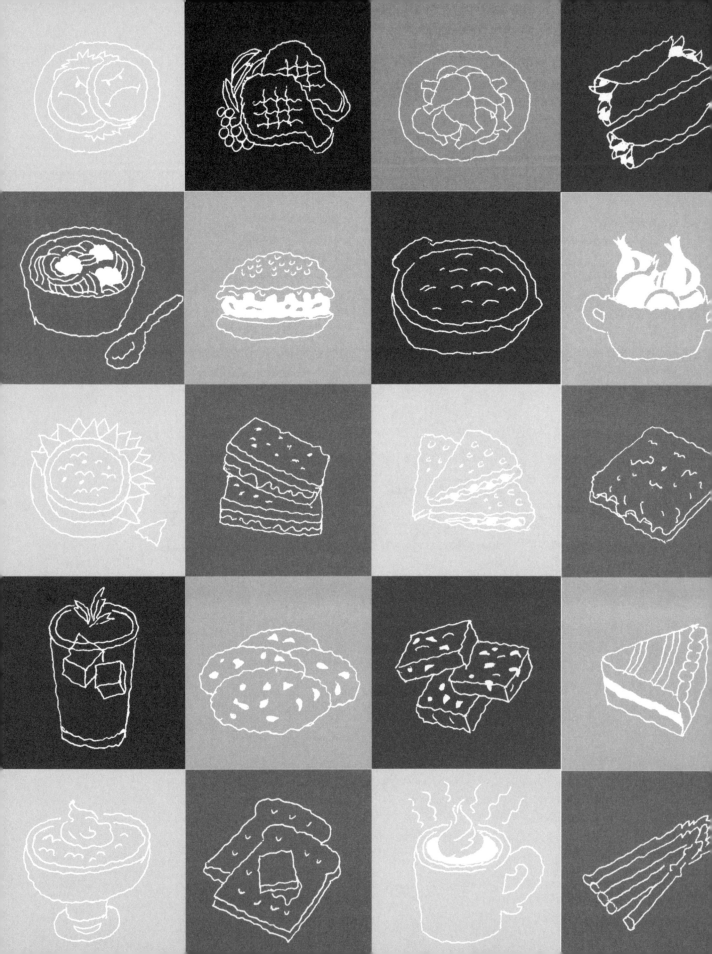

chapter one

What to Feed Your Kids and Why

~ SCALING THE FOOD PYRAMID ~

There's a reason why kids have to be in their late teens to vote, drink, or drive. It isn't until then that they've gained some measure of maturity or self-discipline. That need for good judgment also applies to their nutritional choices. Just as we would never leave a six-year-old unsupervised with a kitchen knife, nor should we leave him with a cupboard packed with candy. Kids of all ages need some healthy eating guidance to ensure that they are getting a nutritious diet. This book will help you help them, providing you with wholesome recipes. Yes, there are also some delicious treats and desserts included, but even the vast majority of these we gave a nutritional makeover so you'll feel better about making them (plus, we feel strongly that kids need to learn moderation, not deprivation). But first, in order to determine what your kids should eat on a daily basis, you need to learn about the basic food groups they should have each day and what constitutes an appropriate portion for their age.

How much kids eat is almost as important as what they eat, and learning about portion control is crucial, even at an early age. The concept of teaching young children about portion control is a relatively new one. Parents used to insist kids clean their plates (some still do) and now we are told that we should allow young children to regulate themselves, eating what they need and leaving the rest on the plate. However, even that modern theory is in dispute. A study of preschoolers published in a 2005 issue of

Appetite magazine found that how much the kids ate correlated strongly with the amount of food placed on their plates.

So, whether you have toddlers or teenagers, it's best to give them the appropriate portions for their ages and sizes. Kids who tend to leave food on the plate should be allowed to do so, unless you feel they are not getting enough protein, calcium, vitamins, and the like. For kids who are natural clean-plate clubbers, give them appropriate portions, and if they ask for seconds, offer them more fruit and veggies first.

It's also never too early for children to learn about healthy and unhealthy foods. The National Heart, Lung, and Blood Institute sponsored a study tracking almost six hundred kids aged eight to thirteen. They found that kids who attended nutrition classes ate a significantly healthier diet, even years later, than those who did not. In response, the institute introduced the idea of "Go Foods," which were healthy everyday foods; "Slow Foods," which you could indulge in a couple of times a week; and "Whoa Foods," which you would have only occasionally. (For more information on this and other health and nutrition information for kids, go to www.realfoodforhealthykids.com.)

What follows is a brief synopsis of the latest government guidelines on what and how much children should eat, broken down by age. It's important to follow these basic tenets for good nutrition, modifying them slightly for your particular child's needs. Obviously, a healthy diet and exercise go hand in hand, something our video-game-playing, computer-glued kids should be reminded of daily. It bears remembering that doctors have concluded that this is the first generation who may not outlive their parents, due to unhealthy weight and its resulting problems such as diabetes and heart disease: Childhood obesity is up 45 percent in the last decade, and at this printing, 16 percent of our children aged six to nineteen are overweight or obese, and another 20 percent are at risk of becoming overweight or obese. There has been a sharp increase in the incidence of Type 2 diabetes and there is a direct correlation between a diet high in sugar and fat and little physical activity.

Daily Nutritional Guidelines

The United States Department of Agriculture created a food pyramid of daily guidelines for kids. (It's available online at www.mypyramid.gov, although the guidelines are only applicable for children aged two and up.) Some nutritionists feel the government should have been more strict, for instance, requiring all, not just some, of the grains to be whole grains, insisting on reduced fat when recommending milk and dairy products, and completely restricting sodas and sports drinks, rather than labeling them as drinks to be used occasionally. Essentially, a child's daily diet should be composed mostly of calories from complex carbohydrates and lean proteins and no more than 20 percent of calories from fat. Here are particulars about each category of food and the specific daily nutritional breakdown for preschoolers, elementary school children, and teenagers, all derived from the U.S.D.A. and the Institute of Medicine.

Daily Foods

Vegetables: Opt for bright and dark veggies: spinach, sweet potatoes, and carrots are great choices. Starchy, whiter foods, such as baking potatoes and corn, are less nutritious.

Fruits: Choose vitamin-rich fresh fruits, such as strawberries, peaches, mangoes, and apples. Fruit juices should be consumed as little as possible. When offering juice, make sure it is 100 percent real fruit juice with no sugar added.

Grains: Use whole or multigrain flours, whole-grain breads, oatmeal, whole-grain low-sugar cereals, brown rice, and whole-wheat pasta. Ban white bread and white rice from your house as much as possible.

Meats and Beans: Serve lean proteins, such as beef, pork, chicken, fish, beans, tofu, or eggs. When preparing any protein-rich food, opt to serve it steamed, baked, or grilled, not fried.

Dairy: Serve lean sources of dairy, such as low-fat milk (check with your doctor to determine whether your child should have whole or reduced-fat milk), low-fat yogurt, ricotta, or cheese.

Oils: Use monounsaturated oil, such as olive—preferably extra-virgin—safflower, and canola oils. They provide vitamin E for healthy skin and the development of cells.

Fats and Sweets: Limit intake of butter, cream, sugary cereals, soda, candy, and the like as much as possible.

Daily Requirements: Preschoolers

Generally, preschoolers need 1,000 to 1,400 calories per day. For this age group, roughly five or six mini-meals throughout the day are preferable to keep their energy up.

Vegetables	1 cup
Fruits	1 cup
Grains	3 ounces
Meats and Beans	2 to 3 ounces
Dairy	2 cups
Oils	3 teaspoons
Fats and Sweets	Limit as much as possible

Daily Requirements: Elementary-School Students

Complex carbohydrates and protein are particularly important for five- to eleven-year-olds, who need 1,400 to 2,000 calories a day. If they are very active, their calorie intake can be in the upper range and if they are fairly inactive, they should have a little less.

Vegetables	2 cups	
Fruits	1½ cups	
Grains	5 to 6 ounces	
Meats and Beans	5 ounces	
Dairy	3 cups	
Oils	4 teaspoons	
Fats and Sweets	Limit as much as possible	

Daily Requirements: Middle- and High-School Students

Generally, teenagers need anywhere from 1,600 calories per day to 3,000 calories for very active boys. Often, teenagers need more calcium and protein than they take in.

Vegetables	3 cups
Fruits	2 cups
Grains	6 ounces
Meats and Beans	5 to 6 ounces
Dairy	3 cups
Oils	5 to 6 teaspoons
Fats and Sweets	Limit as much as possible

Size Matters

The American Dietetic Association (their website, www.eatright.org, is very handy) provides a handy visual guide to appropriate serving sizes:

Meat	3 ounces	Deck of cards/kitchen sponge
Pasta/Rice	½ cup	Tennis ball/ice-cream scoop
Bread	1 slice	CD case
Peanut Butter	2 tablespoons	Ping-Pong ball
Vegetables	½ cup	Lightbulb or rounded handful
Cheese	1 ounce	4 dice
Dried Fruit	1 ounce	Egg
Nuts	1 ounce	Ping-Pong ball

Label Conscious

It is crucial to know exactly what ingredients are in the packaged food we buy and what the nutritional information means. This must become a ritual for you. Here is a brief primer on the science of decoding food labels, what you need to read, and what you can ignore. Most nutritional labels from American manufacturers are now uniform, and these categories are the most important to read:

Serving Size and Servings Per Container: Extremely important yet often ignored, it will tell you how large a portion contained within is so you can figure out how many calories are in that piece of cake you just cut.

Calories: The basic benchmark of energy. Anything with twenty calories or less per serving is considered basically no cal.

Total Fat, Saturated Fat, and Trans Fat: While it is the total fat grams that are most important, differentiating between saturated and trans fats is also crucial as it tells you what types of fat, and how much, are in the item. The Food and Drug Administration changed the rules in 2006, so that every package must reveal how much, if any, trans fat is in the food. Trans fat raises low-density lipoproteins in the blood and raises high-density lipoproteins, the exact opposite of what is healthy for the body. Any food that has five fat grams or less per serving is considered a low-fat food.

Total Carbohydrates, Fiber, and Sugar: This is a confusing category. To understand the true carb count of a food, subtract the number of fiber grams from the total carbs. Foods high in fiber are very good for kids, and obviously, the less sugar, the better.

Protein: It's very important to have enough protein for building strong bodies, especially for kids who are vegetarians (they should make up for it by having protein in the form of eight ounces of calcium a day).

Vitamins A and C, Calcium, and Iron: Children should take a multivitamin daily, but food should be the main source of nutrition.

Sodium: It's important for anyone, including kids, to have foods without excess salt (sodium); a certain amount of sodium is good for the body, but with all of the manufactured foods containing salt, chances are your kid is already getting more than he or she needs each day.

Percentage of Daily Value: This is how much of a percentage one serving is, based on a 2,000-calorie-a-day diet. This does not pertain to children under five years old.

"Free": There is no such thing as a manufactured food that is "free" of anything. Those manufactured products that are "no sugar added" or "fat free" usually compensate by upping the carbohydrate or calorie count to increase flavor. These items are typically overprocessed and should be avoided.

Ingredients

It is crucial to read the ingredient lists for the packaged foods you buy. Because of factory-made and processed foods, chemicals have become prevalent in many diets. Often ingredients are added to enhance flavor—this is especially true for foods with empty calories and long lists of ingredients. Some additives are questionable, but most are safe, and some add nutrition or help to preserve food naturally. In general, especially for children, caffeine, salt, and sugar (various types) should be limited. Additives to be avoided include high fructose corn syrup, artificial colors and flavors, hydrogenated vegetable oil, partially hydrogenated vegetable oil, saccharin, sodium nitrate, and sodium nitrite.

Artificial "Diet" Sweeteners

Better tests need to be performed on aspartame, which causes reactions like headaches and dizziness in some individuals but has not been proven "unsafe" by the Food and Drug Administration. In 1977, the FDA considered banning saccharin because it had been shown that it caused cancer in laboratory rats, but Congress intervened and proposed adding a warning label to products containing the sweetener. In 2000 the Department of Health and Human Services took saccharin off its cancer-causing list, and soon after, the warning labels disappeared. Using artificial sweeteners in general is not a good practice. There is a natural herb used as sugar called Stevia, but the FDA is not convinced this is completely safe. You can read pertinent articles and find more information on food additives and ingredients from the Center for Science in the Public Interest (www.cspinet.org).

A Word on Organics

Consumer Reports magazine did a study in 2006 concluding, "It's worth paying more for organic apples, peaches, spinach, milk, and beef to avoid chemicals found in the conventionally produced versions of those items." Other foods that are easy for pesticides to leach into include potatoes, pears, raspberries, strawberries, cherries, and grapes. Foods that you *don't* have to buy organic, ones that are less likely to retain any pesticide exposure, include asparagus, broccoli, avocados, bananas, corn, kiwis, mangoes, onions, papayas, pineapples, and peas. Be sure to wash either type of produce.

Organic food has become a multibillion-dollar business, rising by 20 percent on average every year in the last decade. Now two-thirds of Americans buy organic foods and beverages. However, the definition of organic has become somewhat muddled, due to the tremendous amount of pressure food conglomerates have put on the government, and so manufacturers are labeling everything organic, including high-sugar cereals.

Generally, organic meat contains no antibiotics or growth hormones, and feed made from animal by-products was not given to the animal during its lifetime, while organic produce is grown without pesticides. Organic items can be up to 50 percent more expensive than nonorganic. However, as big box stores such as Wal-Mart and Costco sell more organic foods, prices will continue to come down. Farmers' markets are terrific places to buy organic, or you can become a member of a Community-Supported Agriculture group (CSA), where you buy shares of a farm and receive a weekly basket of produce. (See "The Experts File" for websites that list CSAs, farmers' markets, and organic companies.) There's nothing better than buying organic food that is local.

~ DISHING WITH KIDS ~
The Benefits of Cooking with Kids

Getting kids into the kitchen to cook with you is a win-win situation, no matter how old they are and no matter what you make. By interacting with you in the kitchen, your child will gain more than just learning how to cook. First and foremost, you will have the opportunity to foster a greater sense of intimacy between you and your child. Here are a few other positive results from interacting together in the kitchen, which are then further broken down into age groups:

- Reading and following recipes improves math, science, and reading comprehension skills.
- Eating dishes from other countries enables learning about other cultures, foreign languages, and geography, and provides a culinary vocabulary.
- Learning about food preparation enhances organizational and cleanliness skills.
- Chances are greater that your child will eat the healthy food you are making if he helps.
- Cooking together strengthens feelings of responsibility and being a valued member of the team, which will form a lifetime of good memories and help to strengthen bonds.

Preschool: Fine motor skills are enhanced with motions such as pouring and stirring; counting ingredients and amounts teaches simple math skills; and working as a team reinforces socializing, learning how to share, and taking turns.

Elementary: Math, science, and reading skills are practiced and improved; an understanding of other cultures and traditions can be taught; the rudiments of nutrition can be learned; and basic cooking skills are learned.

Teenagers: Cooking skills and techniques are refined and knowledge of global cuisine can be enhanced; a sense of success and accomplishment is gained by making a dish or a whole meal.

How can you get the kids more involved in the kitchen? Here are five steps to a successful time together:

1. Ask them what they'd like to make to give them a sense of control and self-worth.
2. Read the recipe first together so that you know what happens and in what order.
3. Take out all of the ingredients ahead of time and have the proper tools ready and grouped in the order in which you're going to use them.
4. Have towels at the ready.
5. Practice patience and have a sense of humor—the two most valuable tools!

House Rules: On Table Etiquette, Cooking, and Eating

These are the rules that we have developed and that our families (generally) live by in all matters pertaining to eating, cooking, and dining.

Our Rules for Table Etiquette

The average American family sits down together to have a meal about four times a week. That frequency is up from the 1990s, but still, that's not very much togetherness time. When you're dining together, you don't want to spend half the meal lecturing your kids on how to act more like royalty than rock star at the table. So, the earlier you can teach them the fundamentals, the better off everyone will be. Kids from six on can understand and quickly learn all of these rules, while younger ones should be taught the first three.

First, some rules for adults: Be sure to compliment the kids on the things they do correctly at the table; make good manners a game, not something that feels like punishment. Remember that they will take their cues from you, so you must be a good role model. Finally, have fun—mealtime is supposed to be enjoyable.

1. Chew each bite with your mouth closed.
2. Hold and use the fork and knife properly. Try to use fingers only for foods such as corn on the cob, tacos, and sandwiches.
3. Use napkins—not clothes—for wiping hands and mouth. Keep the napkin on your lap. Place it neatly next to the plate when you are done.
4. Wait for everyone to be seated and ready before starting to eat.
5. Don't take food from another's plate unless you are invited to do so.
6. Do not speak negatively of your fellow diners' food or culinary preferences.
7. Don't reach across the table to get something. Ask for it to please be passed.
8. No burping or crude talk.

Our Rules for Cooking

1. Before you begin a recipe, read it all the way through and make sure you have the ingredients and the necessary equipment.
2. Prepare the ingredients in the ingredients list—chop the onion, pat the meat dry, peel the carrot, melt the butter.
3. Clean up as you go.
4. The estimated cooking time is an important guide to tell when you've reached a certain point in the recipe, but the way the food looks—Is the onion soft or golden? Is the ground beef crumbled and browned?—is a better indicator.
5. The internal temperature of meats and poultry taken with a thermometer is the ultimate guide to their doneness.

Our Rules for Feeding Children

1. Don't feed kids something you wouldn't eat yourself.
2. Start everyone off with a little "appetizer" of raw veggies—sugar snap peas, edamame, carrots, or snow peas. At breakfast time, start them off with fresh fruit.
3. Don't use food as a punishment or a bribe. Don't say, "If you eat your vegetables, you can have dessert." That sentiment reinforces the notion they must be eating something yucky in order to get dessert.
4. Encourage slow eating: It takes about twenty minutes for the stomach to tell the brain that you are full, so eating slowly is best for both digestion and preventing overeating.
5. Anyone who wants seconds needs to wait a few minutes for the stomach to feel full. Then offer some more veggies or fruit before giving an additional quarter portion of the main dish.

On Food Psychology: Picky Eaters and the No-Thank-You Bite

We all begin with the best intentions. In an effort to make sure our Jacks and Jills have a nutritious diet, we schlep to the market and spend more time and money than we want or have, selecting organic produce, grass-fed meats, and artisanal breads and cheeses. We spend an hour assembling a healthy lasagna. And, at dinner, the pronouncement comes. The world's most ornery food critics—kids—will take one look at the plate, declare they don't like the look of those "bits of green," and ask for a slice of pizza.

Another common scenario: You take the family out to a restaurant that does not have bright plastic chairs as its main decor and for once everyone's hair is combed. Entrees come, and your fourteen-year-old daughter declares she is not hungry anymore. What do you do? Institute some ground rules as soon as you can.

Some kids are picky eaters from the moment they are no longer attached to bottle or breast and many worn-down parents give in. But unless you are fighting a case of malnutrition, throwing in the kitchen towel sends little ones the wrong message from the get-go. Indeed, there have been studies that show half of all two-year-olds are picky eaters, and that their preferences, or lack thereof, continue for years. It's important to realize that a child does not necessarily dislike a dish but could be hesitant to try new things, or hasn't tried something enough. According to recent studies, the magic number is twelve times before a kid's palate gets used to a new taste. Or he may just be trying to exert control and test authority. Of course, she could also just happen to hate broccoli or whatever it is, and you need to substitute something nutritionally comparable.

Older kids who have been picky eaters for a long time need to be handled differently. Do not make it a power play, where you shame, cajole, or bribe. Rather, talk about how much pleasure they are missing. Here are some tips culled from the experts on winning both the battle and the war.

Smells Like Team Spirit: Get your kids involved. Have them make some of the choices for the meal or name the dish. Make them feel like they have some real say in what they eat, but without handing over all of the power to them. Cook some of the food together. Anyone who is invested in choosing or making the dish is more likely to eat it.

Practice What You Preach: In order for your child to eat healthfully, you must eat like that in front of him. Make sure he sees you eating salads, fruits, and vegetables in abundance and with great relish. Conversely, don't let him see you gleefully polishing off an entire bag of Doritos. In this case, imitation is the worst form of flattery.

Join the Beautiful Plate Club: Every successful chef knows that one vital key to winning over a diner's palate is to make a dish look inviting. Children and teenagers are even more visually driven and will be turned off easily if food looks scorched, mushy, or indistinct. Keep the plate looking bright, with a variety of colorful vegetables. Studies have shown brighter colors make food seem more appealing. For older kids, using fine or funky tableware might help.

Ban Membership in the Clean Plate Club: Kids should eat until they feel full and not a bite more. Despite your guilt about other people's children starving, do the right thing—serve your kids a suitable portion size (see Daily Nutritional Guidelines, page 8) and make a donation (money or food) to your local soup kitchen or food bank.

No-Thank-You Bites Are the House Rule: It can take kids over a dozen tastes of a new food until they will actually like and eat it. Make sure your child takes one bite of the new food item each time you make it. Do not force him to eat more than a bite, as it can quickly escalate into a battle of wills. To get older kids interested, tell them what it is, where it's from, and what restaurant serves something similar. Getting kids involved in the creation of the dish also helps them to be open to new tastes.

Get Sneaky: If you are concerned that your child is not getting enough calcium, fiber, or protein, work nutrient-rich ingredients in on the sly. For instance, if your little guy doesn't like plain milk, whip up a calcium-rich rice pudding or a protein-laced, frosty peanut butter–banana smoothie.

Keep Snack Attacks Healthy: If your young child eats only a little of his lunch but then wants a snack, hand him some cut-up fresh fruit, mini-carrots, or cheese sticks. If you don't have the bad stuff around, no one will demand it. Offer healthful snacks in small portions so when mealtime comes, the child is actually hungry. With older kids, you can't really force them to eat a particular food or portion size, but you can ensure they have a myriad of healthy choices to choose from. Have a supply of air-popped popcorn, baked pita chips, dried fruit and nuts, yogurt, exotic fruits, and wholesome dips, which are great paired with sugar snap peas and carrots. (See our "Snack Attacks" chapter, page 97, for specific suggestions.)

Look at the Forest, Not the Trees: Maybe little Jimmy did not get all of his vegetables today, but you know that you will be serving more to him in some regular form all week.

Take Down the "Diner Is Open" Sign: Do not make different meals for every member of the family; you are not a short-order cook. Dinner is dinner, and a child over the age of two can eat at least parts of the same meal you are making for everyone else. If you must relent, only offer a ready-made food such as low-fat cottage cheese, not something that is a treat.

~ FAST-FOOD NOTIONS AND DINING OUT ~

An American Heart Association study done in 2005 revealed that more than 20 percent of Americans said they ate out four times a week or more. Chances are, much of this is fast food. In fact, every day, almost a third of kids are eating a fast-food meal.

Fast-food companies sometimes maintain there is no such thing as bad-for-you food—that the danger lies in overeating. Or they claim they are committed to good nutrition and have reduced items such as trans fats and hormone-injected foods on their menus.

Many establishments have nutritional counts available to consumers. And while this is laudable, more money is spent on marketing efforts than on better ingredients and different cooking techniques to ensure a healthier menu. Fast-food companies spend $15 billion marketing to children through television commercials, product placement, and toy giveaways. The average American kid watches almost five thousand food commercials a year. So how do you fight all of their mesmerizing messaging?

From the earliest age that kids can understand, tell them that French fries are cooked in oil that is used over and over. Inform them how, in order for the food to be fast and cheap, companies have to use inferior, inexpensive ingredients. Explain how chickens live cooped up in tiny pens for just over a month before becoming chicken nuggets. The ultimate test: Bring home a burger from a fast-food place and then make your own homemade version. Have them taste the two side by side in a blind test. This will prove to them how poor tasting fast food really is. When they are ten or older, hand them a copy of Eric Schlosser's *Chew On This: Everything You Don't Want to Know About Fast Food.*

Sometimes, there are no alternatives to fast food, such as when you're on a road trip. Choose places that are more inherently healthy such as Subway or a seafood spot such as Red Lobster, and order the food grilled. If you have to go to a burger joint, keep portions in mind and order small. Start with a green salad and drizzle it with a minimal amount of dressing. Order grilled chicken instead of a hamburger, baked potatoes instead of French fries. Opt for low-fat yogurt rather than premium ice cream.

Typically even those dining at more moderate and upscale restaurants will eat larger portions than they do at home. Be sure your kids don't arrive at a restaurant starving (give them a protein or fiber-rich snack beforehand), order from the adult side of the menu—kids' menus are often junk food—and ask for dressing on the side.

~ SNIFFING OUT FOOD ALLERGIES ~

More than 11 million Americans suffer from life-threatening food allergies and these reactions result annually in more than thirty thousand trips to America's emergency rooms and roughly two hundred deaths. Approximately 90 percent of allergies are to nuts, soy, milk, eggs, fish, shellfish, and wheat.

While you can develop a food allergy at any time, babies and young children usually have a fairly quick reaction, which is why you should introduce babies to a new food one at a time, then wait three days before introducing the next new food. That way, if you see telltale hives or a rash, you know which food it is. Older kids with allergic reactions will produce a reddening of the skin, hives, vomiting, cramps, rashes, or they will feel like they can't breathe. If you suspect your child has an allergy, have her tested. As there is currently no cure, prevention is vital, so follow these tips (for more, go to the Food Allergy and Anaphylaxis Network at www.foodallergy.org):

- Alert your school, camp, and your child's friends' parents of the allergy. Little children should have it not just written in their school medical chart but written out on a card and placed in a wallet or in their backpack.
- Teach your child how to read food labels for the offending ingredient, including vague words such as "spices" or "oils." As of 2006, food manufacturers were required to list eight different allergens on the label, so now your child can search in an easier fashion. If it doesn't have a label, teach your child that when in doubt, skip the food.
- When dining out, explain the situation to the waiter and have him tell the chef your child is allergic to this specific ingredient and nothing in the dish can be made with it or even have touched it. If you are abroad in a foreign-speaking country, bring an index card with a sentence explaining the allergy written in the foreign language and be sure the waiter shows it to the chef.
- For serious allergies, have your doctor prescribe an EpiPen, a penlike shot with epinephrine (adrenaline), to be carried by your kid at all times. If you don't have an EpiPen and an allergy strikes, take your child to an emergency room right away.

~ KITCHEN 101 ~

Comprehensive yet concise, these simple yet effective strategies will keep your kitchen efficient, clean, and kid-safe.

Creating a Kid-Friendly Kitchen

While small children definitely require a kitchen in lockdown status, no matter what the age of your child, there are a few things every parent should do to keep the kitchen safe.

- **Danger with a Capital D:** While age-appropriate equipment and tools should be in a place where your child can easily reach them, dangerous items such as knives, kitchen scissors, matches, igniters, and anything with sharp blades, such as food processors, should be kept out of reach. Depending on the child's level of maturity, this can apply to households with teenagers as well. Also, a small child needs a slip-free step stool.
- **Clean-Up Time Is All the Time:** Nontoxic cleaning supplies, a broom, and a mop should be easily accessible to your kids so that cleaning up becomes an integral part of the cooking/eating process. Get a few fun, funky aprons to have on hand.
- **Keep Them Inspired:** Cookbooks, nutritional guides, food magazines,

bookmarked food websites, and other inspirational materials should be easily available to kids.

❖ **Stock Wisely:** "Sometimes foods" (cookies, candy, etc.) should be placed higher in the cupboard so that they cannot easily be reached or be within the line of sight. Healthier snacks, such as fruit, pretzels, nuts, raisins, and mozzarella sticks, on the other hand, should be easily reachable.

Measuring Basics

Before you make any recipe, you need to make sure you are using the correct measurement. Liquids should be measured in a see-through glass measuring cup. Keeping the cup even, look straight through and add liquid to the desired line on the cup. When measuring most dry ingredients, such as flour and sugar, use the scoop and scrape method: scoop the dry measuring cup into the ingredient, and then scrape across the top of the cup with a knife to level the measurement. When using flour, give the container of flour a stir before measuring, as flour can settle as it sits. Here is a handy basic guide to measuring.

Basic Volume and Liquid Measurements

1 tablespoon	3 teaspoons	½ fluid ounce
¼ cup	4 tablespoons	2 fluid ounces
⅓ cup	5 tablespoons plus 1 teaspoon	3 fluid ounces
½ cup	8 tablespoons	4 fluid ounces
1 cup	16 tablespoons	8 fluid ounces
2 cups	32 tablespoons	16 fluid ounces/1 pint
3 cups		24 fluid ounces/1½ pints
4 cups		32 fluid ounces/1 quart
8 cups		half gallon

Pantry and Refrigerator Must-Haves

To aid in your daily effort to minimize time and maximize flavor, keep your pantry well stocked with these basics. See "A Heated Discussion on Freezing," page 23, for storing tips.

Canned Goods: beans (garbanzo, cannellini, black beans); broth (low-sodium chicken, beef, and vegetable); chiles (dried chiles, chipotle in adobo); coconut milk (light, unsweetened); cooking spray (a pure oil variety); pumpkin puree; tomatoes (peeled whole, pureed, crushed, and paste); light tuna (preferably packed in water or olive oil)

Bottled Goods: anchovy paste; barbecue sauce; Asian chili sauce; extra-virgin olive oil; fish sauce (Thai or Vietnamese); hoisin sauce; honey; hot sauce; jams; ketchup; mayonnaise, regular and low fat; molasses; mustard (Dijon, whole grain, and honey); olives (black and green); olive oil (extra virgin); marinara sauce; peanut butter (natural); salsa; soy sauce (low sodium); sesame tahini; sun-dried tomatoes; Tabasco; vinegar (white wine, balsamic, and malt); Worcestershire sauce; vegetable oil; pure vanilla extract

Frozen Items: bacon; bananas (very ripe); berries; breads and English muffins; butter (unsalted and European style); chicken (boneless skinless breast halves); corn (cut white or yellow); cornmeal; edamame (shelled); flat breads and wraps; ground beef and turkey; ice cream and sorbet; nuts and seeds (walnuts, pecans, peanuts, pine nuts, pumpkin seeds, sesame seeds); pizza dough; ravioli; sausages; shrimp (deveined); spinach; tortillas (fresh corn and flour varieties); wonton wrappers

Refrigerator: butter (unsalted and European style); mayonnaise; natural peanut butter; organic large eggs; cheeses (preferably organic; such as Cheddar, Havarti, Monterey Jack, Parmesan, Swiss, mozzarella); organic milk (whole and fat free); heavy cream; cottage cheese; cream cheese; sour cream; organic plain yogurt

Produce: apples; avocados; bananas; broccoli; butternut squash; carrots; cherries; garlic; lemons; limes; mangoes; yellow and red onions; oranges; pears; potatoes (russet and red); spinach; sugar snap peas; snow peas; other fruit and vegetables in season

Pantry Goods: active dry yeast; baking powder; baking soda; bread crumbs (Japanese style and plain dried); canned fruit; chocolate bars and chips (unsweetened and semisweet); crackers (including graham crackers); unsweetened cocoa powder; couscous (instant and Israeli); cornstarch; flour (unbleached all-purpose, whole-wheat, traditional and white whole-wheat, and plain cake flour); grits; honey; lentils; oatmeal; pasta; polenta (instant); raisins; rice (Arborio, brown varieties); sugar (granulated, confectioners', dark and light brown); tea (black, chamomile, green)

Dried Herbs, Spices, and Flavorings: allspice; black peppercorns; cayenne pepper; Chinese five-spice powder; cinnamon; chili powder (preferably ancho); cloves; coriander; crushed red pepper flakes; cumin (ground); curry powder (Madras); ground ginger; herbes de Provence; nutmeg; oregano; paprika; salt (kosher and fine table varieties); thyme; turmeric

The Essential Equipment

Here is our list of the most valuable tools and appliances to have for a well-stocked kitchen:

Small Appliances: blender or immersion handheld blender; food processor; microwave; toaster oven; handheld mixer; heavy-duty standing mixer

Tools: box grater; cake tester; can opener; cherry pitter; fine-mesh sieve; forged carbon steel knives (we like Wüsthof, Henckels, Global, and Lansom Sharp) in these styles: paring knife, serrated bread knife, and an 8-, 9-, or 10-inch chef's knife; instant-read thermometer; ladle; measuring spoons and cups (a set of dry and liquid in cup, pint, and quart sizes); offset spatulas (large and small); oven mitts and pot holders; oven thermometer; ovenproof meat thermometer; parchment paper; potato masher; spice rack; salad spinner; rasp (plane grater); rolling pin; slotted spoon; spatulas (metal and rubber); tongs; wooden spoons; whisks (a long narrow one for sauces and a small one for mixing dressings); vegetable peeler

Equipment: baking sheets (17- by 11-inch shallow heavy); cast-iron skillet (10 inch); cutting boards (plastic and wooden); colander (stainless steel); Dutch oven casserole (8 quart); mixing bowl set; muffin pans (½-cup capacity); nonstick skillets (9- and 12-inch); 3-quart pasta pot; saucepans (1-, 3-, and 4-quart sizes, stainless steel–lined); stainless steel–lined skillet (9-inch); springform cake pans; steamer basket

Nonstick Cookware

In general, we recommend heavy cookware lined with stainless steel, but it makes sense to have one good nonstick skillet, a pan that requires little fat for cooking. Presently nonstick cookware is under some scientific scrutiny, but the Environmental Protection Agency has stated that these products are safe for home use. Perfluorooctanoic acid, or PFOA, a chemical used in processing to make the coating adhere to the pans, has environmental ramifications, but cookware companies claim that the chemical is absent from the pan by the time you buy it. We opt for using nonstick only when necessary. In many cases a well-seasoned cast-iron skillet is your best friend, but if you do choose to use a nonstick skillet, here are some tips:

❖ Be sure to read the care booklet that comes with the pan. It will tell you to wash the pan thoroughly in hot soapy water with a sponge or a dishcloth and rinse with hot water and dry before its first use.

❖ No matter what the recipe says, cook at no higher than a medium heat setting to prevent overheating and burning. It is inadvisable to preheat the pan. (The pan will be ready in the time it takes to melt a little butter.)

- Use a wooden spatula or other specifically nonstick utensils to prevent scratching. (Never cut in the pan with a knife!)
- Avoid using cooking sprays; they usually contain soy lecithin, which makes the pan hard to clean and compromises its nonstickability.

A Heated Discussion on Freezing

We keep well-stocked freezers. Tracey likes to keep leftovers in the refrigerator, for fast reheating of subsequent servings, but she freezes fresh meats and breads and batches of chili, stews, and soup to have on hand for later. Tanya likes to freeze individual portions so when she comes dashing in from work at 7:00 P.M., or after a Saturday soccer game, there is something healthful and tasty to pop in the microwave to feed a hungry and weary kid just minutes later. We both freeze our home-cooked recipes (see "How to Freeze" and "How to Thaw" on page 24) and keep a minimal stash of processed organic foods. Here is all you've ever wanted to know about freezing—and more.

Ten Things to Have in Your Freezer

1. Cooked Pasta: Cook a pound—bow ties and rotelle are best for this purpose—until barely al dente (so that when you reheat, the pasta will not be mushy) and then freeze (unsauced) in a freezer-ready container for adding to a hot sauce or microwaving later. (Do not rinse the pasta.)

2. Homemade Pasta Sauce: Make a batch on Sunday afternoon (see Quick Skillet Tomato Sauce, page 213; Grilled Tomato Sauce, page 212; or Spaghetti and Meatballs, page 169) and store in containers (be sure to leave a little space at the top for expansion). Cream sauces do not freeze well.

3. Very Ripe Bananas: For an instant protein-rich smoothie, store ripe bananas in the freezer, peeled, in freezer bags and blend them with skim milk and soy protein powder.

4. Pizza Dough: It thaws quickly at room temperature. Also, when you want pizza, cook an extra pie or two, let cool without cutting, wrap, and freeze for later. Just pop the pizza into a 400°F oven until hot, then cut and serve.

5. Vegetable Protein Burgers: When in a pinch, defrost some GardenBurgers, cook them in a cast-iron skillet, slide them between a whole-wheat hamburger roll, and pile on the lettuce and tomato.

6. Shelled Edamame: Buy them frozen in the supermarket, boil them for a few minutes, and serve them in a bowl, lightly salted. These buttery soy kernels are nutritious and surprisingly fun to eat.

7. Bacon: Raw bacon, wrapped side-by-side in pairs in parchment or waxed paper and then enclosed in foil, is great for keeping portions on hand.

8. Peeled Deveined Shrimp: Thaw shrimp quickly under cool running water to make a tasty meal in a snap (see Easy-Bake Scampi, page 129).

9. Frozen Potatoes: Look for organic shoestring, shredded, or crinkle-cut fries or hash browns without additives. You can cook them quickly in the oven or in a skillet and top with browned ground beef and cheese or serve them with eggs.

10. Soups and Stews: Simmered and braised dishes freeze well. Many of our recipes provide a large enough yield that you can freeze at least a quart to serve later. Thaw overnight in the refrigerator.

How to Freeze: You can freeze myriad foods: cake, cheese, bacon, berries, and other fruit. Sauces, broth, and pureed baby food can be stored in ice-cube trays and frozen. Here are some tips on how to ensure your foods don't end up tasting of freezer burn.

- ❖ Slice breads before you freeze for easier removal.
- ❖ Freeze in small portions, so you can defrost a serving fast and easily.
- ❖ Wrap well. Use containers and wraps that were designed specifically for the freezer. Make sure there is no excess air in bags and wraps. If you are storing sauce or soup, keep room at the top of the container for expansion of the liquid.
- ❖ Be sure to label the package with the name of the item and the date of preparation and storage.
- ❖ Place newer things in the back of the freezer and use older items in front.

How to Thaw: Overnight thawing in the fridge is best, but if time is of the essence, you can immerse foods in cold water—bag or container and its contents—and keep changing the water once it reaches room temperature. Transfer soups, sauces, or stews to a saucepan and heat slowly, covered, until the mixture comes to a boil; be sure to stir often. For other individual portions, defrost uncovered in the microwave and cook and serve as soon as possible.

Safety First

It is important to keep your kitchen clean and bacteria free, particularly if your child has a compromised immune system. Besides cleaning your hands with hot soapy water frequently while cooking, here are a few tips to keep your kitchen, equipment, and tools as clean as possible and your food stored properly to prevent bacterial growth.

On Cleaning

Top places for bacteria growth in your kitchen include sponges, cutting boards, and countertops. When cleaning countertops, use paper towels with hot soapy water. Clean cutting boards (both plastic and wood) and utensils with hot soapy water in between each step of your cooking or in the dishwasher. This is particularly true if you are preparing meat, chicken, fish, or raw eggs. If a kitchen towel is wet, use another, dry one to wipe up any moisture on clean plates and so on. Do not put cooked meat or poultry on a plate where the raw food was.

On Storing for Safety

Obviously, meat, chicken, and fish should be cooked thoroughly for children in order to kill any lurking salmonella, E. coli, and other virulent strains of bacteria. Likewise, recipes with raw eggs should be avoided. While most parents know this, they don't realize there is a risk involved in how food is stored.

The key to keeping bacteria at bay after thoroughly cooking food is to get it into the refrigerator as quickly as possible. Within an hour of eating, room temperature food should be wrapped and stored in serving-sized portions and placed in the refrigerator or freezer (see "How to Freeze," page 24, for more tips).

~ A FEW WORDS ON OUR RECIPES ~

We have tried to think of everything, from writing recipes so that you make the most of your valuable time, to telling you exactly what kind of butter or flour to use to ensure success and optimum nutrition.

There are information boxes throughout, and many recipes have Cooks' Notes, which will provide everything from substitutions to hints on how to make a perfect omelet. You will also notice that we offer variations as much as possible, so that if you like a dish but want to tweak it to make it feel new, we offer ideas on how to make it with different ingredients. We also offer suggestions on foods to serve with the recipes to give you a full meal and take out the guesswork.

Every recipe in the book has cooking times and nutrition counts ("First Foods," the baby food chapter, does not have any analyses, but every recipe in that chapter provides optimum nutrients). The time is broken down into preparation, which is roughly the time it should take you to chop, slice, mix, or add, and cooking or baking, which is roughly the time something takes to cook, sauté, bake, or roast. When recipes take less than an hour, that is indicated by a "Speed Limit" symbol and an "MPR" (minutes per recipe) rating, which is the approximate total time the recipe will take, start to finish. Obviously, people cook at their own speed, and ovens and stovetops differ, so these times are to be taken only as guides.

We have also included nutritional analysis for each recipe, breaking it down into the most essential information you need to know: calories, carbohydrates, fat (which includes saturated fat), protein, and fiber. We mention when something has a lot of vitamins or other important health benefits.

The headnotes below each recipe title contain important information and serving suggestions, so always read them. It's also important to read the recipe through completely before starting it.

We rarely give specific ingredient brands but in general we like to cook with kosher salt except when baking, when we prefer to use table or fine salt; we always use unsalted butter, and extra-virgin olive oil is our preferred variety; and in general we like cooking with filtered water, which means water that is screened from harmful additives and does not come straight from the tap. So use water generally from a pitcher with a filter or from a tap with a filter on it, or bottled water unless you feel very confident in the water from your tap. There are companies that test your water for lead and other additives. For more information on getting your water tested, contact the National Lead Information Center. If you do use water from your tap, make sure it is always cold water from a tap that has run for a minute first.

Finally, you will note that many of our recipes have a little chef's hat icon, , which denotes a good recipe to make with your child. Because this book is for any kid six months to sixteen years of age, some recipes are better for older kids to cook up, while other recipes (and tasks, such as stirring or adding things) are easy for even a two-year-old. We have merely pointed out recipes that don't require a scalding hot oven or grill, a whole lot of pointed knives, or tricky ingredients like chiles. Only you know what your child is capable of, but when you're making these recipes, most can employ in some form the talents and skills of your kid, even if it's nominal. One of the most important points of *Real Food for Healthy Kids* is to get you into the kitchen with your child to make wholesome foods and wonderful memories.

chapter two

Breakfast for Champions
The Morning Meal

We've all read how breakfast is the day's most important meal, one that can help turn you into a champion, but this isn't just a marketing gimmick; rather it's an old *wise* tale. There have been litanies of studies that have demonstrated the importance of breakfast for kids: Those who have a nutritious breakfast concentrate and perform better in school, are more physically active, and tend not to overeat later in the day. Indeed, in general, those who eat breakfast are less likely to be overweight. And yet, almost half of all girls and a third of all boys in America are skipping breakfast before school. Those who are eating often choose the grab-and-go breakfast, usually cereal bars, a doughnut, a frozen waffle, or a bagel. These things are easy to eat but filled with empty calories, trans fats, and carbs. They are what we call good-for-nothing foods.

On weekends, breakfast can be a more leisurely affair, and if you don't have time to have dinner together often, sitting down to breakfast as a family is a great alternative. As long as you are having a meal and a chat and sharing a moment of pleasure, it doesn't matter what time of day it is. And yet, few parents seem to expand beyond frozen waffles, cold sugary cereals, or overly sweetened packages of oatmeal even on weekends.

So, what can you make your kids on the weekdays that requires minimum effort for maximum nutrients and flavor? We've developed recipes that solve that dilemma in the "School Daze" section. And we've supplied wholesome, fun-to-make dishes that are perfect for a weekend. We've also included a section entitled the "Breakfast Bakeshop" with recipes that are good for making the night before for a weekday or in the morning for a weekend breakfast. (You can also make and freeze some for anytime.) Think of these as your House Krispy Kremes, but without the added trans fats, calories, expense, and hassle of getting them.

The key to breakfast is to expand your mind beyond the usual. Really, just about anything healthy is appropriate for a morning meal.

school daze: the world beyond cereal

It's very important that a sustaining school-day breakfast consist of two things for kids' brain-power and energy: protein and complex carbohydrates. Also, ideally, kids should have a little more than one-third of their daily vitamins from breakfast. Here are some fast fixes that are nutritious and delicious.

Hole-y Eggs!

Microwave Pizza Frittata

Toaster Oven Use-Your-Bean Taco

Spinach and Bean Taco

Broccoli 'n' Cheese Breakfast Burrito

Carrot Cake Oatmeal

Apple-Maple Oatmeal

Strongman's Oatmeal

Tomorrow's French Toast

Good Day Pear Crisp

Good Day Summer Crisp

Good Day Fall Crisp

Sunshine Parfait

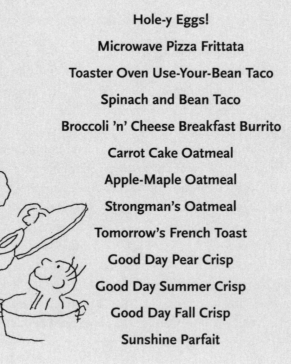

Hole-y Eggs!

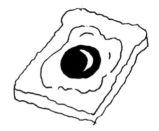

Extra-virgin olive oil is preferable to use in this simple dish (and most others) because of its health qualities (see Cooks' Notes for more information). If desired, sprinkle diced fresh tomatoes on top of the finished egg. For added fun, use different cookie cutters to cut out the center of the bread.

1 slice whole-wheat or multigrain bread
2 teaspoons extra-virgin olive oil or butter
1 large egg
Pinch each of kosher salt and freshly ground black pepper

1. Cut a 3-inch round out of the slice of bread with a cookie cutter, a glass, or a small bowl and reserve the circle and crust section.

2. Warm the oil in a medium nonstick or cast-iron skillet over medium heat until hot. Add both sections of bread separately to the pan and then crack the egg and add to the hole. Season lightly with salt and pepper. Cook until the egg is set on the bottom and the bread is golden, about 1½ minutes. Flip the egg and round with a spatula and cook, uncovered, for about 1 minute or to the desired doneness. Serve the round on the side for dunking into the egg.

PREP: 1 minute
COOKING: 3 minutes
SPEED LIMIT: 4 mpr

Makes 1 serving

PER SERVING:
228 calories,
15g fat (3g saturated),
14g carbohydrates,
2g fiber, 9g protein

Cooks' Notes

❖ Get your kid to love extra-virgin olive oil. Begin with a mild olive oil and work from there. Your goal is extra-virgin, cold-pressed, because it retains more health properties than the more processed milder olive oils.

❖ Think of salad for breakfast! A side of tender greens is a natural with fried eggs and adds fiber and vitamins. And many cultures have savory foods such as fish and meat for breakfast.

"My favorite part was dipping the circle of bread into the egg yolk,"
says ten-year-old Connor G., of Oxford, Mississippi.

Microwave Pizza Frittata

Some kids love savory flavors in the morning. This recipe makes enough for two in a wide shallow soup bowl. When you sprinkle on the cheese, add the kids' favorite pizza toppings, such as thawed frozen vegetables and crumbled cooked turkey bacon. If you have a few extra minutes, serve with toasted Italian bread brushed with olive oil.

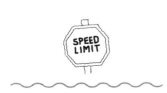

PREP: 2 minutes
COOKING: 4 minutes
SPEED LIMIT: 6 mpr

Makes 2 servings

PER SERVING:
200 calories, 12g fat
(3.5g saturated),
9g carbohydrates,
.5g fiber, 13g protein

Extra-virgin olive oil, for greasing the bowl
3 large eggs
1½ tablespoons water
Pinch of kosher salt and freshly ground black pepper
½ cup shredded (packed) part-skim mozzarella cheese (2 ounces)
    or 2 slices fresh mozzarella
2 tablespoons prepared tomato sauce or Quick Skillet Tomato Sauce
    (page 213)
¼ teaspoon dried oregano, crumbled

1. Lightly grease a 1-cup shallow soup bowl with extra-virgin olive oil. Add the eggs, water, and salt and pepper and beat with a fork until blended. Place in the microwave and cook at medium (50%) power for 2 minutes. Stir with a fork and cook at medium power 1 minute more. (The eggs should be set but very moist at this point.)

2. Sprinkle the cheese on top and spoon on the sauce. Season with oregano and microwave at medium (50%) power for 1 minute (the cheese should be melted and the eggs cooked through). Cut in half and serve.

Cooks' Notes

❖ Add any cheese to top your frittata or stir in cubed cheese when the eggs are half cooked. Try adding cooked diced potato, meats, or vegetables in the eggs as well.

❖ All jarred sauces are not alike. Look for organic tomato sauce that does not contain sweeteners.

Toaster Oven
Use-Your-Bean Taco

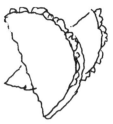

The toaster oven is one of our favorite appliances for quickies like this protein-packed soft taco breakfast with low-fat refried beans and cheese. If you want to make a bunch at once (or if you don't have a toaster oven), place them on a baking sheet and bake in a preheated 500°F oven.

One 7-inch whole-wheat tortilla
3 tablespoons low-fat refried beans
¼ cup sliced or shredded (1 ounce) Monterey Jack, Pepper Jack, or
*   Cheddar cheese, or 1 small stick mozzarella*
1 to 2 pinches of chili powder
2 teaspoons plain low-fat yogurt

1. Lay the tortilla on a work surface and spread the beans on the top half. Sprinkle the cheese and chili powder on the other half and cook in the toaster oven on the medium-dark setting.

2. Spread the yogurt on top of the beans and fold the tortilla in half to make a taco.

Cooks' Note

❖ Substitute corn tortillas for the whole-wheat. They tend to be smaller in diameter, so less filling is needed.

Spinach and Bean Taco: If you have some cold leftover cooked spinach, try this recipe. Warm ¼ cup in the microwave at high (100%) power for 30 seconds and distribute on top of the filling before toasting the tortilla.

PREP: 1 minute
COOKING: 4 minutes
SPEED LIMIT: 5 mpr

Makes 1 serving

PER SERVING:
287 calories, 11g fat
(6g saturated),
31g carbohydrates,
4.5g fiber, 12g protein

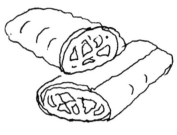

Broccoli 'n' Cheese Breakfast Burrito

PREP: 2 minutes
COOKING: 3 minutes
SPEED LIMIT: 5 mpr

Makes 1 serving

PER SERVING:
*405 calories, 23g fat
(10g saturated),
26g carbohydrates,
3.5g fiber, 21g protein*

Here's a fast burrito. For more protein, add a tablespoon of chopped ham to the burrito. You can also substitute the same amount of any cooked vegetable for the broccoli. If Junior likes things a little spicy, substitute Pepper Jack cheese or hand this over with a bottle of hot sauce. If you're on the go, wrap the burrito in a napkin. Take another napkin along—just in case.

One 7-inch whole-wheat tortilla
¼ cup chopped leftover cooked broccoli or thawed frozen broccoli
1 teaspoon mild olive oil or vegetable oil
1 large egg, beaten with a teaspoon of water and a pinch each of kosher salt and freshly ground black pepper
⅓ cup shredded (packed) Cheddar cheese (1½ ounces)

1. Toast the tortilla in the toaster oven at the medium setting or cook in a dry skillet over medium heat until warm, about 1 minute.

2. Meanwhile, place the broccoli and oil in a small skillet over medium-high heat and cook, stirring, until heated through. Pour in the egg and scramble until set, 1 to 2 minutes.

3. Place the tortilla on a plate and sprinkle the cheese on top. Spoon the hot egg mixture down the center and roll up.

Cooks' Note

❖ Broccoli is packed with calcium and vitamin K for strong bones and teeth. Cooking florets takes only a few minutes (see our "Sidekicks" section, page 191) and frozen broccoli is great in a pinch. Whatever you choose, try to buy organic.

Fifteen-year-old Paul-Michael M., of Royal Palm Beach, Florida, ate a breakfast burrito on his way to football practice and said, "Hey, Mom, we got a winner with this one!"

Carrot Cake Oatmeal

Oatmeal has never tasted better. Flecks of grated carrot add beta-carotene, vitamin A, and gentle sweetness, while currants and chopped pecans add crunch and even more fiber. Serve with a splash of milk and a sprinkling of brown sugar, if desired.

1 medium carrot, peeled and finely shredded
2 cups water
¼ teaspoon kosher salt
Pinch of cinnamon
¼ cup currants or raisins
⅔ cup rolled oats
⅓ cup oat bran (see Cooks' Note)
3 tablespoons chopped pecans

1. In a small saucepan, combine the carrot, water, salt, and cinnamon and bring to a boil. Reduce the heat, add the currants, and simmer until the currants are plumped and the carrot is tender, about 3 minutes.

2. Stir in the oats and oat bran and cook, stirring, until thickened, about 5 minutes. Transfer the oats to two bowls and sprinkle the nuts on top.

Cooks' Note

✤ If you don't have oat bran on hand, substitute ⅓ cup more rolled oats.

Apple-Maple Oatmeal: Substitute ½ cup finely diced peeled apple for the carrot and add 2 tablespoons apple butter and ½ tablespoon pure maple syrup to the finished oatmeal.

PREP: 3 minutes
COOKING: 9 minutes
SPEED LIMIT: 12 mpr

Makes 2 servings

PER SERVING:
*287 calories, 11g fat
(1g saturated),
46g carbohydrates,
8g fiber, 9g protein*

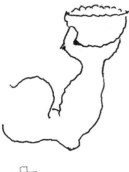

Strongman's Oatmeal

PREP: 5 minutes
COOKING: 4 minutes
SPEED LIMIT: 9 mpr

Makes 1 serving

PER SERVING:
*314 calories, 11.5g fat
(4g saturated),
40g carbohydrates,
5g fiber, 14g protein*

Rolled and steel-cut oats are great on their own, but kids need protein. Mixing an egg into oatmeal adds custardlike creaminess and creates a wholesome breakfast. The trick is to make sure the egg is thoroughly cooked but not scrambled. To ensure this, warm the egg sufficiently in the shell before proceeding with the recipe. Once the oatmeal is ready to eat, add a splash of milk, if desired.

1 large egg
½ cup rolled oats
½ cup water
1 tablespoon oat bran or toasted wheat germ
Pinch of kosher salt
½ tablespoon honey
1 teaspoon unsalted butter

1. Place the egg in the shell in a small bowl and fill with very hot tap water; wait about 30 seconds, then pour out the water and repeat, letting the egg stand in the water until you're ready to add to the hot oatmeal.

2. Combine the oats, water, oat bran, and salt in a shallow soup bowl. Place in the microwave and cook for 3 minutes at 80% power. Immediately crack the egg and add to the oatmeal, mixing with a fork. (The mixture should register 150°F on an instant-read thermometer.) Cover loosely with foil and let stand for 2 minutes to cook the egg. Stir in the honey and butter and serve.

Cooks' Notes

❖ The oatmeal can also be cooked in a small saucepan over medium heat.

❖ Eggs are nutrient-dense. The average egg provides various amounts of almost all of the needed vitamins. Each large egg is only 75 calories and contains over 6 grams of protein and 5 grams of fat, most of which is unsaturated. For the best flavor, buy healthful local organic eggs (antibiotic and hormone free) from uncaged hens.

Tomorrow's French Toast

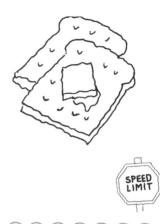

Put this together the night before, pop the baking dish in the oven in the morning, and turn it on before you start the coffee. Serve with a light drizzle of pure maple syrup or a dusting of confectioners' sugar and some fresh fruit.

3 tablespoons unsalted butter
2 slices soft whole-wheat or multigrain bread
1 large egg
¼ cup reduced-fat (2%) milk
Pinch each of cinnamon and kosher salt

1. Place the butter in a medium bowl and heat in the microwave for 45 seconds at medium (50%) power (or 30 seconds at high power); stir until melted.

2. Lightly brush an 8-inch-square glass baking dish with butter. Brush the remaining butter on both sides of each slice of bread and lay the slices in the prepared pan.

3. In the same bowl, beat together the egg, milk, cinnamon, and salt with a fork and then pour over the bread. Cover with plastic wrap and chill overnight.

4. In the morning, place the pan in the oven at 425°F. Set the timer for 15 minutes and bake until the toast is puffed and golden, up to 18 minutes total. Loosen the French toast slices with a flexible metal spatula and serve.

Cooks' Note

❖ Adding salt heightens the flavor of any sweet or savory dish. We like kosher salt for its pure salt flavor, but in baking we always use fine table salt.

PREP: 5 minutes (not including chilling overnight)
BAKING: 18 minutes
SPEED LIMIT: 23 mpr

Makes 1 serving

PER SERVING:
545 calories,
42g fat (24g saturated),
31g carbohydrates,
4g fiber, 14g protein

Upon tasting it, Kelsey S., age ten, from Rye, New York, exclaimed, "I loved it so much. It's so fluffy!"

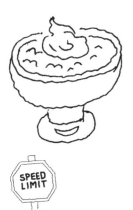

PREP: 5 minutes
BAKING: 20 minutes
SPEED LIMIT: 30 mpr
(includes cooling)

Makes 1 serving

PER SERVING:
*162 calories, 7g fat
(3g saturated),
23g carbohydrates, 3g fiber,
3g protein*

Good Day Pear Crisp

Pie for breakfast? Not quite, but the fragrance of this dish is so good that even the groggiest grouch will be lured out of bed. Look for ripe pears without bruises, and keep at room temperature overnight. Cut the butter in a thin slice off the stick for melting evenly.

Half of a ripe Bartlett pear
1 small lemon wedge
1½ teaspoons dark brown sugar
1 tablespoon rolled oats
½ tablespoon chopped walnuts or pecans
1 teaspoon unsalted butter
Pinch of cinnamon
1 rounded tablespoon cottage cheese or plain whole milk yogurt,
for serving

1. Preheat the oven to 400°F.

2. Halve the pear half and core; cut crosswise into slices and place in a 6-ounce custard cup. Squeeze the lemon on top, add the sugar, oats, nuts, butter, and cinnamon, and bake for 20 minutes, until bubbly and golden and the pears are soft.

3. Let cool for 5 minutes and add a dollop of cottage cheese or yogurt.

Good Day Summer Crisp: In late summer, follow this recipe substituting a ripe nectarine, a plum or two, or a juicy pluot (plum and apricot hybrid), pitted and sliced, for the pear.

Good Day Fall Crisp: In autumn, use a small sweet-tart Royal Gala apple, but peel, quarter, and core the apple before slicing. Add dried cranberries, dried sour cherries, or raisins, as desired.

"Healthy dessert—for breakfast? I love it!"
That's the statement from seven-year-old
Jackson F., of Brooklyn, New York.

Sunshine Parfait

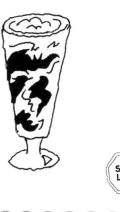

This breakfast sundae is tropical in nature, but you can think of other tempting combos. If you can't find mango, substitute berries, pineapple, or sliced banana. Cutting the fruit just before using is best, but for ease, you can purchase cut-up fruit from the market or cut the fruit the night before. Have a kid who won't touch cottage cheese? Substitute plain whole milk yogurt.

> ½ cup finely diced fresh mango
> ⅓ cup cottage cheese
> ½ tablespoon unsweetened coconut milk
> 2 tablespoons prepared Extreme Granola (page 50) or store-bought
>   granola

Spoon half of the mango into a footed parfait glass. Spoon the cottage cheese and the remaining mango on top. Drizzle with the coconut milk, top with the granola, and serve.

Cooks' Notes

❖ Cottage cheese, a great source of protein, is good to have on hand for meals and snacking because it mixes well with both sweet and savory flavors.

❖ Now you can buy unsweetened (light) coconut milk in handy 5.5-ounce cans. We love it in desserts, drinks, and Asian dishes.

❖ When using store-bought granola, buy organic, no-fat, low-sugar varieties.

PREP: 5 minutes
SPEED LIMIT: 5 mpr

Makes 1 serving

PER SERVING:
173 calories, 5g fat
(3.5g saturated),
25g carbohydrates,
2.5g fiber, 10g protein

rise to the occasion:
breakfast morning, noon, and night

These dishes are a little more involved but they will have your kids jumping out of bed and keep them full of steam for hours. Many of these dishes work at any other time of day and are even suitable for dinner.

Best Eggs on Earth

Green Eggs-in-Ham Quiche Cups

Cheese Omelet

Perfect Poached Eggs

Breakfast Skillet Surprise

Belgian Waffles

Blue Ribbon Pancakes

Blueberry Blue Ribbon Pancakes

Strawberry Blue Ribbon Pancakes

Protein Power Pancakes

Brioche French Toast

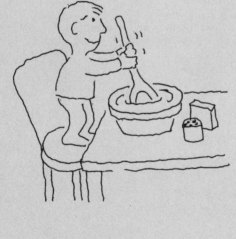

Best Eggs on Earth

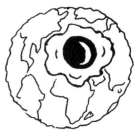

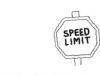

Fried eggs are high on Tracey's comfort food list, along with grilled cheese and a cheese omelet. One day, when she couldn't choose between them, she made these cheesy eggs. They are so good that perhaps your kids will clean their rooms in order to have them. We use two eggs each, but if you are cooking for little ones, 1 egg each and ½ of the remaining ingredients will be more than enough.

½ tablespoon unsalted butter
4 large eggs
¾ cup shredded (packed) extra-sharp Cheddar cheese (3 ounces)
1 ripe medium tomato, cut into ⅓-inch dice
Kosher salt and freshly ground black pepper

1. Preheat the broiler with the rack set in the highest position.

2. Melt the butter in a medium nonstick or well-seasoned cast-iron skillet over medium heat. Crack the eggs and add to the pan, spacing as best you can. Sprinkle the cheese and diced tomato on top around the yolks. Cook until the bottom of the eggs is just firm enough to slip a spatula under, 1 to 2 minutes.

3. Transfer the skillet to the broiler and cook until the cheese is bubbly and the tops of the eggs are just set, 2 to 3 minutes (depending on the intensity of your broiler). Season with salt and pepper.

Cooks' Notes

❖ To keep the yolks a little runny, broil the eggs as soon as they are set on the bottom. For six to eight eggs, use a larger skillet and a little more butter, cheese, and tomato. The cooking time will be about the same.

❖ There is nothing wrong with adding a crumbling of bacon with the cheese—and don't forget toast for dunking.

PREP: 5 minutes
COOKING: 5 minutes
SPEED LIMIT: 10 mpr

Makes 2 servings

PER SERVING:
360 calories,
27g fat (14g saturated),
5g carbohydrates,
.5g fiber, 23g protein

Five-year-old Maddison M., of Traverse City, Michigan, said, "They ARE good! I like the tomatoes and the yolk—I like it all!"

Green Eggs-in-Ham Quiche Cups

PREP: 15 minutes
BAKING: 25 minutes
(includes cooling)
SPEED LIMIT: 40 mpr

Makes 4 servings

PER QUICHE CUP:
243 calories, 17.5g fat
(9.5g saturated),
9.5g carbohydrates,
2g fiber, 13g protein

These individual quiches are fun to make and delicious to eat. Thin slices of prosciutto can be a little sticky to work with, but the packaged imported variety tends to have even slices that are easy to separate. Serve with your favorite toast.

> 1 tablespoon unsalted butter
> 1 small onion, finely chopped
> One 5-ounce bag washed and dried baby spinach
> 8 thin slices imported prosciutto
> 2 large eggs
> 1 cup half-and-half
> 2 pinches of freshly ground black pepper
> 2 ounces imported Swiss cheese, shredded ($\frac{1}{2}$ cup packed)

1. Preheat the oven to 400°F.

2. Melt the butter in a medium well-seasoned cast-iron or nonstick skillet. Add the onion and cook, stirring occasionally, until the onion is softened and begins to brown, about 3 minutes. Add the spinach and turn occasionally until wilted, about 3 minutes. Remove from the heat.

3. Crisscross 2 slices of prosciutto on a work surface, piecing the ham together if necessary, lay on top of a custard cup, and then fit inside the cup as a crust, letting any excess hang over the side. Repeat with the remaining prosciutto and place the cups on a shallow baking sheet.

4. Beat together the eggs, half-and-half, and pepper with a fork in a medium bowl. Add the spinach mixture and cheese and mix again. Spoon the egg mixture evenly into the prosciutto-lined cups. Bake for about 20 minutes, until the filling is puffed and golden. Let stand for 5 minutes before eating (the filling will continue cooking slightly).

Omelet 101

We prefer omelets simply done with just a bit of cheese, and maybe a smidgen of lean meat or vegetable, because that way you can cook the omelets quickly without danger of browning the egg. If you like your eggs packed with other goodies, see Microwave Pizza Frittata (page 30).

The trick to perfect omelets is adding a little water to make the eggs steam as they cook. It is best to cook them quickly over medium heat, scrambling continually until they are half cooked, then stop, removing the pan from the heat, and spread in an even layer before adding the cheese. (If you have an electric stove, let the burner heat up a little before you start cooking, and then let it cool before putting the pan back.) Once the eggs are set on the bottom and the cheese is slightly melted, fold the omelet over. The cheese will melt in about 30 seconds.

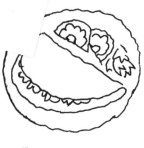

Cheese Omelet

We love omelets with almost anything. See below for some ideas.

4 large eggs
1½ tablespoons cold water
2 pinches of kosher salt
Pinch of freshly ground black pepper
½ tablespoon extra-virgin olive oil or unsalted butter
½ cup shredded (packed) cheese of your choice, such as Cheddar, Swiss,
   or Monterey Jack (2 ounces)

PREP: 2 minutes
COOKING: 3 minutes
SPEED LIMIT: 5 mpr

Makes 2 servings

PER SERVING:
292 calories,
23g fat (9.5g saturated),
1g carbohydrates,
0g fiber, 19.5g protein

1. Combine the eggs, water, salt, and pepper in a small bowl; beat with a fork until well blended.

2. Add the oil to a 9-inch well-seasoned cast-iron or nonstick skillet over medium heat. Pour in the eggs and cook, scrambling constantly with a fork, a silicone spatula, or a wooden spatula until the eggs are half cooked, about 2 minutes. Remove from the heat.

3. Spread the eggs in an even layer and sprinkle the cheese on top. Place the pan over very low heat and let stand for 1 minute. Once the eggs are set on the bottom, fold the eggs over to form an omelet and let stand for 30 seconds to melt the cheese.

Cooks' Note

❧ To make the omelet more substantial, cook some finely chopped onion, diced ham, or thinly sliced small mushrooms in ½ tablespoon additional oil before adding the egg to the pan. Add cooked crumbled bacon to the egg when beginning to cook.

Perfect Poached Eggs

Once you know how to make poached eggs, you can make them even more special by adding a little of our lightened-up Blender Hollandaise (page 210) on top.

1 teaspoon kosher salt
2 teaspoons white vinegar
4 large eggs

1. Place 8 cups water and the salt in a 10-inch skillet and bring to a boil over medium-high heat. Add the vinegar and swirl the water around in a circle with a slotted spoon. Crack 1 egg gently and add to the center of the pan. Once it begins to coagulate, add the other eggs to the water one at a time. Reduce the heat slightly and simmer gently until the eggs are set but the yolks are still wobbly, about 3 minutes.

2. Fold a paper towel in half twice. Gently remove the eggs one at a time from the water with a slotted spoon and blot above and below with the paper towel to remove any excess water, and then transfer the eggs to cups or serve as desired. Repeat with more eggs as necessary.

Cooks' Note

❖ Be creative with your poached egg presentation. Serve the eggs atop toast, split English muffin halves, a toasted croissant, or a piece of French baguette. Add a layer of creamed spinach, grilled tomato slices, sautéed mushrooms, pan-fried ham, Canadian bacon, or sausage patties. For the crowning touch, add a spoonful of Blender Hollandaise (page 210) or Eat-Yer-Veggies Cheese Sauce (page 214).

PREP: 5 minutes
COOKING: 3 minutes
SPEED LIMIT: 8 mpr

Makes 4 eggs

PER EGG:
74 calories,
5g fat (1.5g saturated),
0g carbohydrates, 0g fiber,
6g protein

Breakfast Skillet Surprise

Adding the word *surprise* to a dish leaves it open to infinite possibilities. Versatile eggs are the basis for this recipe, and here we deliciously get protein, vegetable, and starch in one dish. We used zucchini, but you can substitute bell pepper, steamed spinach, or cooked broccoli. For an Italian version, serve the eggs on soft rolls with warmed marinara sauce and a sprinkling of mozzarella or Fontina cheese.

PREP: 10 minutes
COOKING: 22 minutes
SPEED LIMIT: 32 mpr

Makes 6 servings

PER SERVING:
557 calories, 34g fat
(13g saturated)
34g carbohydrates
3g fiber, 27g protein

2 small potatoes, diced
8 ounces fresh chorizo or other sausage, removed from casings
1 small zucchini, halved lengthwise and thinly sliced
1 tablespoon olive oil
6 large eggs
1 tablespoon cold water
3 ounces sharp Cheddar cheese, shredded (³/₄ cup)
3 ounces queso fresco (Mexican) cheese, crumbled (³/₄ cup)
Whole-wheat flour tortillas, warmed
Green salsa or other hot sauce, for serving

1. In a large pot of water, cook the potatoes until tender, about 8 minutes. Meanwhile, place the sausage in a large cast-iron nonstick skillet over medium heat. Cook, stirring occasionally, until the meat is crumbly and beginning to crisp, about 6 minutes. Add the zucchini and cook, stirring, until softened, about 2 minutes. Scrape the sausage and zucchini out onto a paper towel–lined plate.

2. Add the potato and oil to the skillet and cook over medium heat until golden and crisp, about 4 minutes. Return the sausage and zucchini to the pan. Combine the eggs and water in a bowl and beat well with a fork; pour into the pan and scramble over medium-high heat until cooked through but still moist, about 2 minutes. Sprinkle the cheeses onto the hot eggs and then spoon into the warmed tortillas. Serve with salsa or hot sauce if desired.

Cooks' Note

❖ To warm the tortillas, wrap them in aluminum foil and place in a moderate 350°F oven for about 10 minutes.

"These are really good when they are spicy,"
says Tanya's son William.

Belgian Waffles

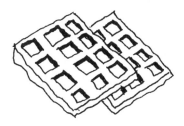

These yeasted waffles are light, crispy on the outside, and slightly gooey (not cakey) on the inside. Although they take a little bit of planning, they are heavenly. Serve with warmed pure maple syrup. If you don't have a Belgian waffle iron (see Cooks' Note), use a regular iron, which will only result in thinner waffles.

½ cup warm water (105°F to 115°F)
2 teaspoons sugar
One ¼-ounce packet active dry yeast
2 cups whole milk
1⅓ cups unbleached all-purpose flour
⅔ cup whole-wheat flour
½ teaspoon fine salt
6 tablespoons unsalted butter
2 large eggs, at room temperature (see Cooks' Note)

1. Fill a glass measuring cup with hot water; insert an instant-read thermometer in the water and add more hot or cool water as necessary until the temperature registers between 105°F and 110°F. Pour out enough water to end up with ½ cup. Stir in the sugar and yeast and set aside until foamy, about 5 minutes.

2. Meanwhile, microwave the milk at high (100%) power for 1½ minutes to warm. Rinse out a large mixing bowl with hot water and wipe dry. Add the milk and the yeast mixture. Add the flours and salt and whisk to blend. Cover with plastic and set aside in a warm place until doubled in bulk, about 1 hour.

3. Plug in a Belgian waffle iron. Melt the butter in the microwave and whisk into the batter along with the eggs until well blended.

4. When the iron is ready, add about ½ cup batter per 4-inch waffle and cook according to the manufacturer's instructions. Serve the waffles as they are ready.

Cooks' Note

❖ To warm the eggs: Place whole eggs (in the shell) in a small bowl and fill with hot tap water, wait about 30 seconds, and pour out the water and repeat.

PREP: 10 minutes plus 1 hour rising
COOKING: about 20 minutes

Makes ten 4-inch waffles

PER WAFFLE:
190 calories, 9.5g fat (5.5g saturated)
21g carbohydrates
1g fiber, 5.5g protein

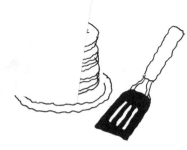

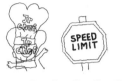

Blue Ribbon Pancakes

The vanilla low-fat yogurt, which adds tang and sweetness, makes these whole-wheaty flapjacks a truly nutritious way to start (or end) your day.

2 large eggs
2 tablespoons unsalted butter
¾ cup unbleached all-purpose flour
¾ cup whole-wheat flour
1 teaspoon baking soda
½ teaspoon salt
1½ cups vanilla low-fat yogurt
¾ cup whole milk
½ cup pure maple syrup, warmed, for serving

PREP: 5 minutes
COOKING: 15 minutes
SPEED LIMIT: 20 mpr

Makes 4 servings (about 14 five-inch pancakes)

PER SERVING:
448 calories, 11g fat (6g saturated), 75g carbohydrates, 3g fiber, 14.5g protein

1. Place the eggs in a small bowl and add hot tap water to cover. Place the butter in a small microwavable bowl and microwave at medium (50%) power for 1 minute; stir until melted.

2. In a large bowl, whisk together the flours, baking soda, and salt. Make a well in the center and add the yogurt, milk, and eggs and whisk until blended. Place a large nonstick skillet or griddle over medium heat. Add the melted butter to the batter and stir with a rubber spatula.

3. Measure out pancakes with a ⅓-cup measuring cup and spoon into the hot pan, leaving enough space between cakes. Cook until bubbles appear on the surface, 2 to 3 minutes, flip, and cook until springy to the touch and golden underneath. Transfer to plates and serve with warm maple syrup.

Cooks' Note

❖ Serving tip: Pour a little puddle of syrup on the plates instead of on top of the cakes—this will cut down on the amount of syrup used.

Blueberry Blue Ribbon Pancakes or Strawberry Blue Ribbon Pancakes: Add 1 cup whole blueberries or sliced strawberries to the batter just before cooking. You can also add ½ cup finely chopped walnuts or pecans; 1 cup diced ripe fresh pear; or ½ cup dried fruit such as currants, apples, or dates.

"My daughter, Lua, age fourteen months, couldn't eat these fast enough," says Holly L., of Amagansett, New York. "Not having a full range of vocabulary yet, she said, 'Mmmmm!'"

Protein Power Pancakes

These are a healthy modification of a recipe Tanya's friend Laura used to whip up after a late night of dancing. Serve these tender and delicious pancakes with warm pure maple syrup, a teaspoon of yogurt or sour cream sprinkled with sugar, or a dab of your favorite jam.

2 large eggs
¾ cup reduced-fat (2%) milk
1 tablespoon unsalted butter
1 cup whole milk ricotta, preferably organic
½ cup unbleached all-purpose flour
⅓ cup whole-wheat flour
1 tablespoon sugar
1½ teaspoons baking powder
¼ teaspoon salt
½ teaspoon cinnamon (optional)

1. Place the whole eggs (in the shell) in a bowl, add very hot water to cover, and let stand. Meanwhile, place the milk in a glass mixing bowl and microwave at high (100%) power for 1 minute. Add the butter and whisk until melted. Whisk in the eggs and ricotta.

2. Add the flours, sugar, baking powder, salt, and cinnamon, if using, and then whisk until the batter is smooth.

3. Heat a large nonstick or well-seasoned skillet or griddle over medium heat until hot. Spoon 2 tablespoons of batter for each pancake into the skillet, leaving enough space between the pancakes. Let cook until bubbles appear on the surface and the cakes are golden underneath, about 2 minutes. Flip and cook for 1 to 2 minutes, until the cakes are springy to the touch. Serve at once.

PREP: 5 minutes
COOKING: 20 minutes
SPEED LIMIT: 25 mpr

Makes about 22 small pancakes

PER PANCAKE:
53 calories, 2.5g fat
(1.5g saturated),
5g carbohydrates,
.5g fiber, 2.5g protein

"Yum, yum, yum, yum, yum," says two-year-old Taven M., of Traverse City, Michigan.

Brioche French Toast

This is a great way to make use of fresh or day-old sliced brioche or challah bread; the thick slices of golden toast are like puffy cinnamon-vanilla soufflés. Top with warmed maple syrup or sautéed fresh fruit.

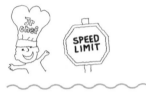

PREP: 5 minutes (includes soaking)
COOKING: 8 minutes
SPEED LIMIT: 13 mpr

Makes 4 servings

PER SLICE (WITH 2 TABLESPOONS MAPLE SYRUP):
410 calories, 14g fat (6g saturated), 57g carbohydrates, 1.5g fiber, 13g protein

4 large eggs
¾ cup low-fat milk
½ teaspoon cinnamon
Dash of pure vanilla extract
Four 1-inch-thick slices brioche or challah bread (8 ounces)
2 tablespoons unsalted butter

1. In a large, wide bowl, combine the eggs, milk, cinnamon, and vanilla. Add all of the bread slices, turning to coat and stacking in two layers. Let soak for about 2 minutes, turning and restacking the slices.

2. Meanwhile, melt 1 tablespoon of the butter in a nonstick large skillet over medium heat until the butter begins to sizzle. Carefully remove the bread slices from the bowl and place them in the skillet. Let cook on medium heat until golden brown underneath, about 4 minutes.

3. Turn the slices, add the remaining tablespoon of butter to the center of the skillet, and cook until the toasts are nicely golden on the other side and springy to the touch, about 3 minutes longer. Serve at once.

Fiona G., of New York City, "loved the vanilla smell"
of the French toast.

breakfast bakeshop: homemade and wholesome

Home-baked goods, like quick breads and muffins, are wonderful on-the-go treats for wholesome breakfasts and are easy to make ahead for weekdays.

Extreme Granola

Yankee Doodle Corn Bread

Ba-Ba Banana Bread

Chocolate Chip Banana Bread

Bursting Berry Muffins

Kiss-of-Honey Wheat Biscuits

Extreme Granola

The Seaman and Steel families are addicted to this homemade granola with dried blueberries and sweet dates. Serve it with a splash of milk or a spoonful of yogurt or ice cream, sprinkled on pancakes, or in a smoothie.

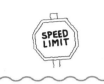

PREP: 10 minutes plus cooling
BAKING: 40 minutes
SPEED LIMIT: 50 mpr

Makes about 7 cups

PER ½ CUP:
298 calories, 16g fat
(4.5g saturated),
34g carbohydrates,
4.5g fiber, 6.5g protein

¾ cup pecans
½ cup natural almonds
4 cups old-fashioned rolled oats
¼ cup sesame seeds (optional)
1 stick (8 tablespoons) unsalted butter
⅓ cup pure maple syrup, cane syrup, or honey, at room temperature
¼ teaspoon fine salt
¾ cup chopped dates
½ cup dried blueberries or raisins

1. Preheat the oven to 375°F. Line a large shallow baking sheet with foil. Spread the pecans and almonds on the sheet and roast for 8 to 10 minutes, until lightly toasted. Transfer the nuts to a board, let cool, and chop the nuts. Set aside.

2. Reduce the oven temperature to 300°F. Pour the oats and sesame seeds, if using, in a mound on the same baking sheet. Melt the butter in a small bowl in the microwave; stir in the maple syrup and salt and drizzle on top of the oats. Stir well with a rubber spatula and then spread out the oats in an even layer.

3. Bake the oats for 30 minutes, stirring once with the spatula halfway through, until the oats are lightly colored. Let cool; the mixture will crisp as it cools. Add the dates, blueberries, and reserved nuts and toss.

Cooks' Notes

❖ Store the granola in covered glass jars at room temperature for up to one month.

❖ Double the fun! Make two batches of granola by doubling the ingredients and using two baking sheets—one in the upper third and one in the lower third of the oven. Package in cellophane bags tied with ribbon for a tasty gift.

Yankee Doodle Corn Bread

This not-too-sweet corn bread is best served soon after baking, split and spread with a bit of soft salted butter. Serve the bread with eggs, soup, or barbecued meats.

6 tablespoons unsalted butter

1⅔ cups yellow cornmeal

1⅓ cups unbleached all-purpose flour

⅓ cup sugar

2 teaspoons baking powder

½ teaspoon crushed red pepper flakes (optional)

¾ teaspoon kosher salt

3 large eggs

1½ cups milk

1. Place the butter in a 10-inch cast-iron or other ovenproof skillet, transfer to the oven, and turn the oven to 375°F.

2. Combine the cornmeal, flour, sugar, baking powder, crushed red pepper flakes, if using, and salt in a large bowl and whisk to blend. Make a well in the center and add the eggs. Beat the eggs well with a fork and add the milk. Stir with a fork until the batter is smooth.

3. When the butter in the skillet is melted, pour it into the batter, leaving enough butter in the pan to coat it well. Stir the batter until the butter is just incorporated.

4. Scrape the batter into the skillet, smoothing the top. Bake for about 25 minutes, until the bread is firm to the touch and a cake tester inserted into the center comes out clean. Let cool for at least 15 minutes before cutting into wedges.

PREP: 10 minutes plus cooling

BAKING: 25 minutes

SPEED LIMIT: 35 mpr

Makes 8 servings

PER SERVING:
312 calories, 13g fat (7g saturated), 43g carbohydrates, 2g fiber, 8g protein

"I could eat this every day of my life," says Tanya's son Sanger.

Ba-Ba Banana Bread

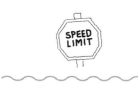

PREP: 8 minutes plus cooling
BAKING: 1 hour

Makes 12 servings

PER SLICE (TOTAL 12 SLICES):
205 calories,
7g fat (1g saturated),
35g carbohydrates,
4g fiber, 5.5g protein

This quick bread comes from an old English recipe Tanya's grandmother used, but Tanya has made it more nutritious. She replaced the usual two sticks of butter with buttermilk and a bit of oil, and the white flour with whole-wheat flour, making it great for breakfast or a lunch box dessert. For best results, use very ripe bananas.

2 cups whole-wheat flour
2 teaspoons baking powder
$\frac{1}{2}$ teaspoon baking soda
$\frac{1}{2}$ teaspoon salt
$\frac{3}{4}$ teaspoon cinnamon
$\frac{1}{4}$ teaspoon nutmeg
2 large eggs
$\frac{3}{4}$ cup sugar
4 very ripe medium bananas, coarsely mashed with a fork
$\frac{1}{3}$ cup buttermilk
1 tablespoon vegetable oil
$1\frac{1}{2}$ teaspoons pure vanilla extract
$\frac{2}{3}$ cup chopped walnuts

1. Preheat the oven to 350°F. Lightly grease a 9- by 5-inch loaf pan. Whisk together the flour, baking powder, baking soda, salt, cinnamon, and nutmeg in a medium bowl and reserve.

2. Beat the eggs and sugar in the bowl of an electric mixer until fluffy, about 2 minutes. Add the bananas, buttermilk, oil, and vanilla and mix at low speed until blended.

3. Add the flour mixture and mix at low speed just until blended. Stir in the nuts and then scrape the batter into the prepared pan. Bake for about 1 hour, until a cake tester inserted into the center comes out clean.

4. Let the bread cool for 15 minutes in the pan on a rack, then turn out and let cool completely. Cut into twelve $\frac{2}{3}$-inch-thick slices.

Cooks' Note

✤ This banana bread makes an awesome sandwich with peanut butter and your favorite go-withs.

Chocolate Chip Banana Bread: Fold $\frac{1}{2}$ cup mini-semisweet chocolate chips into the batter just before baking.

"This is a banana blast for my monkey mouth," says seven-year-old Rye, New York, resident Jack B.

Bursting Berry Muffins

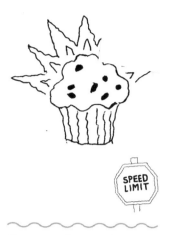

You can enjoy these muffins any time of the year, because they are made with frozen berries. If you like, before baking you can sprinkle the muffin tops with cinnamon sugar for added crispiness. To make two dozen, simply double the recipe and bake in two muffin pans, one in the upper third and one in the lower third of the oven.

> 1 stick unsalted butter, softened
> ¾ cup sugar
> 2 large eggs, at room temperature
> 2 teaspoons baking powder
> 1 teaspoon pure vanilla extract
> ¼ teaspoon fine salt
> 1 cup unbleached all-purpose flour
> ½ cup whole milk
> ⅔ cup whole-wheat flour
> ⅓ cup unprocessed wheat bran or additional white whole-wheat flour
> One 10-ounce bag frozen blueberries (do not thaw)

PREP: 15 minutes plus cooling
BAKING: 30 minutes
SPEED LIMIT: 45 mpr

Makes 1 dozen

PER MUFFIN:
190 calories, 9g fat (5g saturated), 26g carbohydrates, 2g fiber, 3.5g protein

1. Arrange an oven rack in the lower third of the oven and preheat the oven to 375°F. Lightly grease the top of a 12-muffin (½-cup capacity) pan. Line the cups with paper cupcake liners and set aside.

2. Beat the butter and sugar with an electric mixer at high speed until fluffy, at least 3 minutes, scraping down the sides of the bowl as necessary. Beat in the eggs one at a time, beating until fluffy after each addition. Add the baking powder, vanilla, and salt and mix at medium speed to blend. Add the all-purpose flour and the milk and mix at medium speed until just incorporated. Add the whole-wheat flour and bran and mix just until blended. Add the frozen berries and stir.

3. Spoon the batter, piling high, into the muffin cups. Bake for 30 minutes, until golden on top and springy to the touch. Let cool for 15 minutes before serving.

Brendan D., from Rye, New York, age nine, said, "These are amazing. Pretty much the best muffin I ever tasted. It really is really good." Eight year-old sister, Catherine, agrees: "I don't like blueberries, but I like these muffins."

Kiss-of-Honey Wheat Biscuits

A sprinkling of cinnamon sugar makes these generous golden biscuits a special treat for breakfast, and they are quick to mix up. Serve them warm with a smidgen of cream cheese and fresh fruit.

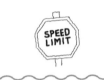

PREP: 10 minutes
BAKING: 13 minutes
SPEED LIMIT: 23 mpr

Makes 7 biscuits

PER BISCUIT:
270 calories,
11g fat (7g saturated),
37g carbohydrates,
2.5g fiber, 5g protein

⅔ cup sour cream
⅓ cup milk
3 tablespoons honey
1 cup whole-wheat flour
1 cup plain cake flour (not self-rising), plus a little more for dusting
1½ teaspoons baking powder
½ teaspoon baking soda
¼ teaspoon salt
4 tablespoons cold unsalted butter, cut into small dice
1½ teaspoons sugar mixed with ¼ teaspoon cinnamon, for sprinkling

1. Preheat the oven to 425°F.

2. Stir the sour cream, milk, and honey together in a small bowl with a rubber spatula.

3. Combine the flours, baking powder, baking soda, and salt in a large bowl. Whisk to blend. Add the butter and work into the dry mixture with your fingertips until crumbly.

4. Pour the sour cream mixture into the dry mixture and stir just until the dough almost comes together in a ball.

5. Lightly flour a work surface, turn the dough out, and knead once or twice to blend. Pat into a ¾-inch-thick circle and then use a glass with a 2½- to 3-inch rim to cut 5 biscuits; place on a shallow baking sheet so that the sides of the biscuits are barely touching. Briefly knead the scraps together, pat again, and cut 2 more biscuits. Sprinkle the cinnamon sugar on top of the biscuits.

6. Bake for 13 minutes, until the biscuits are golden and springy to the touch. Let cool a few minutes before serving.

Cooks' Note

❖ Buyer bee-ware! If you can, use local honey, as it may contain properties that help the immune systems of the inhabitants in the area in which it is produced. Also, Gold Medal whole-wheat flour is the best kind to use here, as it has the perfect texture.

store-bought breakfast foods we like

Here are a few packaged breakfast foods we think are fairly healthy for your kids. For more suggestions, log on to www.realfoodforhealthykids.com.

Kashi Heart to Heart, Organic Promise Autumn Wheat,
and Go Lean cereals
Nature Valley cereals
Bare Naked cereals
Cascadian Farm cereals
Back to Nature cereals
Van's Hearty Oats Waffles and Organic Waffles
Lifestream Buckwheat Waffles

chapter three

On the Rise
Fearless Baking with Yeast

t is surprising how many people are intimidated by baking with yeast. And yet few things are more satisfying than kneading dough and baking bread. Plus, by baking your own bread you are assured that you are giving your children a wholesome loaf that is all natural and made with TLC. Another reason to bake one of these loaves is that they are fun to make with kids, who will love getting their hands on the dough, slapping, punching, and smashing it. Just choose a day when you're not all racing from one place to another because the dough needs to rest and rise before going in the oven. Here are our foolproof tips on how to make magnificent loaves. Be sure to read the recipe through before beginning (there are many helpful hints throughout).

What You Will Need

To make any or all of these recipes, you will need to have basics on hand—unbleached flour, whole-wheat flour, plain cake flour, butter, olive oil, salt, sugar, yeast, and a few other ingredients for flavoring and added texture. Also, get nonaluminum baking powder (see the section on wheat sensitivity for more recipes) because no one needs extra aluminum in his or her life.

Yeast is sometimes available in cake form, but more often you will see dry active yeast in triple packets or in a jar in the baking aisle. For breads and biscuits, we call for regular dry active yeast, not the instant variety, but we do use instant yeast for pizza dough. Check the expiration date stamped on each packet or jar. Store any remaining unopened packets at room temperature in the spice rack or store an opened jar of yeast in the refrigerator.

Yeast Affection

A thermometer is the key to successful bread making; having the water at the perfect temperature, 105°F to 115°F, will produce a happily foaming yeast mixture, which means it's alive. We usually include a bit of sugar to help the process along.

The Proof Is in the Rising

Proofing is the method of activating yeast. First, measure the required amount of filtered water in a glass measuring cup and heat it in the microwave for 1 minute. Take its temperature with an instant-read thermometer: If the water is too cold, heat it a little more and retake the temperature; if the water is too hot, add cold water to lower the temperature. Pour off any extra water (to get the amount you need) and stir in the sugar, if included. Sprinkle the yeast on top, stir it in, and then let the mixture stand while you measure the dry ingredients or make other preparations. The yeast-water mixture should start to froth in a few minutes, which indicates that the yeast will be effective. (If the water is too hot, the yeast will be destroyed and the dough will not rise at all.)

All Mixed Up

If your yeast is alive you're halfway home. Next, you will combine some dry ingredients in a bowl, make a well—or indentation—in the center, and pour in the yeast mixture and any other wet ingredients. (If you are adding oil, milk, or eggs, add them at room temperature. If adding butter, be sure it is soft enough for easy spreading.) Stir everything together with a wooden spoon or a rubber spatula. You can also use the paddle attachment on the mixer. Once the mixture forms a mass, you're ready to begin kneading.

The Need to Be Kneaded

There is a special kind of protein in wheat flour, which is why it is so abundantly found in breads. Once the flour is mixed with liquid, a network of gluten is created. This network is sort of elastic and plastic in nature; it is stretchy but becomes stronger the more it is handled. Kneading exercises the gluten, making it more elastic, while it eventually makes the dough pleasantly smooth. Once the dough reaches that point, it needs to rest; during that time the activated yeast will produce carbon dioxide gases, which push against the "fibers" of gluten and cause the dough to rise.

Man or Machine?

You can knead dough by hand or in a standing mixer. For the nervous novice, using a mixer is a good idea because you will see what a finished dough should look like. The more you handle the dough the better, so have no fear of overhandling. Keep in mind that making bread is much less precise than making a piecrust, which needs a more delicate hand. Generally yeast dough is kneaded between 7 and 10 minutes. Timing will be on the shorter side in a machine, and often in the machine you can use a little less flour.

A Clean Vessel

When the dough is ready to rise, oil a clean large bowl, add the dough, turn to coat in the oil, and then cover the top of the bowl with plastic wrap. This will prevent a skin from forming on top of the dough.

Where Should My Dough Rise?

The perfect room temperature for dough to rise is 75°F to 80°F, but that may not be possible, especially in winter. Seek out a draft-free corner in the kitchen or put the covered bowl of dough in a warm bathroom. If you have a combination oven-cooktop, try turning the oven on as low as it will go (these days some electric ovens begin at 170°F); place the bowl of dough on top of the stove and let it rise there. If your room temperature is lower, don't panic; the dough might just take a little more time to rise.

Slow Rise

You can also let most doughs rise overnight in the refrigerator. To do this, rinse the bowl with warm water (instead of coating with oil) and do not dry. Add the kneaded dough, cover the bowl with plastic wrap, and refrigerate overnight, or for up to 36 hours. When ready to bake, turn the dough out onto the counter and proceed with forming the dough into loaves. Let rise until doubled; because the dough is cold this may take up to twice as long as normal again, so you have to keep watch. Bake as directed.

Maple-Apple Sandwich Bread

Raisin Bread

Cinnamon-Swirl Bread

Skillet Whole-wheat Pita

Special Occasion Biscuits

Pizza Dough

Rosemary Focaccia

Maple-Apple Sandwich Bread

These tender loaves, which are not particularly sweet, will stay moist for several days due to the addition of grated apple. We like the bread best made with a combination of hard red whole-wheat flour (such as King Arthur Traditional) and the milder white whole-wheat flour (from winter wheat), but you can use your choice. For ease, make the dough in a standing electric mixer with the dough hook attached.

PREP: 20 minutes
RISING: About 1½ hours
BAKING: 40 minutes

**Makes two 9-inch loaves
(about 12 slices per loaf)**

PER SLICE:
137 calories, 2.5g fat
(.5g saturated),
26g carbohydrates,
2.5g fiber, 4g protein

1 cup warm filtered water (105°F to 115°F)
¼ teaspoon sugar
One ¼-ounce packet active dry yeast
1 cup whole milk
¼ cup pure maple syrup, at room temperature
2 tablespoons olive oil, plus more for greasing the bowl and the pans
3 cups whole-wheat flour
About 3¼ cups unbleached all-purpose flour
1½ teaspoons fine salt
1 medium eating apple, such as Royal Gala or Golden Delicious
1 tablespoon unsalted butter, melted

1. Place the warm water in a pint-sized glass measuring cup. Stir in the sugar, sprinkle the yeast on top, stir to mix, and reserve.

2. Pour the milk into a small bowl and microwave at high (100%) power for 1 minute to warm. Add the maple syrup and oil to the milk.

3. Combine the whole-wheat flour, 3 cups of the all-purpose flour, and the salt in a bowl of a standing mixer fitted with a dough hook and mix for 1 minute at low speed to blend. Pour in the yeast and milk mixtures and then mix at low speed until the dough comes together.

4. Increase the speed to medium and knead the dough in the mixer, adding about ¼ cup more all-purpose flour (or more as necessary), until the dough is slightly sticky, smooth, and elastic, 7 to 8 minutes.

5. Transfer the dough to a work surface. Wash, dry, and then lightly oil the bowl. Add the dough and turn to coat in the oil. Cover the top of the bowl snugly with plastic wrap and then let the dough rise in a warm place until doubled in bulk, 45 minutes to an hour.

6. Lightly oil two 9- by-5-inch loaf pans. Turn the dough out onto the work surface. Peel the apple, finely shred on a box grater (discarding the apple

core), and then coarsely chop. Press the dough out to ½-inch thick. Sprinkle the apple on top of the dough, fold over, and knead briefly to incorporate throughout. The dough will become moist and sticky. Cut the dough in half, knead each piece into a thick cylinder, and place in the loaf pans. Cover loosely with a kitchen towel and let rise in a warm place until doubled, about 45 minutes.

7. Arrange a rack in the lower third of the oven and preheat the oven to 350°F. Bake the loaves for about 40 minutes, until nicely puffed and golden. Let cool for 10 minutes in the pans on a rack and then cut around the edges of the loaves with a small sharp knife and turn out. Brush the tops with the melted butter. Let the loaves cool completely on the rack before slicing with a serrated knife.

Cooks' Notes

❖ Brushing the top of the loaves with melted butter softens the top crust.

❖ Store the cooled bread wrapped in foil at room temperature. Any bread that will not be used within two days should be sliced, wrapped, and frozen—individually, if desired.

Raisin Bread: Make the dough through step 5, and while the dough is rising, place a cup of raisins in a small bowl, add hot water to cover, and let soak until the dough has risen. Drain the raisins and pat dry. Omit the apple; instead, add the raisins to the pressed-out dough and knead to incorporate. Halve the dough and proceed as directed. (Makes 2 loaves.) The bread is great spread with cream cheese or soft Brie topped with a sliced ripe pear.

Cinnamon-Swirl Bread: Make the dough through step 5. Remove the dough from the bowl and cut in half before pressing out. Omit the apple, and, one at a time, roll out each piece of dough (you shouldn't need to add flour) to a 9- by 18-inch rectangle. In a cup, stir together ⅓ cup sugar and 1½ teaspoons cinnamon. Sprinkle *half* of the cinnamon sugar on top of *each* rolled-out rectangle. Roll up the dough jelly-roll style and place each in a pan. (Makes 2 loaves.)

Skillet Whole-wheat Pita

These tender flat breads are nothing like the usual dried-out thin store-bought variety made of white flour. If this is your first time making bread, this is a great recipe to try. It was inspired by Jeffrey Alford and Naomi Daguid, who wrote *Flatbreads and Flavors*. The breads cook quickly in a cast-iron skillet on top of the stove; the kids will love kneading the dough and then watching the small breads puff. The dough will keep for days in the refrigerator, so you can bake the flat breads all at once or as you need them over a four-day period.

PREP: 30 minutes
RISING: About 1 hour and 10 minutes
COOKING: 2 minutes per pita

Makes sixteen 8-inch pita breads

PER PITA:
173 calories, 4g fat (.5g saturated), 32g carbohydrates, 3g fiber, 5g protein

2½ cups warm water (105°F to 115°F)
One ¼-ounce packet active dry yeast (not instant)
4 cups whole-grain whole-wheat flour
2½ teaspoons fine salt
2 tablespoons extra-virgin olive oil, plus more for cooking
About 2 cups unbleached all-purpose flour

1. Prepare the sponge for the dough: Measure the warm water in a 1-quart glass measuring cup, sprinkle the yeast on top, stir with a fork until dissolved, and let stand for 5 minutes. Place 3 cups of the whole-wheat flour in a large mixing bowl. Pour in the yeast mixture and stir for 2 minutes with a wooden spoon. Cover the top of the bowl with plastic wrap and let stand for 30 minutes at room temperature. The mixture will be bubbly.

2. Sprinkle the salt and drizzle 1 tablespoon of oil on top of the sponge and stir to incorporate. Stir in the remaining cup of whole-wheat flour. Add 1 cup of the unbleached all-purpose flour and stir until almost incorporated (the dough will become difficult to stir). Using the spoon, turn the dough out onto a work surface and knead, dusting with about ½ cup or more of the remaining all-purpose flour, until the dough is smooth and slightly sticky, about 8 minutes. (Reserve the remaining flour for rolling out.)

3. Wash and dry the bowl. Pour in the remaining tablespoon of oil, add the dough, and turn to coat in the oil. Cover the bowl snugly with plastic wrap and let stand in a draft-free area until the dough is doubled in bulk, about 40 minutes.

4. Roll out and bake the pita: Place a 10-inch cast-iron skillet or a griddle over medium heat. Turn the dough out onto a work surface and cut in half. Return one piece of dough to the bowl. Cut the remaining dough into 8 equal pieces and roll, using a cupped hand, into balls. Lightly flour the work sur-

face. Flatten a dough ball with your hand and then roll out with a rolling pin to a thin 8-inch circle.

5. Add about a teaspoon of oil to the skillet and spread around with a crumpled-up piece of paper towel to coat. Set a timer for 2 minutes and carefully lay the dough round flat in the pan. Cook for about 20 seconds, until bubbles appear on the surface. Flip with a metal spatula; the bread will begin to puff. When it stops growing, flip again and it will puff more. Continue cooking, flipping once or twice more until the timer goes off. Transfer the cooked pita to a kitchen towel and wrap to keep warm. (You may need to adjust the temperature of the pan, depending on the heat of your stove. The heat needs to be hot enough for the pitas to puff, but you don't want them to burn.) Repeat rolling out and cooking with the remaining 7 dough balls, making sure to oil the skillet before cooking each pita, and then repeat the process with the remaining half of the dough, making 16 pitas in all.

Cooks' Notes

❖ To easily heat the water: Pour into a glass measuring cup and microwave for 1 to 1½ minutes. Insert an instant-read thermometer—if the temperature is not 105°F to 115°F, microwave again briefly, or let cool until the temperature drops.

❖ If you want to save some dough for later, after returning any dough to the bowl, cover snugly with plastic wrap and then chill until ready to use. Let the dough stand at room temperature for 30 minutes before rolling out; cook as directed.

❖ Wrap any leftover baked pita breads in foil and keep at room temperature for up to 2 days. Toast lightly before serving.

Special Occasion Biscuits

These are the best biscuits you will ever eat. You have to plan ahead a little to make them, but they are gorgeous and foolproof. You can freeze them after baking and rewarm. Kids love to help roll out the dough and cut out the biscuits.

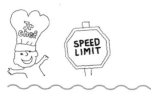

PREP: 30 minutes plus rising
BAKING: 15 minutes
SPEED LIMIT: 45 mpr

Makes about 2 dozen 3-inch biscuits

PER BISCUIT:
207 calories, 8g fat
(5g saturated),
29g carbohydrates,
1g fiber, 4g protein

2$\frac{1}{4}$ cups whole milk
1 tablespoon distilled white vinegar
6 cups plain cake flour (not self-rising)
2 tablespoons sugar
One $\frac{1}{4}$-ounce packet instant yeast
1 tablespoon baking powder
1 teaspoon fine salt
2 sticks ($\frac{1}{2}$ pound) cold unsalted butter, cut into small cubes

1. Place the milk and vinegar in a medium bowl and let stand at room temperature for 10 minutes.

2. Meanwhile, in a large bowl, whisk together the flour, sugar, yeast, baking powder, and salt. Add the butter cubes into the flour mixture with your fingertips or a pastry blender until the mixture is crumbly. Stir in the milk mixture with a fork just until blended. Cover the bowl snugly with plastic wrap. Chill in the refrigerator for 1 hour or up to 3 days.

3. Line a large baking sheet with parchment paper. Scrape the dough out of the bowl onto a lightly floured surface. Dust with flour and then pat with your hands into a 12-inch square. Fold the dough onto itself twice, as you would a business letter. Pat the rectangle of dough until $\frac{1}{2}$ inch thick and repeat folding to make a square. With a rolling pin, roll the dough out to a 12-inch square about $\frac{1}{2}$ inch thick. Cut biscuits out of the dough with a 3-inch round cookie cutter or drinking glass; place the biscuits on the baking sheet with the sides barely touching. Knead the scraps together, roll out to a $\frac{1}{2}$-inch thickness, and cut more biscuits. Cover the biscuits with a kitchen towel and let rise in a warm place for 1 hour.

4. Preheat the oven to 425°F. Bake the biscuits for about 15 minutes, until nicely puffed and golden brown on top. Serve warm.

Cooks' Note

❖ Leftover baked biscuits freeze nicely for up to 2 months: Wrap well in foil. Reheat frozen biscuits, unwrapped, in a 350°F oven for about 10 minutes.

"They taste like pizza crust without the sauce and cheese," says twelve-year-old Martin C., of the Bronx, New York.

Pizza Dough

Use this dough as a base for grilled pizza (page 133), focaccia (recipe follows), and more. For more ideas, see www.realfoodforhealthykids.com. Knead the dough by hand or in a standing mixer with a dough hook.

2¾ cups unbleached all-purpose flour
One ¼-ounce packet instant active dry yeast
1½ teaspoons coarse (kosher) salt
1 teaspoon sugar
1 cup warm water (105°F to 115°F)
3 tablespoons extra-virgin olive oil

PREP: 15 minutes
RISING: 1 hour or up to 3 days in the refrigerator

Makes about 1 pound

PER SERVING (BASED ON 8 PORTIONS):
238 calories, 5g fat (1g saturated),
42g carbohydrates,
1g fiber, 6g protein

1. Combine 2¼ cups of the flour, the yeast, salt, and sugar in a large bowl (or in the bowl of a standing mixer) and stir together with a rubber spatula. Pour in the water and oil and stir until a dough forms.

2. Knead the dough with your hands on the counter (or knead in the mixer with the dough hook at medium speed), adding up to ½ cup more flour a little at a time, until the dough is smooth, slightly sticky, and elastic, 7 to 10 minutes.

3. Return the dough to the bowl, cover the bowl with plastic wrap, and let the dough rise in a warm place until doubled in bulk, about 1 hour. Roll out to the desired thickness when ready to use.

Cooks' Notes

❧ On a humid day you may need to add more flour than you would on a dry day.

❧ To get the right temperature for the water, use an instant-read thermometer: Fill a 2-cup glass measuring cup with hot tap water, insert the thermometer, and then add or pour off hot or cooler water as necessary to get the right temperature and amount of water.

Rosemary Focaccia

Serve this soft, hearty Italian flat bread cut into cubes at dinner, with a little dish of extra-virgin olive oil for dipping, or better yet, cut it into large squares and split it in half horizontally with a serrated knife for the most delicious sandwiches.

PREP: 10 minutes plus dough preparation
RISING: 50 minutes
BAKING: 20 minutes

Makes enough bread for 8 sandwiches or 12 dinner portions of bread

PER SERVING (BASED ON 8 PORTIONS):
228 calories, 10g fat (1g saturated), 31g carbohydrates, 1g fiber, 4.5g protein

1 recipe Pizza Dough (page 65)
2½ tablespoons extra-virgin olive oil
1 teaspoon coarsely chopped fresh rosemary or ½ teaspoon dried
¼ to ½ teaspoon kosher salt

1. Prepare the pizza dough through the rising step (2).

2. Pour 1 tablespoon of the oil into a 15- by 10-inch jelly-roll pan and spread over the bottom of the pan with your hand. Scrape the risen dough out of the bowl onto the pan and press with your hands to spread in the pan until the dough is ½ inch thick. (The dough will not quite fill the pan.) Cover loosely with plastic wrap and let rise in a warm place until doubled, about 50 minutes.

3. Preheat the oven to 400°F. Remove the plastic wrap and drizzle the dough with the remaining 1½ tablespoons of oil. Using a finger, dimple the dough at 2-inch intervals. Sprinkle the rosemary and salt on top and bake for 20 minutes, until the top is golden and the focaccia sounds hollow when you tap it with your finger. Transfer the pan to a rack and let cool for 15 minutes. Transfer the focaccia to a board and cut with a serrated knife into cubes or larger squares.

chapter four

Lunch (En)Counter
Midday Meals for School Days and Weekends

The daily conundrum of what to feed our kids for lunch every day can be mind numbing. On school days, the key is to concentrate on portability, freshness, seasonality, and guaranteed nutritious hits that can be made faster than kids can say, "Mom, I hate crunchy peanut butter—please only give me smooth." On weekends, lunch is a more relaxed affair and the perfect time to try something new; this way, you can make sure he or she is not throwing away any food before trying it, and hopefully, both of you are in the right frame of mind to be a little experimental—and cook together! On weekends, we both love making big lunches for our families and having smaller breakfasts and dinners. Sometimes, it's the only time of the week that a family can all sit down together.

Because lunch requires two different approaches, we have divided this chapter into two sections: "Let's-Do-Lunch Box," focusing on school-day lunches that can stay fresh despite sitting out of the refrigerator for hours, with an array of suggestions and game-plan tips; and "Hot Lunch for Weekends," centering on (mostly) hot midday meals that can also double as great dinners. Whichever ones you choose, these well-rounded meals will keep your troops happy, satiated, and ready to be at their best, whether it's for their ninth period A.P. U.S. history course, at soccer practice, or even for fueling up for a vigorous round of video games.

let's-do-lunch box

Bento Box Chef's Salad

Peanut Butter Berry-wich

Bacon Banana-Rama

Crunchy Asian Chicken Salad

Egg Salad Double-Decker Sandwiches

Roast Beef Siberians

California-Style Tuna Salad Rolls

Turkey Pinwheels

Country Ham Gems

Classic Tabbouleh

Fruit Tabbouleh

Edamame Succotash Salad

Black Bean and Rice Salad

Choppy-Choppy Salad

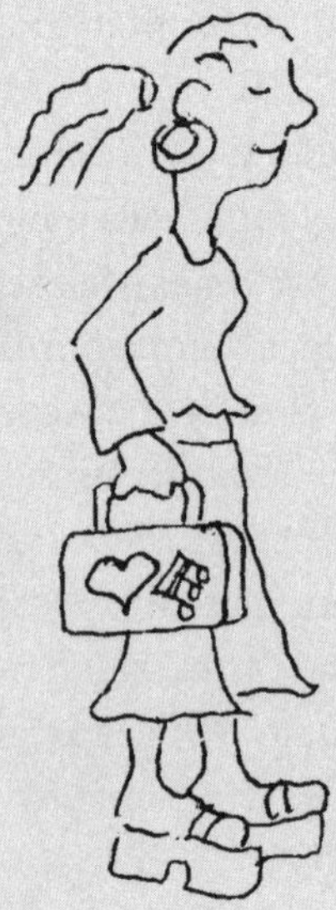

Have you ever visited your kid's school lunchroom? There are more deals going on than on Wall Street's trading floor. Chances are, your child is not always polishing off the organic sprouts with farm-raised breast of chicken on forty-eight-grain bread that you sent him off with. Perhaps he's throwing it away for a plasticlike sandwich containing an artificially colored piece of "cheese"—exactly what you were trying to avoid. So, what is a parent to do? The answer is to think like a kid but act like a chef with a nutritionist's degree. Luckily, we've done that for you and have provided some simple lunch solutions to ensure that Junior is eating the right stuff at school.

On those days when you simply don't have the time to make a wholesome delicious brown-bag meal, educate your kids on the healthiest choices available in the school cafeteria; most important, work with your school board to get more nutritious items offered. (And check out our list of packaged goods that are good store-bought alternatives, particularly for snacking during the school day.) The proof is in the healthy pudding: Wisconsin's Appleton Central Alternative High School, featured in Morgan Spurlock's documentary *Super Size Me,* reported that as a result of a reformed nutritious lunch menu, the students' energy and concentration increased and fewer behavior problems occurred.

When selecting lunch options, remember that the average schoolchild only has about twenty minutes to eat it. Also, few schools have microwaves handy to reheat foods, so choices are limited. If you want your child to have something warm, it must be heated throughout right before being stored in a warmed-up Thermos; it should also be something that is safe to leave cooling slowly, like pasta or soup. Finally, besides speed and portability, weekday lunches need to be balanced, with items loaded with lean protein, calcium, and complex carbohydrates.

~ MENU MATTERS ~

Designing a weekday lunch menu is like creating a workday outfit: You use what you've got from the classics section of your wardrobe and then zip it up with this season's accessories. So look to see what you have in the refrigerator or freezer and build upon that one item, supplementing it with seasonal produce. Try to always have a variety of colors and textures (and something fresh) in the lunch. If you shop once for the week, plan the lunches ahead so that the most perishable items, such as lettuce, tomatoes, and certain fruits, are used in the first half of the week and leftovers and frozen and dried items are used in the second half. For more lunch menu-planning ideas, see the "Snack Attacks" chapter (page 97), which has suggestions on how to use some of the snacks as lunch box stars.

Lunch for Grade-School Kids

Younger kids need complex carbohydrates, protein, and, generally, things that they know and feel comfortable with. They need the same food groups from the U.S.D.A.'s food pyramid as adults, but serving sizes are one-half to two-thirds of an adult's, depending on age and weight.

Sample Grade-School Lunch Box Menu:

Roast Beef Siberian (page 77)

Tree House Trail Mix (page 100)

Tangerine or clementine (choose the no-seed variety)

Organic mini-milk

Lunch for Teenagers

With their active and demanding lives, teens need extra protein and calcium (neither of which they usually get enough of) and require anywhere between 1,600 and 3,000 calories a day, so they should be getting one-quarter to one-third of those calories at lunchtime.

Sample Teen Lunch Box Menu:

Turkey Pinwheel (page 79)

Blue on Blue Dressing (page 218) with cut-up vegetables

Ultimate Oatmeal Cookie (page 274)

Berry Delicious Iced Tea (page 226)

Lunch for Finicky Eaters

Kids who are hard to please need to have foods on school days that provide comfort, yet have a bit of a twist in order to keep quietly broadening their horizons. The other key to feeding finicky eaters? As many choices as possible.

Sample Choosy Children's Lunch Box Menu:

Country Ham Gem (page 80)

Bursting Berry Muffin (page 53)

Sugar snap peas

Mini-100% pure juice box

Blueberries

Unbuttered light popcorn

Lunch for Vegetarians

Kids who practice a vegetarian diet need an extra boost of protein, fiber, and iron.

Sample Vegetarian Lunch Box Menu:

Peanut Butter Berry-wich (page 74)

Edamame Succotash Salad (page 82)

Boardwalk Fresh Lemonade (page 225)

Dried apricots
Chocolate Chip Flying Saucer (page 271)

Assembly Required

When you make a brown-bag lunch for the next day, it doesn't matter if you are doing it for one child or seven (and if you are doing it for that many, well, God bless you). The key is to take a tip from the toques and set up your *mise-en-place* first—that's just a fancy name for getting everything out and in its proper spot to speed assembly and packing. For instance, if you are making turkey wraps, get out the wraps, turkey, mayo, spinach, and everything else you'll need before you begin, as well as the utensils, and packing products. In the beginning, this will take you a moment of thought, but pretty soon you'll do this automatically and it will reduce your mileage around the kitchen.

Lunch Box 101

Presentation is more important than parents realize. If the food entices the eye and the nose, the child will be more inclined to eat it. Here are some steps to ensure that Junior's lunches are as attractive as they are delicious:

1. Let your child choose his or her insulated lunch box (www.lunchboxes .com has a great selection for all ages) before the school year starts. Steer away from the vinyl lunch boxes, as some of those have tested positive for lead. Select items such as funky sandwich containers, a cup with a straw built in, a fun insulated thermal container, and brightly colored plastic wraps and bags.

2. To keep foods cold and fresh, you can freeze a water bottle or a juice box to double as a cold pack (although some studies claim that the plastic leaches into the water); or better yet, get a small freezer pack and use that—just remind your child not to throw it out. For warm soup or stew, before packing the kids off to school, warm the Thermos with hot water and let it sit while you heat up the food. Once it's hot, dump out the water and replace with the hot soup or stew. It will keep warm until lunchtime.

3. Vary the menu. Serve a few different foods that your child likes every day even if the child insists on the exact same lunch. If there is one cherished food, include it, but then vary other items. For little kids, use cookie cutters to make fun sandwich shapes.

4. Empower your child—get her involved in choosing, making, and packing the lunch.

5. Don't introduce new foods into the lunch box. They'll probably just get thrown away.

6. Include healthy snacks for anytime, like our Extreme Granola (page 50) or Tree House Trail Mix (page 100). See the "Snack Attacks" chapter for more suggestions.

7. No matter the age of the child—whether too young to read or older and too-cool-for-school—sneak in a loving and inspirational note, a joke, or a picture of the family or family pet in his lunch box. It will give your kid a smile and remind him how much he is loved.

Must-Have Lunch Box Foods

Here are some lunch box items to have stocked in your kitchen (with a few brand names thrown in when important). For more ideas, log on to www.realfoodforhealthykids.com.

Drinks: mini-bottles of water; mini-cartons of organic cow's, soy, goat's, or rice milk; mini-cartons of pure 100% fruit juices; individual yogurt smoothies

Snacks: mini-bags of soy chips; whole-wheat pretzels; baked pita chips; baked sun crisps; whole-wheat bread sticks; low-calorie popcorn; Stretch Island organic fruit leather; flavored rice cakes; baked low-salt tortilla chips

Sweets: trail mix; low-fat granola bars; low-fat whole-grain cereal bars; yogurt-covered nuts; fig bars; organic animal crackers

Veggies and Fruits: mini-bags of organic carrots; red bell pepper strips; sugar snap peas; shelled edamame; grape tomatoes; small bags of clementine sections; red grapes; hulled strawberries; red grapes; dried fruit

Protein: sliced turkey; sliced ham; microwave bacon; light tuna packed in water or olive oil; frozen chicken tenders; frozen shrimp; frozen turkey burgers; sliced cheeses, such as Swiss, provolone, and Muenster; skim-milk mozzarella sticks

Carbs: rice pudding; low-fat yogurt; low-fat granola; cream cheese; bran muffins; whole-wheat pitas; whole-wheat hero buns; frozen mini-bagels; whole-wheat wraps; tortillas

~ HOMEMADE LUNCHABLES ~

The sammies, wraps, and salads in this chapter are portable and stay fresh for hours. They form the center from which the rest of the school lunch takes its cues.

Bento Box Chef's Salad

This composed salad lunch, which is a spin on boxed lunches popular in Japan, is fun for adults and kids alike. Feel free to add hard-cooked eggs and any other vegetables. Include a small bag of whole-grain or baked tortilla chips and a container of our Berry Delicious Iced Tea (page 226)—and don't forget to pack a fork.

1 tablespoon prepared dressing, such as Rockin' Ranch (page 219) or Blue on Blue (page 218)

1 thin slice meat (1 ounce), such as ham, turkey, or roast beef

1 thin slice cheese (1 ounce), such as Cheddar or Havarti

1 cup thinly sliced romaine lettuce

5 grape tomatoes, halved, or 8 seedless grapes, halved

½ tablespoon raisins

1 teaspoon toasted salted sunflower kernels or pumpkin seeds (pepitas; optional)

2 carrot sticks

2 celery sticks

PREP: 5 minutes

Makes 1 serving

PER SERVING:
353 calories, 21g fat (8g saturated), 28g carbohydrates, 8g fiber, 17g protein

1. Place the salad dressing in a corner of a 3- to 4-cup shallow plastic storage container with a lid.

2. Stack the meat and cheese on a board and cut into thin strips (you will have about ⅓ cup). Arrange on top of the dressing. Place the lettuce in the opposite half of the container. Arrange the tomatoes, raisins, sunflower kernels, carrots, and celery next to the meat and cheese.

bento box bonanza

The Japanese take boxed lunches to work, to school, and on picnics. Half of the typical Japanese bento consists of rice. The rest of the box includes other vegetables and some kind of protein, such as meat, fish, and/or egg. You can purchase bento boxes online.

Peanut Butter Berry-wich

Peanut butter goes well with more than just jam, and this interesting combination proves it. This is delicious with whatever fruit is in season.

PREP: 5 minutes
SPEED LIMIT: 5 mpr

Makes 1 serving

PER SANDWICH:
307 calories, 13g fat
(2.5g saturated),
40g carbohydrates,
5g fiber, 11g protein

2 slices whole wheat bread or Ba-Ba Banana Bread (page 52)
1 tablespoon natural peanut butter
1 tablespoon softened Neufchâtel (reduced-fat) cream cheese
2 medium strawberries, hulled and sliced
1 teaspoon honey

1. Lay the bread slices on a work surface. Spread the peanut butter on one slice and the cream cheese on the other.

2. Arrange strawberry slices in an even single layer on top of the peanut butter. Drizzle the honey on the berries and then place the other slice of bread with the cream cheese on top. Cut into halves or quarters.

Bacon Banana-Rama: We love sandwiches made with our Ba-Ba Banana Bread, especially peanut butter and bacon—a meaty sweet-and-salty treat! Just crumble two strips of cooked bacon on top of the peanut butter and omit the cream cheese. Perfect for a kid who needs extra protein and calories.

You can also add just about any fruit to a peanut butter sandwich: bananas, apples, raisins, prunes, pears.

Crunchy Asian Chicken Salad

Kids and adults alike will enjoy this lunch. Store this tasty salad in a wide-mouthed thermal container, use several Bibb or Boston lettuce leaves to wrap around the salad instead of bread, and pack the nuts separately in a little plastic bag for sprinkling. For those who can take the heat, add a splash of Chinese hot oil or hot sesame oil to the salad.

SALAD

1½ cups finely diced cooked chicken (6 ounces, about 1½ breast halves)
6 canned peeled water chestnuts, rinsed and chopped
1 carrot, peeled and shredded
1 small celery rib, finely diced
½ cup diced apple, such as Gala or Golden Delicious (about ½ apple)

DRESSING

1 tablespoon natural peanut butter or sesame tahini
1 tablespoon seasoned rice vinegar
¾ tablespoon soy sauce
2 tablespoons mayonnaise
1 tablespoon minced fresh chives (optional)
¼ cup roasted soy nuts or coarsely chopped unsalted peanuts
1 teaspoon hot sesame oil (optional)

1. Combine the chicken, water chestnuts, carrot, celery, and apple in a bowl and stir to mix.

2. Whisk together the peanut butter, vinegar, and soy sauce until smooth. Whisk in the mayonnaise and chives, if using, spoon the dressing over the salad, and mix well. Sprinkle with soy nuts just before serving.

PREP: 10 minutes
SPEED LIMIT: 10 mpr

Makes 3 servings (3 cups)

PER SERVING:
235 calories, 13.5g fat
(1.5g saturated),
11g carbohydrates,
2g fiber, 17.5g protein

Nine-year-old Mark L., of Rye, New York, said, "I'm surprised by how I like the apple with the chicken. It somehow works."

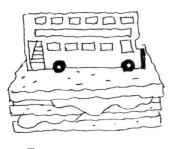

Egg Salad Double-Decker Sandwiches

These are a step up from the traditional egg salad sandwiches. If you want to forgo the bacon, season the egg salad mixture with salt to taste. Add coarsely chopped watercress if you want to add a little bit of a bite. Be sure to keep this cold, stored next to a cold pack or a cold bottle of water.

PREP: 10 minutes
COOKING: 10 minutes
SPEED LIMIT: 20 mpr

Makes 2 servings

PER SERVING:
554 calories, 31g fat
(6g saturated),
44g carbohydrates,
6g fiber, 28g protein

4 large eggs
2 ½ tablespoons mayonnaise
½ teaspoon whole-grain mustard
Freshly ground black pepper
⅓ cup cooked crumbled bacon or real bacon crumbles (such as Hormel),
   recrisped in the microwave
6 thin slices (about ¼ inch thick) whole-wheat sandwich bread

1. Hard-cook the eggs: Place the eggs in a single layer in a small saucepan and add cold water to cover. Bring to a boil, turn off the heat, cover with a lid, and let stand for 10 minutes. Pour off the water from the pot, cover the eggs with cold water, drain, and then cover with icy cold water and let stand until cold, about 3 minutes.

2. Peel the eggs, rinse them, and pat dry. Slice the eggs crosswise and then lengthwise in an egg slicer or finely chop the eggs; transfer to a small bowl. Add the mayonnaise, mustard, and pepper and mash them all together with a fork. Stir in the bacon.

3. Stack all of the bread slices together and cut off the crusts with a serrated knife; lay the bread slices out on a work surface. Spread one-quarter of the egg mixture on each of 4 of the slices. Stack 2 egg-coated slices on top of the other 2 egg-coated slices and then top with the remaining 2 plain slices. Press on the two sandwiches with your hand to compress the layers and slice into halves or quarters.

Ten-year-old Adam M., of Bridgton, Maine, says, "Yes, these are very good! I think I'll try a few more." He then put three more slices on his plate and ate them all.

Roast Beef Siberians

This is the Reuben sandwich reinvented. We like to make the sandwiches small, using the narrow ends of the rye loaf or slices of party rye.

4 small slices rye bread (about ¾ ounce each) or 2 regular slices rye
2 teaspoons honey mustard or Russian dressing
2 thin slices medium-rare roast beef or 4 thin slices steak (2 ounces)
2 slices Havarti cheese (2 ounces), torn into pieces
About ¼ cup Rainbow Slaw (page 205), or other prepared coleslaw

1. Lay the bread slices on a work surface and spread each with honey mustard.

2. Fold the roast beef and arrange on 2 of the bread slices. Place the Havarti and slaw on top. Cover with the remaining 2 bread slices and serve.

PREP: 5 minutes
SPEED LIMIT: 5 mpr

Makes 2 small sandwiches or 1 typical sandwich

PER MINI-SANDWICH:
*253 calories, 12g fat
(6.5g saturated),
22g carbohydrates,
2g fiber, 13g protein*

California-Style Tuna Salad Rolls

These roll-ups are great for school and burst with tuna and veggies. If your child likes wasabi's heat, add an extra ¼ teaspoon to the tuna mixture.

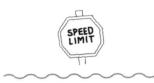

PREP: 10 minutes
SPEED LIMIT: 10 mpr

Makes 4 servings

PER SERVING:
247 calories, 10g fat
(2g saturated),
24g carbohydrates,
3g fiber, 15g protein

1 can (6 ounces) light tuna fish, preferably packed in water, drained and flaked
3 tablespoons mayonnaise
¼ teaspoon wasabi paste or freshly ground black pepper to taste
Two 10-inch flour tortillas
2 medium leaves Boston lettuce
1 Kirby cucumber, peeled and coarsely shredded lengthwise (without seeds)
1 medium carrot, peeled and coarsely shredded
½ of a ripe avocado, peeled, pitted, and sliced ½ inch thick

1. Combine the tuna, 2 tablespoons of the mayonnaise, and the wasabi paste in a small bowl and mix until blended.

2. Lay the tortillas on a work surface. Spread ½ tablespoon mayonnaise on each tortilla and arrange the lettuce on top of both; arrange the cucumber, carrot, and avocado lengthwise in rows near one edge. Spoon the tuna in a line next to the vegetables (away from the edge). Roll each tortilla up snugly into a cylinder. Cut crosswise in half.

Cooks' Note

❖ Wasabi paste is available in the Asian section of the market.

Jackson F., of Brooklyn, New York, is seven years old and declared these to be "great": "I like the crunchiness. This is how I want my tuna sandwiches from now on."

Turkey Pinwheels

All the other kids at school will be jealous when they get a look at these delicious, colorful, healthful wraps.

1 large whole-wheat wrap (11 to 12 inches), or 2 smaller wraps (8 inches),
    or a 12- by 9-inch rectangular lavosh
1 tablespoon mayonnaise
1 lightly packed handful rinsed baby spinach leaves
1 tablespoon dried cranberries
2 medium carrots, peeled and coarsely shredded
2 slices Swiss cheese, such as Jarlsberg (2 ounces)
2 thin slices store-bought roasted turkey breast (2 ounces)

1. If necessary, warm the wrap in a 350°F oven for 2 minutes to soften before filling.

2. Lay the wrap on a work surface and spread the mayonnaise all over. Sprinkle the spinach leaves, cranberries, and carrots evenly on top. Arrange the Swiss cheese and turkey in even layers over the vegetable layer. Fold in the side edges and then roll up snugly from the bottom.

3. Cut crosswise into 4 even pieces and wrap up tightly in plastic.

Cooks' Note

❖ This is a great way to make use of holiday turkey leftovers.

PREP: 5 minutes
SPEED LIMIT: 5 mpr

Makes 2 servings

PER PIECE (½ WRAP):
350 calories, 15g fat
(5g saturated),
36g carbohydrates,
4.5g fiber, 15.5g protein

"This is good and most kids will like it. It's a good choice for a lunch box—it would last really well," says Tehmina P., age nine and a Brooklyn, New York, native. "I might add a layer of tortilla chips inside to keep the lettuce from getting soggy, though."

Country Ham Gems

Make these sandwiches with any cured or smoked ham, but salty country ham is especially good here coupled with the spicy cheese and sweet jam. We like the sandwiches best on our Special Occasion Biscuits (page 64), but you can substitute sliced bread.

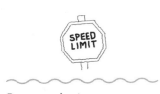

PREP: 5 minutes
SPEED LIMIT: 5 mpr

Makes 4 biscuit sandwiches or 2 regular sandwiches

PER BISCUIT SANDWICH:
208 calories, 12.5g fat
(5g saturated),
15g carbohydrates,
0g fiber, 9g protein

Four 2- to 3-inch biscuits, split, or 4 slices egg bread
2 teaspoons mayonnaise
2 teaspoons peach jam or apricot jam
2 slices (2 ounces) country ham or other cured or smoked ham
2 slices (2 ounces) Pepper Jack cheese or white Cheddar

Lay the biscuits open on a work surface. Spread the cut side of the bottom halves with mayonnaise. Spread the cut side of the top halves with jam. Tear each slice of ham in half and arrange on the bottoms. Tear each slice of cheese in half and place on top of the ham and then top with the jam-coated tops.

Classic Tabbouleh

This mild version of the popular, wholesome Middle Eastern dish is packed with protein and fiber. Serve with Skillet Whole-wheat Pitas (page 62) and baby salad greens.

3 cups water
1 cup bulgur wheat
¼ cup extra-virgin olive oil
2 tablespoons fresh lemon juice
¾ teaspoon kosher salt
¼ teaspoon freshly ground black pepper
2 ripe tomatoes, finely diced (2 cups)
½ cup packed flat-leaf parsley leaves
2 tablespoons minced fresh chives (optional)

PREP: 5 minutes plus cooling
COOKING: 15 minutes
SPEED LIMIT: 20 mpr

Makes 4 cups

PER CUP:
266 calories, 15g fat (2g saturated),
31g carbohydrates,
8g fiber, 5g protein

1. Bring the water to a boil in a medium saucepan. Stir in the bulgur, reduce the heat to medium-low, and simmer, stirring occasionally, until tender, about 15 minutes. Drain in a sieve and let cool for 15 minutes.

2. Transfer the bulgur to a large bowl. Add the oil, lemon juice, salt, and pepper and stir well. Add the tomatoes, parsley, and chives, if using, and toss again.

Fruit Tabbouleh: Omit the tomatoes, parsley, chives, and pepper. Reduce the olive oil to 2 tablespoons, and then add 2 tablespoons honey along with the lemon juice and salt to the cooked bulgur. Add 2 cups finely diced fruit, such as cantaloupe, kiwi, cut-up strawberries, red seedless grapes, and small orange segments.

Edamame Succotash Salad

Make this salad for lunch but serve it hot at dinner first. To give kids extra protein at lunch, add ½ cup finely chopped cold cooked chicken and round it out with Special Occasion Biscuits (page 64) or a small whole-wheat roll and an apple.

PREP: 5 to 10 minutes
(depending on the corn)
COOKING: 12 minutes
SPEED LIMIT: 17 mpr

**Makes 10 servings
(about 5 cups)**

PER ½ CUP SERVING:
130 calories, 5g fat
(.5g saturated),
16g carbohydrates,
4g fiber, 6g protein

2 tablespoons extra-virgin olive oil
1 medium onion, chopped
1 bag (1 pound) shelled edamame (soybeans), thawed
1 bag (1 pound) frozen corn, thawed, or 3 cups fresh-cut corn kernels
   (from about 4 ears)
2 large ripe plum tomatoes, diced
1¼ teaspoons kosher salt
¼ teaspoon freshly ground black pepper
¼ cup minced fresh chives or basil

1. Heat the oil in a 4-quart saucepan over medium heat. Add the onion and cook, stirring often, until softened but not browned, 4 to 5 minutes.

2. Add the edamame and corn and cook, turning often, until heated through, about 7 minutes. Stir in the tomatoes, salt, and pepper. Let cool and then chill if packing in a lunch box. When ready to serve, stir in the chives or basil.

Black Bean and Rice Salad

You can ease the kids into fall (and school) with this Cuban-inspired salad made with sweet late summer corn and protein-packed black beans. To make it even more of a main dish, toss in some shredded cooked chicken, thinly sliced and cut-up grilled steak, or barbecued pork or shrimp. Add a few bits of fresh basil or baby spinach just before packing.

1 cup long-grain brown rice
¼ cup extra-virgin olive oil
1 Cubanelle chile or Italian frying pepper, trimmed and cut into ⅓-inch dice
1 medium red onion, finely chopped
3 garlic cloves, peeled, smashed, and minced
2 cups freshly cut white corn kernels (from 2 ears) or 1 box (10 ounces) frozen corn, thawed
1 teaspoon kosher salt
One 15-ounce can black beans, rinsed well and drained
1 tablespoon distilled white vinegar
Freshly ground black pepper

PREP: 10 minutes
COOKING: 30 minutes
SPEED LIMIT: 40 mpr

Makes 6 cups

PER CUP:
308 calories, 11g fat
(1.5g saturated),
44g carbohydrates,
7.5g fiber, 8g protein

1. Bring a medium saucepan of salted water to a boil. Add the rice and cook, stirring occasionally, just until tender, about 25 minutes. Drain and rinse well with cold water until cool. Transfer to a large bowl.

2. Heat 2 tablespoons of the oil in the same saucepan over medium heat until hot. Add the chile, onion, and garlic and stir until slightly softened, about 3 minutes. Add the corn and salt and cook, stirring, just until heated through, about 1 minute. Transfer the vegetables to the bowl with the rice and toss to mix.

3. Add the beans, the remaining 2 tablespoons oil, and the vinegar and toss well. Season with plenty of pepper and toss again.

Cooks' Notes

❖ Here we cook the rice in plenty of water, like pasta, so that it stays tender after you cool it off.

❖ If your little ones love the spicy stuff, include mini-bottles of hot sauce in their lunch boxes.

Andrew M., six years old, from Rye, New York, really loved this salad, and ate three bowls in one sitting: "I love corn and I love rice and I love these mushy beans and it's all together. Yum!"

Choppy-Choppy Salad

Have kids that don't like to eat veggies? Get them to be big dippers with this salad sure to please the whole family. For ease, prepare the dressing first, blanch the broccoli and cauliflower, and then cut up the veggies (except the tomatoes) up to 12 hours ahead. Layer in a large bowl, cover with plastic wrap, and chill. Add the tomatoes just before packing for lunch.

PREP: 20 minutes
SPEED LIMIT: 20 mpr

Makes 6 servings

PER SERVING (WITHOUT DRESSING):
63 calories, .5g fat
(0g saturated),
12.5g carbohydrates,
6g fiber, 5g protein

2 large stalks broccoli
½ head cauliflower
2 medium Kirby cucumbers
3 carrots, peeled
2 cups grape tomatoes
One 6-ounce bag cut romaine lettuce
About ¾ cup salad dressing, such as Blue on Blue, Rockin' Ranch, or
*   ABC Vinaigrette (see pages 218; 219 and 215)*

1. Prepare the veggies: Cut the broccoli and cauliflower into small florets. Quarter the cucumbers lengthwise, then seed and slice into ¼-inch-thick slices. Coarsely chop the carrots and halve the grape tomatoes.

2. Bring a large saucepan half full of water to a boil. Add the broccoli and cauliflower; reduce the heat and simmer for 2 minutes, drain, and cool with cold running water. Transfer the blanched vegetables to a large salad bowl and add the cucumbers, carrots, tomatoes, and lettuce. (This can be prepared up to 12 hours ahead; cover and chill.) Pack the salad in containers for lunch and pack the dressing on the side.

hot lunch for weekends

Most of these recipes are easy, but a few are slightly more labor intensive and better suited for leisurely weekends, whether it's at noon or closer to midnight.

Old-Fashioned Grilled Cheese Sandwiches

Vegetable Grilled Cheese Quesadillas

Huevos Rancheros

Popeye's Panini Presto

Chicken Salad Melt

Terrific Tuna Melt

Chip'n Nuggets

Mini-Cuban Sandos

South-of-the-Border Pronto Pizza

Chickpea Pita Pockets

Middle Eastern Veggie Burgers

Sesame Sauce

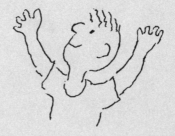

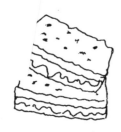

Old-Fashioned Grilled Cheese Sandwiches

PREP: 5 minutes
COOKING: 5 minutes
SPEED LIMIT: 10 mpr

Makes 4 servings

PER SERVING:
455 calories, 22g fat
(11g saturated),
45g carbohydrates,
4g fiber, 18g protein

This is for the purist—a simple combo of cheese and bread. You don't need a special appliance to make a great grilled cheese—just two good heavy skillets. Mellow Yellow Split Pea Soup (page 167) is a natural with these sandwiches, or, to round out the meal, be sure to serve some veggies and fresh fruit alongside.

8 slices multigrain bread
1½ cups (6 ounces) extra-sharp Cheddar cheese, coarsely shredded
2 tablespoons soft unsalted butter

1. Heat a large cast-iron skillet or a griddle over medium heat.

2. Meanwhile, lay the bread on a work surface. Divide the cheese evenly between 4 slices, lightly packing the cheese. Place the remaining 4 slices of bread on top of the cheese-covered slices.

3. Spread half the butter on top of the sandwiches and then invert, butter side down, in the hot skillet. Spread the remaining butter on top of the sandwiches. Place another skillet on top of the sandwiches to compress them, and let cook, over moderate heat, for 2 to 3 minutes, until the sandwiches are golden underneath.

4. Flip, place the skillet on top, and cook about 2 minutes more, until the sandwiches are nicely golden and the cheese is melted. Cut in half and serve.

"Can I have another, please? No, wait; make it two," says Brian S., sixteen, of Boca Raton, Florida.

Vegetable Grilled Cheese Quesadillas

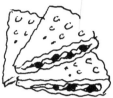

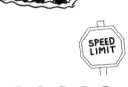

This Mexican version of grilled cheese has become a favorite for all ages. Add diced cooked chicken or cooked drained pinto beans to the filling for an extra protein boost, or if your kids object to broccoli, try spinach. Serve with Chucky Guacamole (page 104) or Sunny Summer Salsa (page 107) and sour cream.

2 tablespoons finely chopped onion
1 cup finely chopped broccoli
1 tablespoon vegetable oil
1 large ripe plum tomato, finely diced
2 teaspoons chili powder, preferably ancho
Eight 6-inch flour tortillas
1½ cups (6 ounces packed) shredded Monterey Jack cheese

PREP: 5 minutes
COOKING: 9 minutes
SPEED LIMIT: 14 mpr

Makes 4 servings

PER SERVING:
373 calories, 22g fat (9.5g saturated), 30g carbohydrates, 1g fiber, 16g protein

1. Cook the onions and broccoli in the oil in a small skillet over medium heat, stirring occasionally, until softened, about 3 minutes. Remove from the heat and stir in the tomato and chili powder.

2. Lay 4 tortillas on a work surface. Top each with 2 large pinches of cheese. Divide the vegetable mixture among the tortillas, spooning on in an even layer. Sprinkle the remaining cheese on top and cover with the remaining 4 tortillas.

3. Preheat the grill (or a skillet, see Cooks' Notes) and grease the rack with oil. Add the quesadillas, cover, and cook until golden and crisp underneath, about 3 minutes. Flip the quesadillas over, cover, and cook until the cheese is melted and the other side is crisp, about 3 minutes more. Transfer the quesadillas to a board and cut into quarters with a large sharp knife.

Cooks' Notes

* You can cook the quesadillas on the stove: Lightly oil a grill pan or a griddle and place over medium heat until hot.

* Cooking for a crowd? Assemble quesadillas several hours ahead: Stack on a plate, cover, and chill until ready to cook. Leftovers can be popped in the toaster oven and toasted on medium.

Nine-year-old Gabriel B., from Oxford, Mississippi, made these quesadillas with his mom, Ginny. "The end product is really yummy, but it takes a while to make."

Huevos Rancheros

Beans are an important source of protein in Mexico. When mashed, the creamy, satisfying texture pairs well with slightly runny medium-fried eggs, warmed tortillas, and Sunny Summer Salsa.

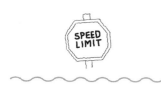

PREP: 15 minutes
COOKING: 10 minutes
SPEED LIMIT: 25 mpr

Makes 4 servings

PER SERVING:
677 calories, 33g fat
(11g saturated),
67g carbohydrates,
13g fiber, 27g protein

4 scallions, trimmed, white part thinly sliced, green part roughly chopped
3½ tablespoons vegetable oil
One 19-ounce can pinto beans, drained and rinsed
Four 11- to 12-inch whole-wheat flour tortillas
1 cup (packed) shredded Monterey Jack or Pepper Jack cheese (4 ounces)
4 large eggs
1 cup Sunny Summer Salsa (page 107) or fresh or jarred salsa

1. Preheat the oven to 350°F.

2. Cook the scallions in 1 tablespoon of the oil in a small saucepan over medium heat, stirring occasionally, until softened, about 2 minutes. Add the beans and mash coarsely with a potato masher. Keep warm.

3. Meanwhile, heat ½ tablespoon oil in a nonstick 12-inch skillet over medium heat. Cook the tortillas one at a time, just until heated through, a little less than 1 minute per side. (For each tortilla, add ½ tablespoon oil.) Transfer the tortillas to a foil-lined baking sheet, spread one-quarter of the beans on each tortilla, and top with 2 tablespoons of the cheese. Transfer the baking sheet to the oven to keep the tortillas warm and melt the cheese.

4. Add the remaining ½ tablespoon oil to the same skillet, crack the eggs, and add to the pan. Sprinkle cheese on top, cover, and cook until the desired doneness. Transfer an egg to each tortilla, and sprinkle some of the scallion greens on top. Serve with salsa.

Cooks' Note

✣ For big eaters, cook 2 eggs per person to serve on top of the tortilla.

Popeye's Panini Presto

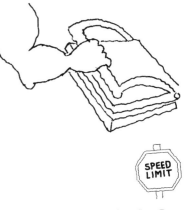

Italian panini presses were a recent rage, but two heavy skillets will work just as well to make these great spinach-cheese sandwiches. Serve with a simple salad of sliced ripe tomatoes drizzled with olive oil.

One 10-ounce box frozen leaf spinach (see Cooks' Notes)
2 tablespoons plus 2 teaspoons extra-virgin olive oil
1 small onion, finely chopped
1 garlic clove, smashed, peeled, and finely chopped
¾ teaspoon kosher salt
¼ teaspoon crushed red pepper flakes
1½ (packed) cups shredded part-skim mozzarella cheese (6 ounces)
Four 3-ounce soft mini-sub (hoagie) rolls (about 6 inches long), split horizontally, excess bread dug out and discarded

PREP: 5 minutes
COOKING: 13 minutes
SPEED LIMIT: 18 mpr

Makes 4 servings

PER SERVING:
409 calories, 22g fat (8g saturated), 34g carbohydrates, 5g fiber, 18g protein

1. Place the spinach in a strainer and rinse with running water until thawed. Squeeze handfuls of spinach to remove as much moisture as possible. Coarsely chop the spinach and set aside.

2. Heat 2 tablespoons oil in a nonstick skillet over medium heat. Add the onion and garlic and cook, stirring, until softened, about 4 minutes. Add the spinach, salt, and crushed red pepper flakes and stir until the spinach and oil are blended. Remove from the heat and stir in the mozzarella (to partially melt the cheese.)

3. Heat a panini press (or a heavy skillet, see Cooks' Notes). Place the split rolls on a board, divide the spinach mixture among the bottoms and spread the filling evenly. Cover the rolls with the tops. Brush the bottoms of 2 sandwiches lightly with oil and add oiled side down to the press. Lightly brush the tops with oil and close the press. Cook for about 4 minutes, until the sandwiches are golden and crisp. Repeat with the remaining sandwiches and oil.

Cooks' Notes

❖ To use a large skillet, place over medium heat, add two sandwiches, oiling as directed. Place a second heavy skillet on top to compress and cook for about 2 minutes on medium-low heat; turn the sandwiches, place the skillet on top, and cook 2 minutes more.

❖ You can substitute fresh spinach (use an entire 1-pound package) if you have it. Just sauté with the onion and garlic and stir until the spinach is cooked through.

Chicken Salad Melt

Got some leftover roasted chicken? Use it on this delicious twist on the classic tuna melt (see the variation), which makes a quick hot lunch.

PREP: 10 minutes
COOKING: 8 minutes
SPEED LIMIT: 18 mpr

Makes 4 sandwiches

PER SERVING:
*405 calories, 20g fat
(8g saturated),
33g carbohydrates,
4.5g fiber, 27g protein*

8 slices whole-wheat or pumpernickel sandwich bread
6 ounces imported Swiss cheese, shredded (1½ cup)
4 slices beefsteak tomato or 8 slices of a smaller tomato
1½ cups coarsely chopped cooked chicken (about 6 ounces, about
   1½ chicken breast halves)
1 medium celery rib, finely diced
2 tablespoons mayonnaise
Freshly ground black pepper

1. Preheat the oven to 500°F. Arrange the bread in a single layer in pairs on a large baking sheet. Distribute ¼ cup cheese on each of 4 slices of bread. Place 1 tablespoon cheese on each of the opposite slices, place the tomato on top, and bake for 6 to 8 minutes, until the bread is toasted and the cheese is bubbly.

2. While the bread is toasting, combine the chicken, celery, and mayonnaise in a bowl and mix with a fork. Season with pepper.

3. Divide the chicken salad among the bread slices with the tomato. Cover with the plain cheese-coated slices. Cut each sandwich in 4 triangles and serve hot.

Terrific Tuna Melt: Substitute Cheddar for the Swiss cheese and a lightly drained 6-ounce can of light tuna (preferably packed in water or olive oil) for the chicken.

Chip'n Nuggets

These crunchy homemade chicken treats can't be beat! Choose lightly salted reduced-fat potato or tortilla chips or lightly sweetened cornflakes and crush very well with a rolling pin or in a food processor. Serve with crudités and Rockin' Ranch Dressing (page 219), Horseradish Dunk (page 103), or ketchup for dipping.

1½ cups well-crushed, lightly salted, reduced-fat potato chips, tortilla chips, or cornflakes

2 large eggs

¼ teaspoon dried thyme, crumbled

¼ teaspoon hot paprika

2 large boneless skinless chicken breast halves (about 1 pound), each halved lengthwise and cut into ½-inch-thick slices

¼ cup extra-virgin olive oil or corn oil, for pan frying

1. Line a large baking sheet with foil and lightly grease. Place the well-crushed chips in a shallow bowl. In a second bowl, beat together the eggs, thyme, and paprika.

2. Add the chicken slices to the eggs one at a time and stir with a rubber spatula to mix. Coat the chicken pieces one at a time in the crumbs and place on the prepared baking sheet. Add the remaining chicken to the eggs and then coat in the remaining crumbs. Preheat the oven to 400°F.

3. Heat the oil in a 10-inch skillet over medium heat until ripples appear on the surface. Add the chicken pieces to the pan and cook until golden underneath, about 2 minutes, then turn with tongs or a spatula and cook 2 minutes more. Transfer the chicken back to the baking sheet. Place the baking sheet in the oven and bake until the chicken is golden and cooked through, about 15 minutes.

PREP: 10 minutes
COOKING: 20 minutes
SPEED LIMIT: 30 mpr

Makes 4 servings

PER SERVING (ABOUT 4 PIECES):
414 calories, 19g fat (3.5g saturated), 29g carbohydrates, 0g fiber, 30g protein

Mini-Cuban Sandos

Use pork from Slow-Roasted Pork Shoulder (page 147) on these messy sandwiches or buy thinly sliced roast pork from the deli. These make a great weekend lunch or super-fast weeknight dinner.

PREP: 10 minutes
COOKING: 5 minutes
SPEED LIMIT: 15 mpr

Makes 4 small sandwiches to serve 2 to 4

PER MINI-SANDWICH:
*228 calories, 9g fat
(3.5g saturated),
24g carbohydrates,
1g fiber, 14g protein*

*8 slices (⅓ inch thick) from a long Italian bread
8 teaspoons Mexican Adobo Dressing (page 217)
Thin pickle slices
2 ounces imported Swiss cheese, shredded (½ cup packed)
½ cup (packed) thinly sliced or pulled roast pork
4 thin slices boiled deli ham or sliced baked ham*

1. Heat a large cast-iron skillet over medium heat (or heat a panini grill or a waffle iron).

2. Meanwhile, lay the bread in 4 pairs on a work surface. Spread about 1 teaspoon dressing on each slice of bread, place pickles on 4 slices, and top all 4 with half of the cheese. Divide the pork among the 4 bread slices with cheese, and place the ham and remaining cheese on top. Cover with the remaining bread.

3. Place the sandwiches in the hot dry skillet, place another skillet on top of the sandwiches to compress them, and let cook for about 3 minutes, until the sandwiches are golden underneath.

4. Flip, place the skillet on top again, and cook about 2 minutes more, until the sandwiches are nicely golden and the cheese is melted.

Cooks' Note

✢ We like to purchase whole pickles and slice them, as they are much fresher. Get them at the deli or buy Claussen brand from the refrigerator section at the market.

South-of-the-Border Pronto Pizza

A wholesome lunch or dinner doesn't get any easier or faster. If you can't find large flour tortillas, this makes enough for six 7- to 8-inch tortillas.

Four 10-inch flour tortillas, preferably whole-wheat
One 15.5-ounce can black beans, drained and rinsed
2 cups (packed) shredded extra-sharp Cheddar cheese (10 ounces)
1 large ripe tomato, diced
¼ cup chopped fresh cilantro
Chunky Guacamole (page 104) or green salsa and plain low-fat yogurt,
   for serving

1. Preheat the oven to 500°F.

2. Place 2 flour tortillas on each of 2 large baking sheets. Divide the beans (a heaping ⅓ cup each) and cheese among the tortillas, sprinkling evenly and leaving a 1-inch border. Bake the pizzas for about 8 minutes, or until the edges are browned and the cheese is bubbly. Transfer the pizzas to a board and cut each into quarters. Sprinkle some tomato and cilantro on top and serve the guacamole or salsa and yogurt on the side.

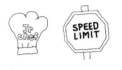

PREP TIME: 5 minutes
BAKING: 8 minutes
SPEED LIMIT: 13 mpr

Makes 4 servings

PER TORTILLA:
550 calories, 25g fat
(13g saturated),
53g carbohydrates,
8.5g fiber, 26g protein

Chickpea Pita Pockets

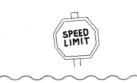

PREP: 15 minutes
PAN FRYING: 6 minutes
SPEED LIMIT: 21 mpr

Makes 4 servings

PER PITA HALF:
373 calories, 15.5g fat
(2g saturated),
49g carbohydrates,
8g fiber, 12g protein

Any devout carnivore will feast on these falafel sandwiches, which are somehow meaty, and rich in protein and fiber. Use our Skillet Whole-wheat Pitas or buy them in the store, but since pita comes in different sizes your number of sandwiches may vary.

One 15-ounce can chickpeas, drained and rinsed
1 small onion, peeled and coarsely chopped
1½ teaspoons ground cumin
⅔ cup dried whole-wheat bread crumbs or Panko-style Japanese bread crumbs
1 large egg
½ teaspoon kosher salt
¼ teaspoon freshly ground black pepper
3 tablespoons extra-virgin olive oil
Sesame Sauce (recipe follows)
Two 7-inch Skillet Whole-wheat Pitas (page 62), warmed and cut in half
2 cups thinly sliced romaine lettuce
2 ripe medium tomatoes, finely diced

1. Place the chickpeas and onion in a food processor and process until finely chopped. Add the cumin, bread crumbs, egg, salt, and pepper and process until blended. Using a tablespoon, form the mixture into 1-inch balls and flatten into ⅓-inch-thick patties (you should have about 24 small patties); place on a plate.

2. Heat the oil in a large skillet over medium heat. Add the patties and cook until nicely browned underneath, about 3 minutes. Turn and cook 2 to 3 minutes more. Transfer to paper towels to drain.

3. Spread 1 tablespoon sesame sauce inside a pita half. Add 3 warm patties in the bottom crease of the pita (it's okay if they break apart). Top with some lettuce and tomatoes, more sesame sauce, and 3 more warm patties.

Cooks' Notes

❖ Prepare the sesame sauce, lettuce, and tomato and warm the pitas before frying the patties.

❖ If your hands get too sticky when forming the chickpea balls, wipe your hands and dust them with a little whole-wheat flour or bread crumbs.

❖ The patties reheat well in the toaster oven.

Middle Eastern Veggie Burgers: Prepare the chickpea mixture as directed, but form into 4 patties about ½ inch thick. Cook in a large skillet, about 4 minutes per side, and serve on warmed whole-wheat burger buns, spread with sesame sauce. Top the burgers with sliced tomato and lettuce.

Sesame Sauce

¼ cup sesame tahini
⅓ cup plain reduced-fat (2%) yogurt
¼ cup water
2 tablespoons fresh lemon juice
½ teaspoon kosher salt
Pinch of crushed red pepper flakes

Combine the tahini and yogurt in a small bowl and stir with a fork to completely blend. Stir in the water, lemon juice, salt, and red pepper flakes.

PREP: 5 minutes

Makes about 1 cup

PER 1 TABLESPOON:
*27 calories, 2g fat
(.5g saturated),
1g carbohydrates,
0g fiber, 1g protein*

*"I'm a vegetarian and this is my favorite sandwich to eat because of the texture of the falafel balls and the sesame sauce,"
says nine-year-old Brenna M., of Port Chester, New York.*

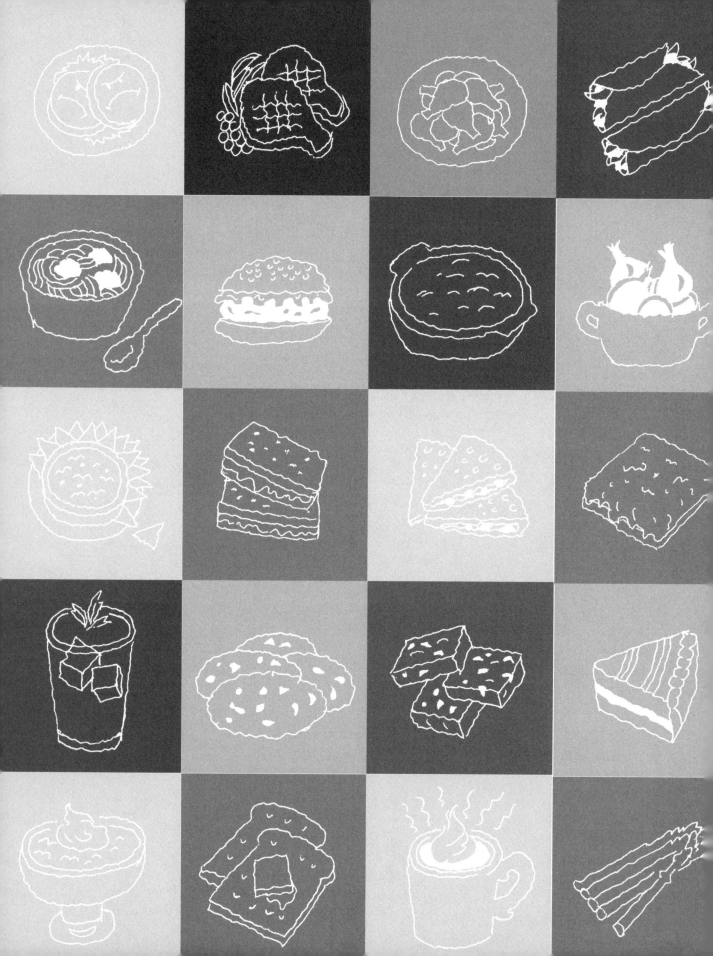

chapter five

Snack Attacks
Homemade Munchies

We are a nation of snackers, but that doesn't necessarily have to be a bad thing. It's all about what you munch on and how you space those mini-meals out in relation to breakfast, lunch, and dinner. In fact, kids who eat small meals throughout the day are actually less likely to overeat at mealtime, according to several studies, and, depending on what they eat, maintain a higher energy level and alertness throughout the day.

There are several tricks to smart snacking: The first is to maintain a regular meal schedule so that kids know the appropriate times to munch and keep the growlies away, and thus aren't so hungry that they reach for the easiest, craved item—that is, junk food. The American Dietetic Association recommends that snackers eat healthy foods at least one hour *prior* to a meal, so figure anywhere from two hours to ninety minutes between meals is the right time for kids to munch.

The second point to healthy snacking is that just as at mealtime, it's best to eat in the kitchen or the dining room, away from televisions, computers, PlayStations, and the like, so that the child notices and appreciates what he or she is eating and feels satiated.

Once you've figured out the when and where for your child, you need to decide the what. To encourage good-for-you munchies, devote an area in the pantry and/or refrigerator to good-for-you snacks or create a snack tray, or three—one for the cupboard, one for the fridge, and even one for long trips in the car. Buy long, narrow sturdy plastic bins and keep them stocked with the snacks mentioned here. You can store individual servings, or if that is too much for you to keep track of, keep larger portions in resealable plastic bags and canisters. Perfect items include the following, as well as the store-bought items listed on page 110:

❖ For the nonrefrigerated trays: granola and granola bars, whole-wheat pretzels, trail mix, raisins and other dried fruit, healthy cereal, baked pita and tortilla chips, nuts, seeds, nut butters, and crackers

❖ For the refrigerated tray: mozzarella sticks, yogurt, individual smoothies, crudités and dips, pieces of fruit, salsas, and hummus

❖ For the freezer: 100% fruit juice pops, red seedless grapes, edamame, sorbets and sherbets, whole-wheat waffles, and peeled and wrapped ripe bananas (for fast smoothies)

Finally, before making dinner, check in with your child to see what snacks he or she ate that day, so these can be taken into account when planning supper. If they've snacked on healthy foods such as carrots and apples, then you don't have to feel that Junior must feast on a mound of produce at dinner, and if they've had a less than healthy snack such as a candy bar, you can increase the veggies and reduce the dessert at dinner.

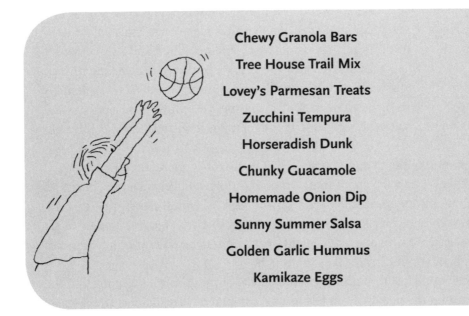

Chewy Granola Bars

Tree House Trail Mix

Lovey's Parmesan Treats

Zucchini Tempura

Horseradish Dunk

Chunky Guacamole

Homemade Onion Dip

Sunny Summer Salsa

Golden Garlic Hummus

Kamikaze Eggs

Chewy Granola Bars

These bars, perfect to tuck into book bags and lunch boxes for a high-energy snack, are thick and soft, with plenty of fiber. We like them made with our Extreme Granola, which has plenty of toasted nuts and dried fruit. If you are making this with store-bought granola, make sure to add raisins and chopped dates. After cutting, wrap the bars and keep them in the fridge.

> 4 cups Extreme Granola (page 50) or 3 cups packaged all-natural granola plus ½ cup each raisins and chopped dates
> 1 cup corn squares cereal, such as Health Valley Corn Crunch'ems, slightly crushed
> ½ cup high-fiber cereal, such as All-Bran
> 5 tablespoons unsalted butter, cut into 5 pieces
> ½ cup packed dark brown sugar
> ¼ cup honey
> ¼ teaspoon salt
> 2 large egg whites

SPEED LIMIT

PREP: 10 minutes plus cooling and chilling
BAKING: 20 minutes

Makes 16 bars

PER SERVING:
165 calories, 5.5g fat
(2g saturated),
28g carbohydrates,
2g fiber, 2.5g protein

1. Preheat the oven to 325°F. Lightly grease an 8-inch square baking pan and line with an 8-inch-wide and 12-inch-long sheet of parchment paper, letting the excess hang over the sides. Lightly grease the paper.

2. Combine the granola and corn and high-fiber cereals in a large bowl and mix well.

3. Combine the butter, brown sugar, honey, and salt in a 2-cup glass measuring cup and microwave for 1 minute at high (100%) power. Stir and microwave 30 seconds more, until the mixture is hot. Stir until smooth and pour in the bowl with the granola mixture. Stir with a wooden spoon until the dry ingredients are well coated. Add the egg whites and stir in until thoroughly blended. Scrape the mixture into the prepared pan and press to compact with a rubber spatula. Bake for about 20 minutes, until set in the center.

4. Transfer the pan to a rack, let cool completely, and then cover with foil and chill overnight to set.

5. Pull the confection out of the pan by grasping the paper and transfer to a board. Cut into sixteen 2-inch squares.

Cooks' Note

❖ If you're using prepackaged granola, look for the Back to Nature or Bare Naked brands or any other organic granola light on sugar.

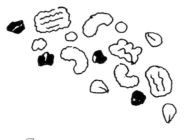

Tree House Trail Mix

Sweet, chewy dried fruit and slightly salty crunchy nuts make a winning combo, whether you're out in the wild or at a soccer game. For best results, buy raw nuts and seeds, roast them yourself, and toss with salt while still warm.

1 cup pecans
1 cup almonds
1 cup raw pumpkin seeds (pepitas)
½ cup sunflower seeds
1 teaspoon extra-virgin olive oil
½ teaspoon fine table salt
1 cup pitted dates
1 cup dried papaya chunks or pineapple chunks
1 cup yogurt-covered raisins

PREP: 5 minutes plus cooling
COOKING: 13 minutes

Makes 1 quart (about 12 servings)

PER SERVING:
354 calories, 24g fat (4g saturated), 30g carbohydrates, 5g fiber, 9g protein

1. Preheat the oven to 375°F. Spread the pecans and almonds on a large shallow baking sheet and roast in the oven for 8 minutes, until fragrant and lightly toasted.

2. While the nuts are roasting, place the pumpkin and sunflower seeds in a medium skillet over medium heat. Cook, shaking the pan, until the seeds are fragrant and begin to pop, 3 to 5 minutes. Remove from the heat, stir in the oil and salt, and transfer to a medium bowl. When the nuts are ready and have cooled, coarsely chop them and add to the seeds and toss. Let cool.

3. Cut the dates and papaya into a small dice and add to the nut mixture along with the raisins. Store in a covered glass jar in a convenient place for snacking.

Ten-year-old Connor G., from Oxford, Mississippi, said, "The trail mix was easy to make and great to eat on the road!"

Lovey's Parmesan Treats

Tracey's earliest food memories include these little cheese toasts, which were her introduction to hors d'oeuvres. Her mom (aka Lovey) made them in the toaster oven before dinner for company. Originally, they were made with white bread, but we love them with whole-wheat. They are simple and kids of any age are happy to make a meal of these, especially if they help mix and spread the topping.

> ½ cup finely grated Parmigiano-Reggiano
> ⅓ cup mayonnaise
> ¼ cup minced fresh onion (about ½ small onion)
> 2 pinches of freshly ground black pepper
> 5 slices Maple-Apple Sandwich Bread (page 60)
>   or 20 thin slices whole-wheat baguette

1. Preheat the oven to 400°F. In a small bowl, combine the Parmesan, mayonnaise, onion, and pepper and stir to blend. Line a baking sheet with foil.

2. Trim the crusts from the bread, cut the slices into quarters (squares or triangles), and place on the baking sheet. Top each piece of bread with a heaping teaspoon of the Parmesan mixture and bake for about 10 minutes, until the topping is puffed and nicely golden. Let cool for a minute or two before eating.

PREP: 5 minutes
BAKING: 10 minutes
SPEED LIMIT: 15 mpr

Makes 5 servings

PER SERVING (4 PIECES):
240 calories, 16.5g fat
(3.5g saturated),
15g carbohydrates,
2g fiber, 8g protein

Three-year-old Jacob S., of Booneville, Indiana, liked this so much he ate half of it uncooked and really loved mixing the spread "like a big boy."

Zucchini Tempura

These golden crispy snacks are sure to become almost as popular as French fries at your house. Our batter is light and simple—a mixture of flour and bubbly soda. You can also make the tempura with green beans or broccoli florets. Serve with zesty Horseradish Dunk.

PREP: 5 minutes
COOKING: 15 minutes
SPEED LIMIT: 20 mpr

Makes 4 servings

PER SERVING
(WITHOUT DIP):
330 calories, 28g fat
(4g saturated),
18g carbohydrates,
1.5g fiber, 5g protein

PER SERVING (WITH DIP):
470 calories, 43g fat
(5.5g saturated),
19g carbohydrates,
1.5g fiber, 5.5g protein

1 quart vegetable oil
⅔ cup unbleached all-purpose flour
⅔ cup seltzer or club soda
½ teaspoon kosher salt
½ teaspoon hot sauce, such as Tabasco
3 medium zucchini (about a pound), trimmed and cut into ⅓-inch-thick diagonal rounds
Horseradish Dunk (page 103) and lemon wedges, for serving

1. Heat the oil in a heavy 4-quart saucepan fitted with a deep-fry thermometer over medium-high heat until the oil is bubbling and the temperature reaches 375°F.

2. Meanwhile, combine the flour, seltzer, salt, and hot sauce in a large bowl and whisk until smooth. Add 8 to 10 zucchini rounds (or other vegetable pieces) to the batter, turning with a rubber spatula to coat. Carefully transfer the rounds one at a time to the hot oil with your fingers (being careful not to burn them) and cook, turning, until golden, 2 to 3 minutes. Transfer with a slotted spoon to paper towels to drain. Continue frying the remainder in batches and let all of them cool slightly before serving with Horseradish Dunk and lemon wedges.

Cooks' Notes

❖ Mix up the dunking sauce before you begin preparing the tempura.

❖ You can easily double the amount of vegetables: Simply increase all of the ingredients except the oil and fry in batches.

"I like the batter—it would be good with fish, too," said Aidan C., twelve years old, from the Bronx, New York.

Horseradish Dunk

Serve this sauce with tempura, steak, and raw veggies, and on hamburgers and sandwiches.

⅓ cup plain whole milk yogurt
⅓ cup mayonnaise
1 tablespoon prepared horseradish
Freshly ground black pepper

Combine all of the ingredients in a small bowl and stir with a fork to blend.

PREP: 5 minutes

Makes about ⅔ cup

PER SERVING:
*146 calories, 15g fat
(2g saturated),
2g carbohydrates, 0g fiber, 1g
protein*

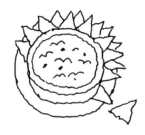

Chunky Guacamole

Serve the guacamole with salted tortilla chips and any of our Mexican dishes.

PREP: 10 minutes
SPEED LIMIT: 10 mpr

Makes 8 servings (about 4 cups)

PER SERVING:
135 calories, 11g fat
(1.5g saturated),
10g carbohydrates,
5g fiber, 2g protein

3 ripe Hass avocados, halved and pitted
3 tablespoons fresh lime juice
1 tablespoon fresh lemon juice
1 large ripe tomato, cored and finely diced
1 small onion, finely chopped
2 large garlic cloves, smashed, peeled, and minced
1 tablespoon minced fresh jalapeño or one 4-ounce can chopped green chiles
½ teaspoon kosher salt

1. Dice the flesh of an avocado half right in the peel (make a checkerboard with a knife) and scoop it out into a bowl with a fork. Repeat with the remaining avocados. Add the lime and lemon juice, tomato, onion, garlic, jalapeño, and salt and mix well.

2. Cover with plastic wrap directly on the surface. Chill until ready to serve, up to 4 hours.

Cooks' Note

❧ We prefer the darker, smaller Hass avocado from California to the larger, less flavorful bright green fruit from Florida.

Homemade Onion Dip

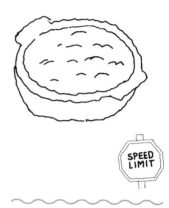

Onion dip has been popular for decades—even the weird freeze-dried kind. Ours takes longer to make than dumping a packet of dehydrated soup mix into a bowl of sour cream, but it's worth the effort. Plus, you can feel great about what the kids are scarfing down, especially if it acts as a conduit to eating carrots and sugar snap peas. Serve the dip in a decorative bowl or a hollowed-out pineapple, winter squash, or bell pepper.

2 tablespoons extra-virgin olive oil

2 medium onions (1 pound total), finely diced

1 package (8 ounces) cream cheese, softened

1½ cups plain yogurt (preferably whole milk)

2 teaspoons kosher salt

⅛ teaspoon ground white pepper or ¼ teaspoon black freshly ground pepper

⅓ cup minced fresh chives

Vegetable crudités and baked potato chips, for serving

PREP: 15 minutes plus cooling and chilling
COOKING: 10 minutes

Makes 3 cups

PER ¼ CUP DIP:
120 calories, 9g fat (4.5g saturated), 6.5g carbohydrates, .5g fiber, 3g protein

1. Heat the oil in a heavy skillet over medium heat until hot. Add the onions and cook, stirring occasionally, until the onions are softened and golden, about 6 minutes. Transfer the onions to a plate and let cool. (You can place them in the fridge to hasten the process.)

2. Place the cream cheese in a bowl; gradually add the yogurt and mash with a fork until smooth. Stir in the salt, pepper, and chives. Stir in the cooled onions and then chill until cold, about 1 hour. Serve with fresh raw veggies.

Cooks' Note

❖ For best flavor, make the dip several hours ahead before serving.

vedgemania

You can make vegetables even more delicious by creating a fun crudités platter. Be sure to cut carrot and celery sticks thin for small mouths—$\frac{1}{4}$ to $\frac{1}{3}$ inch thick is perfect. Add colorful bell peppers, cut into strips, and small cherry tomatoes, Kirby cucumber slices, and tiny cauliflower florets. If adding asparagus, trim and peel the stalks if they are thick, cook for 2 minutes in boiling water, and rinse with cold water until cool. Arrange colorful fresh veggies on your favorite platter or dish. Turn a large square platter into a tic-tac-toe board by arranging vegetables in nine different squares within the square.

Sunny Summer Salsa

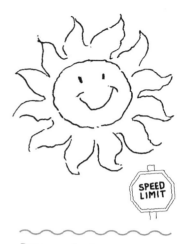

Real, ripe summer tomatoes have so many health benefits, such as lycopene, an excellent antioxidant, and salsa made when tomatoes are at their peak is the ultimate. Since some tomatoes are so juicy, we use a combo of meaty plum tomatoes and slicing tomatoes. If the salsa is too juicy, drain off some of the liquid with a fine-mesh sieve. Serve with lightly salted tortilla chips and your favorite foods.

1 medium jalapeño, trimmed, quartered lengthwise, and seeded (if desired)
1 garlic clove, smashed and peeled
½ cup packed cilantro leaves
½ sweet onion, such as Vidalia, peeled and cut into 1-inch pieces
1½ pounds (2 to 3) ripe beefsteak tomatoes, sliced
1 pound ripe plum tomatoes (about 8), sliced
1½ teaspoons kosher salt
1 tablespoon fresh lime juice

PREP: 5 minutes
SPEED LIMIT: 5 mpr

Makes 6 cups

PER ½ CUP SALSA:
25 calories, 0g fat,
5g carbohydrates,
1g fiber, 1g protein

1. Place the jalapeño and garlic in a food processor and process until the mixture sticks to the bowl. Scrape down the side, add the cilantro, and process to finely chop; transfer to a medium bowl. Add the onion to the processor and process to finely chop; add to the cilantro mixture.

2. Place half of the tomato pieces in the processor and pulse in one-second pulses until evenly but coarsely chopped; transfer to the bowl and repeat with the remaining tomatoes. Season with the salt and lime juice and serve.

Cooks' Notes

❖ Take care when seeding the jalapeño! You can wear disposable gloves, but if you don't have them, cut the chile lengthwise in quarters, hold each piece on the thicker end, and cut out the rib and seeds with the knife. Wash your hands immediately in cold water after seeding and be careful not to put your fingers in your eyes.

❖ The salsa will keep well for a week in a covered jar in the refrigerator.

Golden Garlic Hummus

Our kids love this creamy chickpea spread. Scoop it up with warmed Skillet Whole-wheat Pitas (page 62), plain crispy pita chips, crackers, or fresh veggies.

PREP: 8 minutes
COOKING: 2 minutes
SPEED LIMIT: 10 mpr

Makes 1½ cups (6 servings)

PER ¼ CUP:
*195 calories, 15g fat
(2g saturated),
11g carbohydrates, 3g fiber,
5.5g protein*

One 15-ounce can garbanzo beans, drained and rinsed
3 tablespoons sesame tahini
3 garlic cloves
¼ cup extra-virgin olive oil
¼ teaspoon ground cumin
3 tablespoons water
1½ tablespoons fresh lemon juice
1 teaspoon kosher salt

1. Combine the garbanzo beans and tahini in a food processor and process until the beans look finely ground.

2. Smash the garlic cloves with the side of a large knife. Trim the ends and discard the peel.

3. Heat 2 tablespoons of the oil in a small skillet over medium heat. Add the garlic and stir until fragrant and golden, 1 to 2 minutes. Remove from the heat and add the cumin; stir until toasted, about 5 seconds. Quickly stir in the remaining 2 tablespoons of oil and scrape the mixture into the processor; process until incorporated. Add the water, lemon juice, and salt and process until the mixture is fluffy and smooth, 2 to 3 minutes. Serve chilled or at room temperature.

Cooks' Note

❧ Tahini tends to separate while it sits on the shelf in the store. When you open a fresh jar, pour the oil and scoop the solids into your food processor. Process until smooth and then scrape the tahini back into the jar and keep in the refrigerator until you need it.

genie and the magic lunch

Hummus makes a great sandwich: Spread generously on whole-wheat bread or in halved pita pockets. Add sliced tomatoes and cucumber and sprouts, such as clover or alfalfa.

Kamikaze Eggs

We've added a kick to these deviled eggs with a dab of wasabi paste, but you can substitute a teaspoon of brown or Dijon mustard for a less potent execution.

10 large eggs
2 teaspoons wasabi paste (see Cooks' Notes)
4 tablespoons cream cheese, cut up
½ cup mayonnaise
2 tablespoons minced fresh chives (optional)
Kosher salt and freshly ground black pepper

1. Hard-cook the eggs: Place the eggs in a single layer in a large pot and add cold water to cover. Bring to a boil, turn off the heat, cover with a lid, and let stand for 10 minutes. Pour off the water from the pot, cover the eggs with cold water, drain, and then cover with ice water and let stand until cold, about 3 minutes, or chill overnight in the refrigerator.

2. Peel the eggs and cut in half lengthwise with a small sharp knife. Pop the egg yolks out into a bowl and mash with a fork until crumbly. Add the wasabi paste and cream cheese and mash until no flecks of white remain. Stir in the mayonnaise and chives, if using. Season to taste with salt and pepper.

3. Transfer the yolk mixture to a pastry bag with a small to medium star tip or to a quart resealable plastic bag and snip off ¼ inch of a corner. Arrange the whites in a deviled egg dish, and pipe the yolk mixture into the whites in a circular motion, filling to the top.

Cooks' Notes

❧ Wasabi paste is available in many supermarkets, but to make your own, mix equal parts wasabi powder and water and let stand for 10 minutes to develop the flavor.

❧ You can assemble the eggs up to 12 hours ahead and store in a plastic container with a tight-fitting lid. Cook a few extra eggs to ensure a selection of perfect egg whites for filling. (You can use any leftover eggs in a salad.) To pack for lunch, use a small plastic container with a tight-fitting lid and pack flat in a bag or a lunch box.

PREP: 10 minutes plus cooling
COOKING: 15 minutes

Makes 5 servings

PER SERVING (2 PIECES): *178 calories, 16g fat (3.7g saturated), 1g carbohydrates, 0g fiber, 6g protein*

store-bought snacks we like

Here are a few things we have on hand for our kids. For more suggestions or to tell us about healthy snacks that you like, log on to realfoodforhealthykids.com.

Energy bars, such as Pria and Luna brands

Low-fat vegetable crisps and soy crisps, such as Terra or Genisoy

Baked tortilla chips or potato chips

Unsulfured dried fruit

Motts or Earth's Best unsweetened applesauce cups

Health is Wealth Spinach Munchees

Save the Forest Organic Trail Mix

Amy's Bean and Cheese Burritos

Horizon Organic Yo-Yos

Newman's Own Organics cookies

Semisweet chocolate

Cheddar guppies and cheese puffs from 365 Degrees

Michael Season's potato chips

Green Mountain Gringo tortilla strips

Garden of Eating and Bearitos brand tortilla chips

Healthy Handful Organic Snacks for Kids

Kashi TLC Crackers and Chewy Granola Bars

Graham crackers

Rice cakes

Whole-wheat pretzels

Almond and cashew butters

~ MORE HOMEMADE MUNCHIE SUGGESTIONS ~

Here are some other recipes in the book that make good snacks.

Bursting Berry Muffins (page 53)
Island-Style Smoothie (page 227)
Microwave Pizza Frittata (page 30)
Old-Fashioned Grilled Cheese Sandwiches (page 86)
Cheese Omelet (page 42)
Protein Power Pancakes (page 47)
Sunshine Parfait (page 37)
Toaster Oven Use-Your-Bean Taco (page 31)
California-Style Tuna Salad Rolls (page 78)
Turkey Pinwheels (page 79)
Watermelon Gell-ee (page 267)
Zucchini-Parmesan Pancakes (page 200)

chapter six

What's for Dinner
Satisfying Suppers and Fast Weekday Solutions

What's for dinner? I'm starving!" That's the refrain we hear each day as soon as the clock strikes 6:00 P.M. It's the eternal burning question, and the problem appears on our radar at 4:00 every afternoon with a creeping panic. On weekdays, it's hard to resist pulling into a fast-food driveway or pulling out a frozen pizza. And weekends aren't much easier, filled with lessons, sports, and family outings. But with a modicum of advance planning, and a stocked kitchen, you can whip up a delicious, nutritious dinner that will make your family happy to be at your table.

If you read the Introduction, you know how important it is for the family to take twenty minutes every night to sit down together, break bread (hopefully homemade), and talk about their day. So we have created recipes for every night of the week that are wholesome, delicious, and easily doable.

We know that what to serve depends largely upon what night of the week it is, so we have broken this chapter into several sections. Our first, "Homemade Fast Food," is devoted to quick weeknight dishes, most of which take advantage of superior convenience products and speedy cooking techniques. A bridge between the weekend and weekday can be found in "Double Plays." These recipes for roasts and the like—perfect for making on a Sunday afternoon—are designed to make *two* dinners, the first for Sunday supper and the remaining (we don't use the word *leftover*) meat, poultry, or fish for a fast weeknight dinner. Then we have dozens of recipes for nights when there is time for something a little more involved, whether you are entertaining other families or your own. These are featured in "Blue Plate Specials." "One-Dish Dinners" focuses on soups, stews, and casseroles. "Meat-Free Mains" are vegetarian—not vegan—entrees, while "Sidekicks" offers delicious vegetable and whole-grain sides. With all of these options, you will never go blank when trying to figure out what's for dinner.

homemade fast food: dinner in 30 minutes or less

Skillet Chicken Cacciatore

Peachy Keen Chicken

Chicken Cherries Jubilee
   with Goat Cheese

Cherry Pork Chops

Cherry Steak

Quick Chick Parm

Hail Caesar, Jr.

Chicken Caesar

Shrimp Caesar

Thai Green-Curry Chicken

Thai Beef, Pork, or Shrimp Curry

Not-Your-Basic Turkey Burger

Crispy Jamaican Pork
   with Pan-Fried Bananas

Mexican-Style Pan-Roasted Pork
   with Pineapple

Pork Chops with Fresh Pear Stuffing

Pan-Fried Steaks Chimichurri

Super Steak Fajitas

Quick Confetti Chili

Quick Vegetarian Chili

Fins and Chips

Crabby Cakes

Easy-Bake Scampi

Shrimp Confetti Tostadas

Princess and the Pea Risotto

Grilled Pint-Sized Pizzas

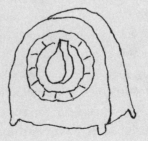

We both embody the typical busy, stressed, working parent who has to get dinner on the table every weekday. On weekends, we enjoy making dishes that take a little more time and care, but Monday through Friday, we put in full days, change gears, and try to get dinner on the table within a half hour.

Whatever your family dynamic, it is important to sit down to dinner together as much as possible. Here are many delicious options (with variations) that will help make it happen. They are innovative and involve as little time and preparation, and as few ingredients, as possible.

The time amounts listed here are a guide. To help speed up the process, keep your pantry stocked with basics (see page 20). When you're ready to start cooking, quickly read your recipe through, and before you heat up the skillet, get out all the necessary equipment and do any chopping and measuring. You will be more relaxed and the cooking process will be smoother. Plus, the more you cook, the better and faster your techniques will become.

Skillet Chicken Cacciatore

Make this chicken cacciatore with boneless chicken thighs and a light, bright vegetable sauce in minutes. Serve with Perfect Rice (page 196) or lightly buttered whole-wheat noodles.

PREP: 10 minutes

COOKING: 25 minutes

SPEED LIMIT: 35 mpr

Makes 4 servings

PER SERVING:
396 calories, 20g fat
(4g saturated),
17g carbohydrates,
4g fiber, 36g protein

1½ pounds skinless boneless chicken thighs (6 pieces)
¼ teaspoon kosher salt
Freshly ground black pepper
2 tablespoons unbleached all-purpose flour
2 tablespoons extra-virgin olive oil
One 10-ounce package medium mushrooms, quartered
1 large onion, sliced
1 yellow bell pepper, cut into ¼-inch-thick strips
2 garlic cloves, smashed and peeled
One 14-ounce can diced tomatoes in juice
One 14-ounce can low-sodium chicken broth
¼ cup chopped fresh basil or flat-leaf parsley

1. Place the chicken in a medium bowl and sprinkle with the salt and pepper. Stir the flour in with a large spoon to coat the chicken.

2. Heat the oil in a 10-inch skillet over medium-high heat. Add the chicken thighs smooth side down flat in the pan, and let cook until golden, about 2 minutes. Turn and cook 2 minutes more and then transfer the chicken to a plate.

3. Add the mushrooms to the same skillet and cook over medium-high heat, stirring often, until golden, about 3 minutes. Add the onion, bell pepper, and garlic and cook, stirring, until softened, about 3 minutes. Pour in the tomatoes and broth and bring to a boil over high heat.

4. Return the chicken thighs and any juices to the skillet, nestling the chicken in the sauce. Reduce the heat to medium-low and simmer until the chicken is cooked through, about 10 minutes. Transfer the chicken, covered, to a clean platter and simmer the sauce about 5 minutes more to thicken. Stir in the basil, season to taste, and spoon the sauce over the chicken.

Peachy Keen Chicken

Although the recipe calls for boneless skinless breasts, you can use chicken tenders or a cut-up chicken with skin, but the cooking time will vary (see Cooks' Note). If you want to use fresh or frozen sliced peaches instead of canned, add 2 tablespoons honey to the marinade. Grilled pitted fresh peach or nectarine halves are great alongside. Serve with potatoes and a crisp green salad. Any leftover sliced chicken is great on a sandwich with a little lettuce, honey mustard, and peach jam.

> One 15-ounce can light sliced peaches (in pear juice), lightly drained
> 1 tablespoon extra-virgin olive oil
> ½ tablespoon honey
> 1½ pounds boneless skinless chicken breast halves or chicken tenders
> Kosher salt and freshly ground black pepper

PREP: 5 minutes plus 15 minutes marinating
GRILLING: 10 minutes
SPEED LIMIT: 30 mpr

Makes 4 servings

PER SERVING:
205 calories, 5g fat (1g saturated),
4g carbohydrates,
0g fiber, 34g protein

1. Place the peaches in a food processor and process to a smooth puree. Add the oil and honey and process briefly to blend; transfer to a large resealable plastic bag. Add the chicken pieces and close, squeezing out the air. Chill for 15 minutes (or you can do it the day before).

2. Prepare the grill (gas grill at medium; charcoal grill arranged for indirect heat), heat a grill pan over medium heat, or preheat the broiler. Remove the chicken pieces from the bag and place on a plate. Season lightly with salt and pepper and transfer to the grill. Cover and cook until charred underneath, 4 to 5 minutes. Turn and cook until charred and firm when poked with a finger, 4 to 5 minutes more.

Cooks' Note

❖ For chicken tenders, cook 3 to 4 minutes on each side; for chicken pieces with bone in, cook for 30 to 40 minutes, turning occasionally, until the juices run clear when pierced with the tip of a knife.

When Alfred M., of Royal Palm Beach, Florida, was asked by his mom how his chicken with peaches was, he said simply, "Sweet!"

Chicken Cherries Jubilee with Goat Cheese

This isn't a combo of dinner and dessert, but it's bound to become a specialty of your house. You can use cherries in season or thawed frozen cherries. Serve the chicken with brown rice and steamed snow peas or sugar snap peas.

PREP: 15 minutes
COOKING: 14 minutes
SPEED LIMIT: 29 mpr

Makes 4 servings

PER SERVING:
414 calories,
21g fat (10g saturated),
21g carbohydrates,
1.5g fiber, 34g protein

4 large boneless skinless chicken breast halves (about 2 pounds total)
4 ounces fresh goat cheese, cut into 4 slices
Kosher salt and freshly ground black pepper
1 tablespoon unbleached all-purpose flour
2 tablespoons extra-virgin olive oil
1 shallot, finely chopped
1 cup canned low-sodium chicken broth
*2 cups fresh dark sweet cherries, pitted (see Cooks' Notes), or thawed
   frozen dark cherries (with their juice)*
*2 tablespoons seedless blackberry, black currant, or raspberry fruit
   spread or jam*
1 tablespoon unsalted butter

1. Carefully cut a horizontal slit through the center of each chicken breast to make a pocket, cutting in as far as possible without cutting through to the other side. Insert a slice of the cheese into each pocket and then press down on the top of the chicken breast to evenly distribute the cheese. Secure the openings with one or two toothpicks to prevent the cheese from leaking out during cooking. Sprinkle the chicken on both sides with the salt and pepper and flour.

2. Heat the oil in a nonstick 12-inch skillet over medium heat. Add the chicken smooth side down and cook until nicely browned, about 2 minutes. Turn and cook 2 minutes more, then cover the pan with foil and cook, turning once or twice, until the chicken is cooked through, about 6 minutes. Transfer the chicken to a plate and cover loosely with foil.

3. Meanwhile, add the shallot and cook, stirring, for 1 minute. Add the broth and cherries and bring to a boil over medium-high heat. Continue boiling until the sauce is reduced by half, about 3 minutes. Stir in the fruit spread and butter and season the sauce to taste.

4. Remove the toothpicks from the chicken pieces and arrange on 4 plates. Spoon the cherry sauce on top and serve.

Cooks' Notes

❖ Inexpensive cherry pitters are available from Sur La Table, Crate & Barrel, and Williams-Sonoma, online and in their stores. The cherries come out whole and it's super-fast.

❖ If you don't have a cherry pitter, discard the stems and put on plastic gloves if desired. Squeeze a cherry between your thumb and index finger to soften and tear in half. Squeeze out the pit with your fingers, reserving the juice.

❖ In a hurry? Skip the goat cheese stuffing if time is of the essence. The chicken will take about the same time to cook.

Cherry Pork Chops: Sauté four $^3/_4$-inch-thick boneless pork chops stuffed with cheese about 4 minutes per side, until lightly golden and cooked through.

Cherry Steak: Grill four 6-ounce filets mignons stuffed with cheese about 4 minutes per side for medium doneness.

Quick Chick Parm

This is a big improvement upon the heavily breaded, greasy, time-consuming original. You can substitute with thin turkey cutlets. Serve with a side of whole-wheat linguini and a simple salad with ABC Vinaigrette (page 215).

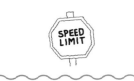

PREP: 10 minutes
COOKING: 18 minutes
SPEED LIMIT: 28 mpr

Makes 4 servings

PER SERVING:
337 calories,
16g fat (4g saturated),
10g carbohydrates,
1g fiber, 36g protein

¼ cup unbleached all-purpose flour
½ teaspoon kosher salt
¼ teaspoon freshly ground black pepper
1 pound thin chicken breast cutlets
3 tablespoons extra-virgin olive oil
1 cup canned low-sodium chicken broth
1½ cups (packed) shredded mozzarella cheese (6 ounces)
½ cup marinara sauce or Quick Skillet Tomato Sauce (page 213)
Finely chopped fresh basil or flat-leaf parsley

1. Combine the flour, salt, and pepper in a gallon-size resealable plastic bag, seal, and shake to mix. Add about one-third of the chicken and shake to coat. Remove the chicken, lightly shaking off any excess flour, and lay flat on a plate. Repeat with the remaining chicken in two batches.

2. Heat 1½ tablespoons of the oil in a nonstick 12-inch skillet over medium heat until hot. Add half of the chicken and cook until browned underneath, about 2 minutes. Turn, cook 2 minutes more, and transfer the chicken to a plate. Repeat with the remaining 1½ tablespoons oil and chicken.

3. Pour off any remaining fat in the skillet and add the chicken broth to the pan. Bring to a boil and cook until reduced by half, about 3 minutes. Return the chicken to the pan and turn to coat in the broth. Arrange the cutlets in an even layer, sprinkle the mozzarella on top, and spoon a little marinara sauce on top of each piece. Cover the pan with a lid or foil and cook until the cheese is melted, 1 to 2 minutes. Transfer the cutlets to plates, spooning any remaining sauce on top of each. Sprinkle some basil on top and serve.

Hail Caesar, Jr.

Introducing kids to a Caesar is a great way to get them to appreciate salad. Our version is mild but flavorful, with bite-sized pieces of lettuce for small mouths. We forgo the croutons, which can be hard for little kids to deal with.

1 medium garlic clove, peeled
Juice of ¼ lemon
1½ tablespoons red wine vinegar
½ teaspoon anchovy paste (optional)
½ teaspoon Dijon mustard
Dash of Worcestershire sauce
¼ cup extra-virgin olive oil
1 small head romaine
2 tablespoons finely grated Parmigiano-Reggiano
Freshly ground black pepper

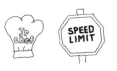

PREP: 10 minutes
SPEED LIMIT: 10 mpr

Makes 4 servings

PER SERVING:
155 calories,
15g fat (3g saturated),
2g carbohydrates, 1g fiber,
2g protein

1. Rub the inside of your big salad bowl (a wooden one works best) with the peeled garlic, and then discard the garlic. Add the lemon juice, vinegar, anchovy paste, if using, mustard, and Worcestershire sauce and stir with a fork to blend. Gradually mix in the oil until incorporated.

2. Slice the romaine leaves crosswise into ½-inch-wide ribbons, and cut in half. (You should have about 10 cups.) Add the romaine to the dressing and toss well. Sprinkle the Parmesan on top, season lightly with pepper, and toss again.

Chicken Caesar: Add 1 small grilled chicken breast, chopped, or ⅓ cup diced cooked chicken to each portion.

Shrimp Caesar: Toss peeled and cleaned extra-large shrimp lightly with olive oil and cook on the grill or in a grill pan over medium heat just until firm and brightly colored. Cut the shrimp into small pieces and sprinkle on top of each portion.

Thai Green-Curry Chicken

This quick stew is chock-full of colorful veggies and tender lean chicken. It is easy to make now that prepared curry pastes are available in the ethnic section of the supermarket. Serve the curry over Perfect Rice (page 196), rice noodles, or whole-wheat pasta.

PREP: 10 minutes
COOKING: 13 minutes
SPEED LIMIT: 23 mpr

Makes 4 servings

PER SERVING:
198 calories, 7g fat
(3g saturated),
16g carbohydrates, 3g fiber,
15g protein

One 13.5-ounce can Thai coconut milk (do not shake)
½ cup canned low-sodium chicken broth
1 to 2 teaspoons green curry paste, such as Taste of Thai brand
2 tablespoons light brown sugar
1½ tablespoons Thai or Vietnamese fish sauce
1 medium onion, halved and cut into thin slices
1 large green bell pepper, cut into ¾-inch dice
2 medium summer squash, ends trimmed and cut into bite-sized pieces
2 large boneless skinless chicken breast halves, cut crosswise into thin slices
2 ripe plum tomatoes, cored and cut into ½-inch dice
½ cup chopped fresh basil

1. Scoop the creamy top off of the coconut milk (about 1 cup) and place in a large saucepan. (Discard the clear watery liquid.) Whisk in the broth and green curry paste and bring to a boil. Reduce the heat to medium; stir in the brown sugar and fish sauce. Add the onion, bell pepper, and squash, and simmer gently, stirring, for 3 minutes.

2. Add the sliced chicken and tomatoes and cook, stirring occasionally, until the chicken is cooked through, about 8 minutes. Stir in the basil and serve.

Cooks' Note

✤ Make sure to buy unsweetened coconut milk, not sweet coconut cream. Fish sauce can be found in your supermarket in the Asian food section.

Thai Beef, Pork, or Shrimp Curry: Substitute 1 pound of sliced beef or pork, or 1 pound peeled and deveined medium shrimp for the chicken.

"I'm not a big fan of peppers, but this was really very tasty and I could have this often," says Tanya's eight-year-old son Sanger.

Not-Your-Basic Turkey Burger

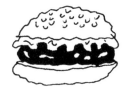

A mixture of both dark and white turkey meat is preferable here, because all white meat is too dry and firm for burgers. We call for Havarti, but you can use Swiss, Cheddar, or mozzarella instead.

2 tablespoons extra-virgin olive oil

1 small onion, finely chopped

1 small zucchini (4 to 5 ounces), trimmed and cut into 1/4-inch dice

1 1/2 pounds ground turkey (white and dark meat)

1/4 cup drained roasted red pepper in olive oil, finely diced

1/2 teaspoon kosher salt

1/4 teaspoon freshly ground black pepper

6 ounces Havarti cheese, preferably creamy Havarti, shredded

6 whole-wheat hamburger buns, split and warmed or toasted (optional)

About 2 cups baby salad greens

About 1/4 cup Rockin' Ranch Dressing (page 219), mayonnaise, or ketchup, for serving

PREP: 10 minutes
COOKING: 12 minutes
SPEED LIMIT: 22 mpr

Makes 6 servings

PER SERVING (WITHOUT DRESSING):
416 calories,
17g fat (7g saturated),
26g carbohydrates,
3.5g fiber, 40g protein

1. Heat 1 tablespoon of the oil in a large cast-iron or other heavy skillet over medium heat. Add the onion and cook, stirring occasionally, until slightly softened and golden, about 3 minutes. Add the zucchini and cook until nearly tender, about 2 minutes. Transfer to a plate and let cool. Rinse out and dry the skillet.

2. Crumble the ground turkey into a mixing bowl. Add the cooled vegetables, roasted red pepper, salt, and pepper. Mix with a wooden spoon until blended. Form into 6 equal balls.

3. Return the skillet to medium heat and add the remaining tablespoon of oil. When the oil shimmers, flatten the portions of the meat mixture into 4- to 5-inch-diameter patties and add to the pan; cook until lightly browned on the bottom, about 3 minutes; turn, cover the pan with a lid, and cook 3 minutes more, or until completely cooked through. Add the cheese, cover, and cook for 1 minute to melt the cheese. Transfer the burgers to the bun bottoms, if using, top with greens, dressing, and bun tops.

Cooks' Note

❖ If you don't need all 6 burgers, wrap any extra uncooked patties and freeze to cook another time. See freezer tips on pages 23–24.

Crispy Jamaican Pork with Pan-Fried Bananas

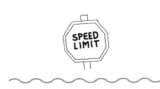

This West Indian–inspired dish is flavored with a hint of Jamaican spices. Adjust the heat of the crumb mixture according to your family's preference. The sweet, soft bananas pair perfectly with the spicy crusted pork. Any leftover pork cutlets can be served for lunch on soft rolls with Rainbow Slaw (page 205).

PREP: 10 minutes
COOKING: 10 minutes
SPEED LIMIT: 20 mpr

Makes 4 servings

PER SERVING:
663 calories,
44g fat (7.5g saturated),
40g carbohydrates,
3g fiber, 31g protein

1 large or 2 small pork tenderloins (about 1 pound total), cut into
   12 pieces
1 cup plain dried bread crumbs, preferably Panko (Japanese-style)
2 teaspoons Asian five-spice powder
1 teaspoon dried thyme, crumbled
1 teaspoon ground allspice
¾ teaspoon fine salt
⅛ to ½ teaspoon ground dried hot pepper, such as cayenne or habanero
3 large eggs
½ cup plus 2 tablespoons vegetable oil, for frying
4 firm but ripe medium bananas, sliced ⅓ inch thick

1. On a work surface, between two pieces of plastic wrap and using the heel of your hand or a mallet, flatten the pork into medallions about ¼ inch thick and set aside.

2. In a shallow bowl, stir together the bread crumbs, five-spice powder, thyme, allspice, salt, and hot pepper. In a second shallow bowl, beat the eggs with a fork. Turn the pork medallions one at a time in the crumbs, then turn in the beaten egg and turn again in the crumb mixture to coat well; transfer to a plate.

3. Heat 2 tablespoons of the oil in a large cast-iron skillet over medium heat. Add half of the pork and cook until golden brown and crisp, 2 to 3 minutes; turn and cook until crisp on the other side, 2 to 3 minutes more. Transfer the pork to a plate and keep warm in a low oven while you repeat with 2 more tablespoons of the oil and the remaining pork.

4. Heat the remaining 2 tablespoons oil in the same skillet over medium-high heat. Add the bananas and pan-fry, tossing occasionally, until golden on both sides, about 4 minutes total. Serve the bananas with the pork.

Mexican-Style Pan-Roasted Pork with Pineapple

Tracey's kids' longtime babysitter is from Oaxaca, Mexico, and through the years, Tracey has incorporated many dishes from that region into her repertoire. Pork slow-roasted with pineapple, onion, and cumin is typical for Oaxaca, but here we pan-fry the meat for a speedy rendition. Serve with Perfect Rice (page 196) or buttered noodles.

1 tablespoon unbleached all-purpose flour
1 teaspoon ground cumin
$\frac{1}{2}$ teaspoon kosher salt
Freshly ground black pepper
1 to 1$\frac{1}{2}$ pounds trimmed pork loin, cut into 8 slices (about $\frac{1}{3}$ inch thick)
2 tablespoons safflower oil
1 medium onion, thinly sliced
$\frac{1}{2}$ teaspoon dried oregano, crumbled
One 20-ounce can pineapple chunks in juice, drained (juice reserved)
1 cup canned low-sodium chicken broth

PREP: 10 minutes
COOKING: 12 minutes
SPEED LIMIT: 22 mpr

Makes 4 servings

PER SERVING:
416 calories, 22g fat
(6g saturated),
24 carbohydrates,
2g fiber, 28g protein

1. Combine the flour, cumin, salt, and several grindings of pepper in a shallow bowl and stir to blend. Turn the pork slices in the seasoned flour to coat lightly and transfer to a plate.

2. Heat the oil in a heavy 12-inch skillet over medium-high heat. Add the pork slices and cook for 2 minutes, until golden brown underneath. Turn and cook until browned on the other side—juices will begin to pool on top—about 2 minutes more. Transfer the pork to a plate and cover loosely with foil to keep warm.

3. Add the onion and oregano to the pan and cook over medium heat, stirring often, until softened, about 5 minutes. Add the pineapple and stir for 1 minute. Add the broth and 2 tablespoons of the reserved pineapple juice. Simmer briskly until the sauce is thickened and the onion and pineapple are nicely tender, 3 to 4 minutes.

4. Return the pork slices and any exuded juices to the pan and turn the slices to coat. Arrange the pork on plates. Season the pan sauce to taste with salt and then spoon the sauce over the pork.

"This was great—salty and sweet at the same time," says eight-year-old Emma S. from Rye, New York.

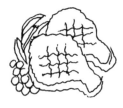

Pork Chops with Fresh Pear Stuffing

If your kids love stuffing, this is a recipe for them—and you. Using half of a piece of fruit might seem silly, but the other half provides a snack while you cook. Take care not to overcook the chops, since pork is so lean. To check for doneness, poke a chop with your finger: Pork that is ready will be firm to the touch.

PREP: 10 minutes
COOKING: 17 minutes
SPEED LIMIT: 27 mpr

Makes 4 servings

PER SERVING:
319 calories, 14g fat
(4g saturated),
11g carbohydrates, 2g fiber,
36g protein

Four 1-inch-thick boneless pork chops (about 6 ounces each)
1 tablespoon extra-virgin olive oil
½ small onion, finely chopped
½ medium Bartlett pear (no need to peel), quartered, cored, and finely diced
2 slices whole-wheat bread, diced
3 tablespoons canned low-sodium chicken broth or water
1 tablespoon chopped fresh parsley
Kosher salt and freshly ground black pepper

1. Place a pork chop flat on a work surface. Cut a horizontal slit through the center of the chop, slicing almost all the way through to make a pocket. Repeat with the remaining chops and set aside.

2. Heat ½ tablespoon of the oil in a heavy ovenproof skillet, preferably cast iron. Add the onion and cook, stirring often, until softened, about 5 minutes. Stir in the pear and remove from the heat. Stir in the bread, broth, and parsley and season to taste with salt and pepper.

3. Lightly salt the inside of the pork pockets. Divide the stuffing among the chops, packing it in lightly. Season the chops on both sides with salt and pepper.

4. Rinse and wipe out the skillet. Add the remaining ½ tablespoon oil and return to medium heat. When the pan is hot, add the chops and cook until nicely browned on both sides and firm to the touch, about 6 minutes per side, turning once. Let the chops stand for a few minutes before serving to let the juices redistribute.

Cooks' Note

❖ You can substitute an apple for the pear.

casting out

A well-seasoned cast-iron skillet is one of the best pans to have around for everything from nicely seared meats to corn bread to biscuits cooked on an outdoor grill. To keep your skillet primed, after you use it always rinse the skillet out, wipe it, and then use kosher salt to scrub the pan with a paper towel. Rinse and wipe dry and add a thin film of oil.

Pan-Fried Steaks Chimichurri

Chimichurri sauce—a South American specialty—is a lively blend of fresh parsley and/or cilantro with garlic, oil, and hot pepper. Our version is tame but you can substitute cilantro for half of the parsley and increase the red pepper flakes. Serve with Super-Mash! (page 206) and a leafy green salad with tomatoes.

CHIMICHURRI SAUCE

4 garlic cloves, peeled and smashed

2 cups lightly packed flat-leaf parsley sprigs (thick stems discarded)

$\frac{2}{3}$ cup extra-virgin olive oil

2 tablespoons fresh lemon juice

2 tablespoons red wine vinegar

$1\frac{1}{4}$ teaspoons kosher salt

$\frac{1}{2}$ teaspoon crushed red pepper flakes

STEAKS

Four 6-ounce filet mignon steaks, about $\frac{3}{4}$ inch thick, or $1\frac{1}{2}$ pounds hanger steak, cut into 4 portions

Kosher salt

Freshly ground black pepper

1 tablespoon unsalted butter

PREP: 10 minutes
COOKING: 10 minutes
SPEED LIMIT: 20 mpr

**Makes 4 servings
(with extra sauce)**

PER SERVING:
460 calories, 33g fat
(8.5g saturated),
2g carbohydrates, .5g fiber,
38g protein

1. Place the garlic in a food processor and process until the garlic is chopped and sticks to the bowl. Add the parsley and process until finely chopped. In a bowl, combine the oil, lemon juice, vinegar, salt, and crushed red pepper flakes and, with the motor running, pour the mixture through the feed tube into the food processor; process until blended (the parsley will still appear chopped). You will have about 1 cup of sauce.

2. Heat a large cast-iron skillet over medium-high heat. Pat the steaks dry and season on both sides with salt and pepper. Add the butter to the skillet and, when it is melted, add the steaks. Cook until the steaks are nicely crusted underneath, about 5 minutes. Turn and cook 7 minutes more for medium doneness.

3. Transfer the steaks to plates and let stand for a few minutes before serving with some of the chimichurri sauce.

Cooks' Note

❖ Chimichurri sauce keeps well in the fridge for about a week. Transfer any remaining sauce to a jar, cover with a thin layer of oil, screw on the lid, and chill. You can use chimichurri on potatoes, eggs, grilled meat, and poultry.

Super Steak Fajitas

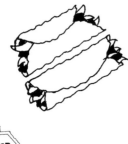

This dish incorporates a colorful mixture of vegetables and butter steak, which is a lean cut from the shoulder. We use reduced-fat thick Greek yogurt instead of sour cream. Even the littlest kids will have fun rolling their own tortillas.

PREP: 12 minutes
COOKING: 18 minutes
SPEED LIMIT: 30 mpr

Makes 4 servings

PER SERVING:
684 calories, 29g fat
(8g saturated),
58g carbohydrates, 5.5g fiber,
42g protein

Eight 7-inch whole-wheat or white flour tortillas
One 1¼-pound butter steak or skirt steak
Kosher salt
Freshly ground black pepper
2 tablespoons vegetable oil
2 medium onions, thinly sliced
1 orange or yellow bell pepper, trimmed, seeded, and sliced into
  ¼-inch-thick strips
3 garlic cloves, peeled, smashed, and chopped
2 teaspoons chili powder, preferably ancho
½ teaspoon dried oregano
2 medium tomatoes, cut into thin wedges or diced
¾ cup plain reduced-fat (2%) yogurt or sour cream

1. Preheat the oven to 300°F. Tear off a 14-inch sheet of foil; place the stack of tortillas on top and enclose in the foil. Place in the oven.

2. Meanwhile, place a 10-inch cast-iron skillet or grill pan over medium heat. Pat the steak dry with paper towels and cut into 2 pieces that will fit in the pan (they don't have to be the same size). Season the steak lightly on both sides with salt and pepper. Add 1 tablespoon of the oil to the skillet and swirl to coat. Add the steak and cook for 6 minutes. Turn and cook 5 minutes more for medium. Transfer the steak to a plate, let stand for 5 minutes, and then slice thinly against the grain.

3. Add the remaining tablespoon of oil to the pan with the onions, bell pepper, and garlic. Add the chili powder, oregano, and ¾ teaspoon salt and cook over medium heat, stirring often, until the vegetables are crisp-tender, 3 to 4 minutes. Add the tomatoes and cook until slightly softened, about 2 minutes. Add the sliced steak, stir to mix, and remove from the heat.

4. Remove the tortillas from the oven and transfer to a plate. Set the skillet on a board at the table and serve the steak mixture and yogurt for rolling up in the tortillas.

Brian L., age thirteen, from Rye, New York, gave this a "thumbs-up" and "really liked the meat and onions in this."

Quick Confetti Chili

Serve this speedy chili with your favorite accompaniments or with our Yankee Doodle Corn Bread (page 51) or Kiss-of-Honey Wheat Biscuits (page 54). This freezes well and, like many soups, stews, and sauces, tastes even better the next day.

2 pounds (85%) lean ground beef
2 tablespoons chili powder
2 teaspoons ground cumin
¼ teaspoon cayenne pepper
1 yellow or orange bell pepper, trimmed, seeded, and finely diced
6 scallions, thinly sliced
2 garlic cloves, peeled, smashed, and finely chopped
One 14.5-ounce can diced tomatoes
One 8-ounce can tomato sauce or 1 cup Quick Skillet Tomato Sauce
* (page 213)*
One 15-ounce can pinto beans, drained and rinsed

PREP: 5 minutes
COOKING: 25 minutes
SPEED LIMIT: 30 mpr

Makes 8 servings (about 1 cup each)

PER CUP:
*209 calories, 6g fat
(2g saturated),
14g carbohydrates,
5g fiber, 26g protein*

1. Heat a heavy 10-inch skillet over medium heat. Add the ground beef and cook, breaking the meat with a wooden spoon and turning occasionally until nicely browned, about 6 minutes. Add the chili powder, cumin, and cayenne and cook, stirring, 1 minute more.

2. Add the bell pepper, scallions, and garlic and cook over medium-low heat for 5 minutes. Stir in the diced tomatoes and tomato sauce and bring to a boil. Reduce the heat and simmer until thickened, about 8 minutes. Stir in the beans and cook, stirring, until heated through, about 5 minutes longer.

Quick Vegetarian Chili: Omit the ground beef in step 1. Heat 2 tablespoons vegetable oil in the skillet before adding the spices in step 1 and the vegetables in step 2. When you add the beans, stir in two 12-ounce packages of soy crumbles.

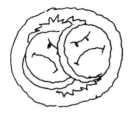

Crabby Cakes

PREP: 15 minutes plus
5 minutes chilling
COOKING: 8 minutes
SPEED LIMIT: 28 mpr

Makes two dozen small crab cakes to serve 6 to 8

PER 3 CRAB CAKES:
*338 calories, 18g fat
(2.5g saturated),
23g carbohydrates,
1g fiber, 19g protein*

Crab cakes are best with as much crabmeat as possible and not much else. These little cakes are easier to pan-fry if you chill them first, and the kids will love them as a main dish or a special appetizer. Serve with Tzatziki or store-bought tartar sauce.

1 pound lump crabmeat (see Cooks' Notes)
⅓ cup plus 2 cups Panko Japanese-style bread crumbs
¼ cup finely chopped celery, about ⅔ of a rib
½ teaspoon hot paprika
⅓ cup reduced-fat mayonnaise
½ teaspoon kosher salt
¼ teaspoon freshly ground black pepper
3 large eggs
¼ cup plus 2 tablespoons extra-virgin olive oil, for pan frying
Lemon wedges and Tzatziki sauce (page 220), for serving

1. Flake the crabmeat into a medium bowl. Add ⅓ cup of the bread crumbs, the celery, paprika, and mayonnaise and stir with a fork to mix.

2. Place the remaining 2 cups bread crumbs in a shallow bowl with the salt and pepper. Toss to mix. Spoon a rounded tablespoon of the crab mixture onto the bread crumbs. Sprinkle the crumbs on top and then flip to coat well and form into a patty, compressing lightly. Transfer to a small baking sheet or a plate. Repeat with the remaining crab and more of the crumbs. Reserve the remaining bread crumbs. Chill the cakes for 5 minutes in the freezer.

3. In a second shallow bowl, beat the eggs with a fork until blended. Turn each crab cake carefully in the eggs and then turn again in the crumbs and transfer to another plate. Repeat with the remaining crab cakes.

4. Heat 3 tablespoons of the oil in a 12-inch skillet over medium heat. Add half of the crab cakes and cook until golden underneath, 2 to 3 minutes. Turn and cook until golden and crisp on the other side. Repeat with the remaining oil and crab patties. Serve hot with lemon wedges and Tzatziki.

Cooks' Notes

❧ You can buy 1-pound cans of jumbo lump crab reasonably priced from a warehouse store. Bumble Bee also sells canned lump crab in 6-ounce cans.

❧ Panko Japanese-style bread crumbs are available in most supermarkets in either the bread section or Asian section. If you have plain dried bread crumbs on hand, you can use them as well.

Easy-Bake Scampi

The idea for this recipe came from our friend Renée Lucadamo from Mill-wood, New York. Serve the scampi with lemon wedges for squeezing.

4 tablespoons unsalted butter

3 garlic cloves, smashed, peeled, and minced

2 tablespoons extra-virgin olive oil

2 pounds thawed frozen peeled and deveined medium shrimp, tail shells removed

1¼ teaspoons kosher salt

½ teaspoon freshly ground black pepper

1 cup Panko Japanese-style bread crumbs or ¾ cup plain dried bread crumbs

½ teaspoon dried oregano

½ teaspoon dried thyme

1. Preheat the oven to 400°F.

2. Combine the butter and garlic in a small saucepan and cook over medium heat, stirring until melted. Stir in the oil.

3. Place the shrimp in a 2-quart baking dish, such as an 8-inch square or a shallow 12-inch oval casserole. Drizzle 2 tablespoons of the garlic butter on top and sprinkle with ¼ teaspoon each of salt and pepper. Toss the shrimp to coat and then spread evenly in the dish.

4. Place the bread crumbs in a small bowl. Add the remaining garlic butter, the remaining teaspoon of salt and ¼ teaspoon pepper, the oregano and thyme and stir to mix. Sprinkle the crumb mixture on top of the shrimp and bake for about 15 minutes, until the shrimp is pink and firm and the crumbs are golden brown. Serve hot.

PREP: 10 minutes

BAKING: 15 minutes

SPEED LIMIT: 25 mpr

Makes 6 servings

PER SERVING:

262 calories, 14g fat (6g saturated), 7g carbohydrates, .5g fiber, 25g protein

Sara H., age eight, of Rye, New York, says, "This shrimp is awe-some! I love the bread crumbs and I made it myself! Can I have it for lunch tomorrow, too?"

Shrimp Confetti Tostadas

For a special occasion serve the shrimp mixture in a clear bowl to show off the colorful mixture of shrimp, avocado, tomato, corn, and edamame.

PREP: 10 minutes
COOKING: 5 minutes
SPEED LIMIT: 15 mpr

Makes about 5 servings

PER SERVING (2 TOPPED
TOSTADAS):
190 calories,
11g fat (3g saturated),
12g carbohydrates,
2g fiber, 11g protein

TOPPING

1 pound thawed frozen peeled and deveined medium shrimp (36 per
  pound) tail shells removed and halved lengthwise
1 ripe Hass avocado
1 tablespoon fresh lime juice
2 ripe plum tomatoes, diced $\frac{1}{4}$ inch thick
1 cup thawed frozen white corn
1 cup thawed frozen shelled edamame (soybeans) or thawed petit peas
4 ounces queso fresco (Mexican cheese) or mild feta, crumbled (1 cup)
$\frac{1}{2}$ small head romaine, trimmed and thinly sliced crosswise

Ten 5-inch tostadas (crisp corn tortillas—see Cooks' Note)
About $\frac{3}{4}$ cup reduced-fat sour cream

VINAIGRETTE

1$\frac{1}{2}$ tablespoons distilled white vinegar
$\frac{1}{2}$ tablespoon finely chopped fresh mint
$\frac{1}{2}$ tablespoon fresh lime juice
$\frac{1}{2}$ teaspoon kosher salt
$\frac{1}{2}$ teaspoon sugar
$\frac{1}{4}$ teaspoon freshly ground black pepper
3 tablespoons extra-virgin olive oil

1. Bring 2 quarts of water to a boil in a medium saucepan. Stir in the shrimp and cook until they curl up and are just firm, 1 to 2 minutes. Drain in a colander, and then cover with 2 cups ice cubes to cool. (You can cook the shrimp 1 day ahead: Place in a bowl, cover, and chill overnight.)

2. Prepare the salad ingredients: Halve and pit the avocado, cut into $\frac{1}{2}$-inch dice, and transfer to a medium serving bowl. Add the lime juice and tomatoes and toss to mix. Add the shrimp, corn, edamame, queso fresco, and romaine in layers; do not toss.

3. Make the vinaigrette: Whisk together the vinegar, mint, lime juice, salt, sugar, and pepper. Gradually whisk in the oil. Drizzle the dressing on top of the lettuce, toss all of the ingredients well, and season to taste.

4. To serve, spread each tostada with about a tablespoon of sour cream, top with the shrimp mixture, and serve with napkins to be eaten out of hand.

Cooks' Note

❖ If you can't find crisp tostadas, you can use taco shells or, to bake your own tostadas, use ten 5-inch fresh corn tortillas: Preheat the oven to 450°F. Arrange 5 tortillas on a large baking sheet. Brush the tortillas lightly with corn oil, turn, and brush the other side. Bake for 6 to 8 minutes, until crisp and a shade darker; transfer the tortillas to a rack to cool; repeat with the remaining tortillas.

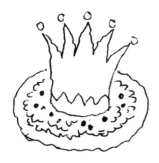

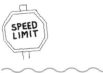

Princess and the Pea Risotto

This dish, reminiscent of the retro Chicken à la King, is a good way to enjoy leftover chicken or turkey. We use frozen shelled edamame (soybeans), which have a distinctive chewy texture and mild flavor.

Prep: 5 minutes
Cooking: 25 minutes
Speed Limit: 30 mpr

Makes 8 servings (about 10 cups)

Per 1¼-cup serving:
390 calories, 10g fat
(4.5g saturated),
52g carbohydrates,
3g fiber, 22g protein

5 cups low-sodium canned chicken broth
3 cups water
4 tablespoons (½ stick) unsalted butter
1 large onion, diced
1 pound Arborio (Italian short-grain) rice
½ cup white wine
2 medium carrots, peeled and finely chopped
1 cup thawed frozen shelled edamame or petit peas
2 cups coarsely chopped cooked chicken or turkey
⅓ cup finely grated Parmigiano-Reggiano
Salt and freshly ground black pepper
¼ cup chopped parsley (optional)

1. Heat the broth and water in a medium saucepan to just below a simmer; keep covered over very low heat.

2. Meanwhile, melt 2 tablespoons of the butter in a 6-quart pot over medium heat; add the onion and cook, stirring occasionally, until slightly softened, about 3 minutes. Add the rice and stir to coat with the butter. Stir in the wine and cook, stirring, until nearly evaporated.

3. Set a timer for 20 minutes. Stir in the carrots and ½ cup of hot broth and cook at a bare simmer, stirring almost constantly. As the broth is absorbed and the rice is slightly thicker, add ½ cup more broth. Continue stirring and slowly adding more broth in ½-cup increments until 20 minutes have passed. Taste the rice—if it is still firm, add more broth and cook 2 to 3 minutes more.

4. When the rice is al dente, stir in the edamame, chicken, and the remaining 2 tablespoons butter. Stir in the cheese and season to taste with salt and pepper. The mixture should be slightly soupy but thick enough to pile up on a spoon. If the risotto seems too thick, stir in ¼ cup more broth. Sprinkle the parsley on top, if using, and serve immediately.

Grilled Pint-Sized Pizzas

Joanne Killeen and George Germon, the owners of Al Forno restaurant in Providence, Rhode Island, started grilling pizza in the late 1980s. It is a fun way to enjoy homemade pizza even in hot weather, and the kids will love to help!

1 recipe Pizza Dough (page 65), prepared through rising
Extra-virgin olive oil
1½ cups warm tomato sauce
¾ pound part-skim mozzarella, shredded
½ cup fresh basil leaves

1. Brush the grill rack clean and then preheat the grill to medium-high.

2. Punch the dough down and cut into 8 pieces. (If you have a small kitchen scale, use it to check to see if they are about equal.) Place the pieces on a lightly greased baking sheet and cover with a towel.

3. Shape and grill the dough: Invert a second baking sheet and coat with 2 tablespoons of oil. Place a piece of dough on top, turn to coat in the oil, and then press and stretch out with your palms into an 8-inch free-form shape, about ¼ inch thick. Lift the dough and carefully lay on the hot grill. Cover and cook for 3 to 4 minutes, until the dough is crisp on the bottom and bubbly air pockets appear on the top. (You can cook several pizzas at once.)

4. Flip the dough with a spatula or tongs, quickly spoon on and spread about 2 tablespoons warm tomato sauce, and sprinkle a handful of cheese on top. Cover the grill and cook until the cheese is bubbly and the crust is golden underneath, about 3 minutes more.

5. Transfer the pizza to a board and top with some basil leaves. Cut into 4 wedges and serve. Repeat with olive oil as necessary and the remaining dough and toppings.

PREP: 15 minutes plus dough preparation
GRILLING: 10 minutes per pizza

Makes 8 personal pizzas

PER SERVING:
363 calories, 17g fat (7g saturated), 35g carbohydrates, 3g fiber, 14g protein

toppings for grilled pizza

You can add any of your favorite toppings—anything from broccoli and sausage to fresh salad greens. Because the pizza cooks quickly, have all of your tasty toppings hot and fully cooked before you begin grilling the dough. Keep them warm until you spoon them on top (which you do right after you add the cheese). Steam and season certain firmer vegetables, such as broccoli and asparagus, and lightly sauté softer vegetables, such as peppers and mushrooms, in a little olive oil before adding to the pizza.

grill tips for pizza

- Before beginning, be sure to brush grill racks clean. There is no need to grease them—there will be plenty of oil on the dough.
- Gas grills can vary. You want the pizza to cook quickly but not burn. Set the flame on your gas grill at medium to medium-high for best results.
- When using a kettle-style grill, after preparing coals and heating until they are ashen, carefully arrange hot coals in a ring, leaving an open circle in the center. Cook the pizzas in the center of the rack, covered, over indirect heat.

store-bought frozen dinner entrees

Here are some frozen dinners that are fairly healthy, whether they are organic, low in fat or calories, or vegetarian. For more suggestions, go to www.realfoodforhealthykids.com.

Kashi Black Bean Mango
Tandoori Pad Thai
Ethnic Gourmet Chicken Pad Thai
Amy's Pizza 3 Cheese, Cornmeal Crust Pizza, Whole-wheat Crust Pizza with Soy Cheese
Linda McCartney All-Natural Pizza Mushroom and Spinach
Health is Wealth Spring Rolls

Moosewood Organic Vegetarian Farfalle and Spinach Pesto Sauce
Ethnic Gourmet Vegetable Korma
Cedarlane Spinach and Feta Pie
Amy's Cheese Enchilada
Cedarlane Black Bean and Tofu Enchilada Meal
Franklin Farms Veggie Burgers
365 Degrees Whole Foods frozen line

double plays: two meals from one roast

We are nothing if not multitaskers. The recipes in this section feature oversized roasts—perfect to make on Sundays—followed by simple recipes that make the most of the leftovers on a following weeknight.

Perfectly Punctual Prime Rib

Roast Beef Hash

Chicken Hash or Turkey Hash

Juanita's Deep Dark Mole

Chicken Enchilada Casserole

Juicy Flank Steak

My Hero!

My Italian Hero

Grilled Wild Salmon

Sumo Salmon Cakes with Salad

Oven-Barbecued Beef

Mexican Beef Salad

Slow-Roasted Pork Shoulder

Pulled Pork

Mexican Tomatoes Rellenos

Good-as-Gold Roast Chicken

Sicilian Roast Chicken

Chicken Provençale

Chinese Roast Chicken

Chicken Fried Stuffing

241

Perfectly Punctual Prime Rib

Prime rib is something usually reserved for holidays and dining out, but a small roast can be cooked relatively quickly and easily, making any Sunday dinner special. You can use any extra meat in our yummy Roast Beef Hash (recipe follows).

PREP: 10 minutes
ROASTING: 1 hour and
20 minutes

**Makes 8 servings or 6
servings with leftovers**

PER SERVING (1 SLICE,
ABOUT 6 OUNCES
COOKED):
*409 calories, 32g fat
(13g saturated),
3g carbohydrates,
1g fiber, 25g protein*

1 tablespoon extra-virgin olive oil
2 large onions, thinly sliced
One 4½- to 5-pound boneless beef rib roast
1 teaspoon dried rosemary
1 teaspoon kosher salt
¼ teaspoon freshly ground black pepper
⅔ cup water

1. Preheat the oven to 450°F. Heat the oil in a medium skillet over medium heat. Add the onions and cook, stirring often, until softened, about 6 minutes. Transfer the onions to a flameproof roasting pan just big enough to hold the beef.

2. Place the roast on top of the onions. Insert an ovenproof meat thermometer horizontally into the center of the roast. Rub the beef all over with the rosemary, salt, and pepper and place in the oven for 20 minutes. Reduce the heat to 350°F and continue roasting 45 minutes to 1 hour longer, until the temperature reaches 135°F for medium. Transfer the roast to a board with grooves; cover loosely with foil and let stand for 10 minutes.

3. Meanwhile, add the water to the onions and juices in the pan, place over medium heat, and cook, stirring up any brown bits stuck to the surface of the pan, until hot. Season to taste with salt and pepper. Carve the beef with a sharp carving knife and serve with the onion gravy.

Roast Beef Hash

Serve this hash for breakfast, lunch, or dinner; it goes perfectly with eggs cooked any style. Serve it with hot sauce or Salsa Verde, if desired.

4 medium baking potatoes (1½ pounds)
2 tablespoons extra-virgin olive oil
1 medium onion, chopped
1 tablespoon unsalted butter
8 ounces leftover cooked prime rib or thinly sliced leftover cooked steak,
   cut into bite-sized pieces
Kosher salt and freshly ground black pepper

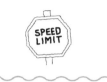

PREP: 5 minutes
COOKING: 20 minutes
SPEED LIMIT: 25 mpr

Makes 4 servings

PER SERVING:
334 calories, 16g fat
(5g saturated),
33g carbohydrates,
3g fiber, 15g protein

1. Peel the potatoes and cut into ¾-inch dice; place in a medium saucepan with cold salted water. Bring to a boil over high heat, reduce the heat, and simmer until the potatoes are almost tender, about 8 minutes. Drain the potatoes and coarsely chop.

2. Heat 1 tablespoon of the oil in a 10-inch cast-iron or other heavy skillet over medium heat. Add the onion and cook, stirring often, until golden, about 5 minutes. Add the butter and the remaining tablespoon of oil. When the butter is melted, stir in the potatoes until coated and then spread the mixture evenly in the skillet. Cook over medium-high heat for about 2 minutes, turn with a metal spatula, and cook, turning once or twice, until golden, about 4 minutes more.

3. Add the cut-up beef, season well with salt and pepper, and cook, turning occasionally, until the meat is heated through, about 1 minute more.

Chicken Hash or Turkey Hash: Substitute 1½ cups torn or chopped poultry for the beef.

Juanita's Deep Dark Mole

In Mexico, mole makes an appearance at special occasions. This version, particular to Oaxaca, has a deep, rich sauce that ranges from reddish brown to black with dried chiles, onion, nuts, seeds, and a bit of cinnamon and chocolate. Instead of browning the ingredients in oil as is traditional, our friend Juanita makes it better (and better for you) by roasting them in the oven—taking care not to burn them. Serve a piece of chicken with some of the sauce and a side of beans and brown rice or fresh corn tortillas. Use leftovers to make a Chicken Enchilada Casserole (recipe follows) later in the week.

PREP: About 2½ hours total

Makes 8 servings plus some leftovers

PER SERVING:
578 calories, 26g fat
(5g saturated),
28g carbohydrates,
5g fiber, 60g protein

2 chickens (3 to 3½ pounds each), quartered

3 quarts water

5 ancho chiles

3 guajillo chiles

1 pasilla chile

1 cup raw sesame seeds

¼ cup pumpkin seeds (pepitas)

¼ cup sliced almonds

1 medium onion

1 small garlic bulb, peeled; cloves separated

1 medium apple, such as Royal Gala or Golden Delicious, quartered and cored

1 medium tomato, quartered and cored

1 tablespoon extra-virgin olive oil or vegetable oil

5 whole cloves

¼ teaspoon dried oregano

1 small piece (about ½ inch) cinnamon stick (see Cooks' Note)

2 slices crusty whole-wheat bread (about 3 ounces)

2 teaspoons kosher salt

2 ounces bittersweet chocolate, chopped

1. Prepare the chicken and broth: Place the chicken pieces in a large 7- to 8-quart pot with all of the water. Bring to a boil, reduce the heat, and simmer, partially covered with the lid, until the chicken is just cooked through, about 40 minutes. Transfer the chicken pieces to a large bowl and when cool, remove and discard the skin. Strain the broth into a large bowl, let stand for 5 minutes, and then skim the fat from the surface. Wash out the pot.

2. Make the sauce: Preheat the oven to 350°F. Tear up the three kinds of dried chiles, discarding the seeds and stems, and place the pieces on a large bak-

ing sheet. Cook in the oven for 7 minutes, until lightly toasted, dried, and fragrant. Transfer the chile pieces to the blender and add 3 cups of the hot chicken broth; let soak for 20 minutes to soften.

3. Meanwhile, increase the oven temperature to 400°F. Spread the sesame seeds, pumpkin seeds, and almonds on the same baking sheet and bake for 7 to 8 minutes, until golden brown. Let cool.

4. Lay a large medium-mesh strainer over the same large pot. Blend the soaked chiles and broth at high speed for 2 minutes and then transfer to the strainer and force through and into the pot; discard the solids. Transfer the seeds and nuts mixture to the blender, add 2½ cups more broth, and blend for 2 minutes. Force through the strainer into the pot, discarding the solids.

5. Roast the vegetables and fruit for the sauce: Trim and quarter the onion. Separate the pieces into their natural layers and place on the baking sheet with the garlic, apple, and tomato. Drizzle on the oil, toss well, and spread the fruit and vegetables in an even layer on the baking sheet. Roast at 400°F for 30 minutes, until softened and browned on the edges.

6. Place the cloves, oregano, and cinnamon in a small skillet over medium heat and cook, stirring, until lightly colored and fragrant, about 2 minutes. Transfer the spices and the roasted vegetable mixture to the blender. Add 2 cups of broth and puree until smooth. Force through the strainer into the pot. Toast the bread until dark, but do not burn. Transfer to the blender with 2 more cups of the broth. Puree and strain into the sauce. (Save any remaining broth for another use.)

7. Place the pot over medium heat and bring to a boil, stirring often. Reduce the heat, stir in the salt and chocolate until melted, and simmer, stirring often, until the sauce is slightly reduced, about 15 minutes.

8. Cut the chicken pieces in half with a large knife and return to the pot. Let cook, simmering gently, until the chicken is hot, about 15 minutes.

Cooks' Note

❖ You can purchase a variety of dried chiles, cinnamon sticks, sesame seeds, and pumpkin seeds in Latin markets and at specialty stores or online from www.kalustyans.com.

Chicken Enchilada Casserole

For ease, we arrange the enchiladas in a baking dish for cooking all at once. But for a single serving, you can roll up one or two enchiladas and then place on a plate, sprinkle some cheese on top, and heat in the microwave.

> *Generous 2 cups shredded cooked chicken*
> *2 cups Juanita's Deep Dark Mole sauce (page 138)*
> *8 fresh corn tortillas*
> *1 cup (packed) shredded Cheddar or Monterey Jack cheese*
> *½ cup thinly sliced onions (optional)*
> *2 cups shredded lettuce*
> *½ cup sour cream, for serving*

1. Preheat the oven to 400°F. Combine the chicken and mole sauce in a bowl and stir well to mix. Lightly oil a 13- by 9-inch baking dish. Spread 1 cup of the chicken-mole mixture in the bottom of the pan.

2. Turn a burner on low heat. Place a tortilla on the low burner, cook for 30 seconds, turn with tongs, and cook 30 seconds more to heat through and soften. Transfer to a work surface. Spoon about ¼ cup of the chicken-mole mixture in a line in the center of the tortilla, roll up, and place in the pan. Repeat the process with the remaining tortillas.

3. Spoon the remaining chicken-mole mixture on top of the enchiladas and spread evenly. Sprinkle the cheese on top, cover loosely with foil, and bake for 25 to 30 minutes, until piping hot. Sprinkle the onions, if using, on top of the casserole. Transfer the enchiladas to plates with a metal spatula and garnish with the lettuce. Serve the sour cream on the side.

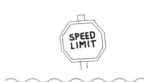

PREP: 15 minutes
BAKING: 30 minutes
SPEED LIMIT: 45 mpr

Makes 6 servings

PER ENCHILADA:
383 calories, 16g fat
(7g saturated),
30g carbohydrates,
3g fiber, 31g protein

Juicy Flank Steak

This kid-friendly, mouthwatering meat recipe only requires a few condiments and quick cooking on the grill or under the broiler. Use leftovers in My Hero! (page 142).

1/3 cup maple syrup
1/4 cup safflower oil or mild olive oil
1/4 cup soy sauce or tamari sauce
2 flank steaks (1 1/2 pounds each)
Kosher salt and freshly ground black pepper

1. Combine the maple syrup, oil, and soy sauce in a large bowl. Add the steaks and turn to coat. Cover and chill, turning the meat occasionally, for 30 minutes or overnight.

2. Prepare the grill or preheat the broiler. Season the steak lightly with salt and pepper and place on the grill. Cook, covered, for about 6 minutes, rotating the steaks once. Turn and cook until nicely charred, about 6 minutes more for medium doneness. Transfer the steaks to a board and let stand for 5 minutes before thinly slicing on the diagonal.

SPEED LIMIT

PREP: 5 minutes plus marinating
GRILLING: 12 minutes

Makes 10 servings

PER SERVING (4 OUNCES COOKED STEAK):
262 calories, 10g fat (4g saturated), 2g carbohydrates, 0g fiber, 38g protein

My Hero!

These are reminiscent of Philly cheese steaks, but they are made with lean flank steak, tossed with tender well-cooked onions and topped with reduced-fat Cheddar.

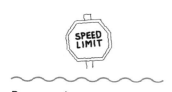

PREP: 5 minutes
COOKING: 15 minutes
SPEED LIMIT: 20 mpr

Makes 4 servings

PER SANDWICH:
*585 calories, 25g fat
(11g saturated),
41g carbohydrates,
3g fiber, 46g protein*

1 tablespoon extra-virgin olive oil
2 medium onions, thinly sliced
1 garlic clove, smashed, peeled, and minced
1 cup canned low-sodium beef broth
Kosher salt and freshly ground black pepper
1 pound chilled cooked flank steak, thinly sliced (3 cups packed)
*1 cup (packed) shredded sharp reduced-fat white Cheddar cheese
   (4 ounces)*
4 hoagie rolls or Kaiser rolls (about 3 ounces each), split

1. Heat the oil in a large skillet over medium heat. Add the onions and garlic and cook, stirring often, until softened, about 8 minutes. Pour in the broth and continue cooking until the onions are tender and the broth has evaporated, about 4 minutes. Season to taste with salt and pepper. Transfer the onion mixture to a serving bowl and keep warm.

2. Place the same skillet over medium-high heat. Add the cold steak, season lightly with salt and pepper, and cook, stirring, just until heated through, about 3 minutes. Sprinkle the cheese on top of the meat and remove from the heat. Fill the rolls with the meat and cheese and top with the onions.

My Italian Hero: Substitute mozzarella for the Cheddar and add a green bell pepper to the onions when cooking. Serve with warmed Quick Skillet Tomato Sauce (page 213) or another marinara sauce.

Grilled Wild Salmon

Look for boneless wild salmon fillets (not steaks), about 1 inch thick, which are rich in omega 3s. Avoid farm-raised salmon, which are given antibiotics, fed pellets that aid their coloring, and may contain cancer-causing PCBs and other toxins. Crispy Grilled Spudniks (page 197) and Edamame Succotash Salad (page 82) are perfect accompaniments for this simple, sumptuous dish. There's enough salmon for leftovers to make Sumo Salmon Cakes with Salad (recipe follows), another fast dinner.

Vegetable oil, for greasing the grill
6 skin-on salmon fillets (6 ounces each)
Kosher salt and freshly ground black pepper
Lemon wedges, for serving

1. Prepare a charcoal grill or preheat a gas grill at medium flame. Brush the hot racks to clean them and lightly grease with vegetable oil.

2. Remove any stray bones from the salmon with tweezers or needle-nose pliers. Season the salmon on both sides with salt and pepper. Add the fillets skin side down on the hot grill (cover only if using a gas grill), and cook for 4 minutes. Turn and cook on the other side until the fish is just opaque in the center, 3 to 4 minutes. Remove the skin if desired before serving with lemon wedges.

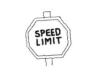

PREP: 2 minutes
GRILLING: 8 minutes
SPEED LIMIT: 10 mpr

Makes 6 servings or 4 servings with leftovers

PER 6-OUNCE FILLET:
307 calories, 15g fat (2.5g saturated), 0g carbohydrates, 0g fiber, 38g protein

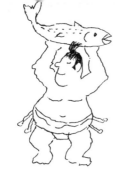

Sumo Salmon Cakes with Salad

Japanese pickled ginger and soothing avocado enhance moist and crispy salmon cakes served with baby greens.

PREP: 15 minutes
plus chilling
COOKING: 5 minutes

Makes 4 servings

PER SERVING:
534 calories, 33g fat
(5g saturated),
30g carbohydrates,
5.5g fiber, 30g protein

CAKES

    12 ounces grilled salmon fillet, skinned and flaked (2 cups)
    1/4 cup plus 1 cup plain dried bread crumbs, preferably Panko Japanese-style bread crumbs
    1 small Kirby cucumber, peeled, seeded, and finely diced
    2 1/2 tablespoons mayonnaise
    1 tablespoon minced fresh chives or flat-leaf parsley
    1 large egg
    Kosher salt and freshly ground black pepper
    3 tablespoons extra-virgin olive oil

SALAD AND GARNISHES

    4 cups lightly packed baby salad greens
    1 tablespoon extra-virgin olive oil
    1/2 tablespoon rice wine vinegar
    Kosher salt and freshly ground black pepper
    1 ripe Hass avocado, peeled, pitted, and thinly sliced
    Pickled sliced ginger, drained, for garnish (optional)

1. Prepare the salmon cakes: Combine the salmon, 1/4 cup of the bread crumbs, the cucumber, mayonnaise, and chives, and stir with a fork to mix well. Chill for 30 minutes to soften the crumbs.

2. Beat the egg in a shallow bowl. Place the remaining cup of bread crumbs, 1/2 teaspoon salt, and 1/4 teaspoon pepper in a second bowl and toss to mix. Form the salmon mixture into 4 patties. Coat each in the bread crumbs, then the egg, and again in the bread crumbs and place on a plate.

3. Heat the oil in a cast-iron skillet over medium heat. Add the salmon cakes and cook until golden underneath, about 3 minutes. Turn and cook until golden on the other side, about 2 minutes more.

4. While the cakes are browning, combine the greens, oil, and vinegar in a salad bowl, season to taste, and toss well. Arrange a pile of greens on each of 4 plates. Divide the avocado slices among the mounds, season lightly with salt and pepper, place a salmon cake on top, and garnish each serving with some pickled ginger, if using.

Big kid Nathan S., who goes to college in San Diego, claimed he hated salmon, but then when cajoled into tasting these, was shocked: "This is, most definitely, the best fish item I've ever eaten."

Oven-Barbecued Beef

Here is a simple way to enjoy a summer favorite all year long. It's a dish that requires almost no attention yet gives great results. Serve the beef with Thick 'n' Spicy Barbecue Sauce (page 211) and typical barbecue fare, such as Cowboy Beans (page 204) and Rainbow Slaw (page 205).

2 tablespoons ancho chili powder
1 tablespoon kosher salt
1 tablespoon sugar
1 tablespoon hot paprika
½ teaspoon freshly ground black pepper
5 pounds lean beef chuck, cut into 2-inch pieces
¼ cup distilled white vinegar
Thick 'n' Spicy Barbecue Sauce or other barbecue sauce, for serving

1. Preheat the oven to 375°F. Combine the chili powder, salt, sugar, paprika, and pepper in a small bowl.

2. Line a shallow baking sheet with heavy-duty aluminum foil and evenly spread the beef on top. Sprinkle the spice mixture over the beef, stir to distribute, and cover the pan snugly with a second sheet of foil. Bake for 2 hours, until the meat is lightly browned.

3. Uncover the meat and turn the pieces over with tongs. Drizzle the vinegar on top. Return the pan to the oven and bake, uncovered, for 1 hour longer, until the meat is tender enough to flake with a fork. Let cool, covered loosely with foil.

4. Working on the baking sheet, shred the meat, and toss with the pan juices. Transfer the meat to a pot, add the barbecue sauce, and stir often over medium heat until the meat is hot.

PREP: 10 minutes
ROASTING: About 3 hours

Makes about 10 cups shredded beef; serves 6 with leftovers

PER CUP (NOT SAUCED):
294 calories, 8g fat (3g saturated), 2g carbohydrates, 1g fiber, 51g protein

Mexican Beef Salad

This light satisfying dish comes from Mexico City via Veracruz via New Jersey from Tracey's babysitter (who is from Oaxaca). Serve the salad with warmed soft corn tortillas, flour tortillas, or unsalted tortilla chips.

PREP: 10 minutes
SPEED LIMIT: 10 mpr

Makes 4 servings

PER SERVING:
437 calories, 30g fat
(10g saturated),
15g carbohydrates,
8g fiber, 29g protein

3 cups cold shredded Oven-Barbecued Beef (page 145); or any shredded well-cooked beef (without sauce)
2 tablespoons red wine vinegar
1 tablespoon balsamic vinegar
1 tablespoon extra-virgin olive oil
1 small head romaine, thinly sliced (4 cups)
2 ripe medium tomatoes, sliced
2 ripe Hass avocados, pitted and sliced
Kosher salt
Freshly ground black pepper
1¼ cups crumbled queso fresco (fresh Mexican cheese) or mild goat cheese, crumbled

1. Chop the beef and place in a microwavable bowl. Cook at hgih (100%) power for 1½ minutes to take the chill off. (Skip this step if your meat is at room temperature.) Stir in the red wine, balsamic vinegar, and oil. Add the lettuce and toss well.

2. Arrange the tomatoes on a round or oval platter. Arrange the avocado slices on top and then season with a pinch of salt and pepper. Season the meat and lettuce mixture with more salt and pepper and mound on top of the avocado. Sprinkle the crumbled cheese on top.

Slow-Roasted Pork Shoulder

Leftovers can be used to make Mexican Tomatoes Rellenos (recipe follows) or Mini-Cuban Sandos (page 92). To make it into Pulled Pork, see the variation. Serve the tender pork with Grasshopper Potato Salad (page 195).

One 8¼-pound pork picnic shoulder (with bone)
2 teaspoons kosher salt
1½ teaspoons dried oregano, crumbled
1 teaspoon Mexican-style hot chili powder
¼ teaspoon freshly ground black pepper
1½ cups canned low-sodium chicken broth
½ cup water
3 tablespoons distilled white vinegar
Kosher salt and freshly ground black pepper

PREP: 5 minutes
plus standing
ROASTING: Long and slow!

Serves 8 with leftovers

PER SERVING (4 OUNCES):
*141 calories, 6g fat
(2g saturated),
0g carbohydrates,
0g fiber, 20g protein*

1. Cut off any tough skin from the pork, but do not trim any fat. Place the pork in a roasting pan. In a small bowl, combine the salt, oregano, chili powder, and pepper; rub the seasoning mixture all over the pork, turn the roast fat side up in the pan, and let stand at room temperature for 1 hour before cooking.

2. Preheat the oven to 325°F. Insert an ovenproof meat thermometer in the thickest part of the pork, inserting it into the meat as far as possible. Roast the pork for 4 to 4½ hours, until the internal temperature reaches 170°F on the thermometer.

3. Transfer the pork to a cutting board with grooves and let stand. Pour the pan juices into a glass measuring cup and skim off the fat. Return the juices to the roasting pan, add the broth, water, and vinegar and bring to a boil over medium heat; deglaze the pan, scraping up any brown bits with a wooden spoon. Season the juices to taste with salt and pepper and reserve.

4. Slice the pork thinly across the grain, working around the bones as best you can and serve with the juices.

Pulled Pork: Wait until the pork is completely cool, then cut the meat from the bone in chunks. Discard the fat and pull the meat into shreds. Stir any remaining pan juices into the pulled pork and chill or freeze until ready to reheat and serve with your favorite barbecue sauce.

Clayton Z., seven years old, from Port Chester, New York, thought this the ultimate comfort food. "It tastes rich and good to us kids, and my parents loved it, too."

Mexican Tomatoes Rellenos

Red, ripe, late-summer tomatoes are heaven as it is, but wait until everyone tries this inspired dish that uses leftover pork. If your tomatoes are in top form, you can spoon the warm pork mixture in and serve them straight away. Less than perfect tomatoes can be warmed in the oven. Serve the tomatoes with steamed brown rice or toasted slices of crusty whole-wheat bread. If you are counting calories, forgo the additional slice of cheese on top.

PREP: 10 minutes
COOKING: 13 minutes
SPEED LIMIT: 23 mpr

Makes 6 servings

PER STUFFED TOMATO:
293 calories, 16g fat
(7g saturated),
10g carbohydrates,
2g fiber, 26g protein

2 poblano chiles or Anaheim chiles
1 tablespoon safflower oil or mild olive oil
1 medium onion, finely chopped
2 garlic cloves, smashed, peeled, and minced
6 large ripe tomatoes
3 cups finely diced Slow-Roasted Pork Shoulder (page 147)
5 ounces (1 1/4 cups packed) Monterey Jack cheese, shredded
Kosher salt and freshly ground black pepper

1. Roast the chiles on the open flame of a gas burner, on a gas grill, or under the broiler, turning often, until charred all over. Transfer the chiles to a heatproof bowl, cover snugly with plastic wrap, and let cool. When cool, rub the skins off the chiles, remove the stem and seeds, and discard. Finely dice the chile and place in a bowl.

2. Heat the oil in a nonstick large skillet over medium heat. Add the onion and garlic and cook, stirring often, until soft, about 6 minutes.

3. While the onion is cooking, prepare the tomatoes: Cut the top quarter off of each tomato. Remove the seeds with your finger and discard. Carefully scoop out the inner flesh with a spoon and then coarsely chop enough of the tomato flesh to get 1 cup; stir into the chile.

4. When the onion is soft, add the pork and chile-tomato mixture, and cook, stirring, until hot, about 5 minutes. Add 3/4 cup cheese and cook until melted. Season the mixture with salt and pepper.

5. Divide the pork mixture and remaining 1/2 cup cheese among the hollowed-out tomatoes. You can bake the tomatoes in a 350° oven for 15 minutes if desired.

Good-as-Gold Roast Chicken

Golden crispy, succulent chicken with homemade gravy is the ultimate American meal, and if you follow our foolproof recipe, you will be worshiped by the recipients, plus you will reap the benefits of an easy future meal or two by using the meat in our Chicken Fried Stuffing (recipe follows) on a simple hot or cold sandwich on one of our sensational breads, or tossed in a Hail Caesar, Jr. (page 119).

CHICKEN

One 7-pound roasting chicken, rinsed inside and out and patted dry
Kosher salt and freshly ground black pepper
2 tablespoons extra-virgin olive oil
1 lemon, halved
½ teaspoon dried thyme
2 small onions, ends trimmed and quartered with the peels left on

PAN GRAVY

2 cups water
One 14-ounce can low-sodium chicken broth
½ cup unbleached all-purpose flour
Kosher salt and freshly ground black pepper

PREP: 10 minutes
ROASTING: 1¾ hours

Makes 8 servings

PER SERVING (4 OUNCES LIGHT AND DARK MEAT):
658 calories, 49g fat (13g saturated), 2.5g carbohydrates, .5g fiber, 49g protein

PER 2 TABLESPOONS GRAVY:
12 calories, 0g fat (0g saturated), 2g carbohydrates, 0g fiber, .5g protein

1. Arrange a rack in the lower third of the oven and preheat the oven to 400°F.

2. Place the chicken in a 13- by 9-inch roasting pan. Sprinkle ¼ teaspoon kosher salt inside the cavity and brush the top and sides of the bird with the oil. Squeeze the lemon halves over the top of the chicken and place the halves in the cavity. Season the bird with ¼ teaspoon salt, thyme, and a few grindings of pepper. If using an ovenproof meat thermometer, insert it now deep into the thigh just below the drumstick, parallel with the thighbone but being careful not to touch the bone. Arrange the onion pieces skin side up in the pan around the bird.

3. Roast the chicken for 1¼ hours, then pour 1 cup of water in the pan. Continue roasting for about 30 minutes, basting the bird with the pan juices after every 15 minutes, until the internal temperature of the chicken reaches 160°F.

4. Transfer the chicken to a platter, cover loosely with foil, and let stand for 10 minutes. (The chicken will continue to cook as it stands.)

5. Meanwhile, discard the peels from the onion pieces, pour the broth into the roasting pan, place over medium-high heat, and bring to a boil, scraping off

the onions and any browned bits from the bottom of the pan. In a cup, gradually mix together the flour and the remaining cup of water with a fork. Whisk into the hot broth in the pan. Cook, whisking constantly, until thickened, about 3 minutes. Season to taste with salt and pepper.

6. Carve the chicken with a sharp carving knife: Cut off the wings and transfer to a platter. Cut along the inside of each leg to release the legs but don't remove. Starting at the top of the bird, cut into the center of the breast and then down along the breastbone on one side, cutting close to the rib cage to remove one breast half. Transfer the breast meat to a board and cut crosswise into slices. Arrange on the platter and repeat on the other side. Cut off the leg quarters and cut each leg section through the joint to separate the drumstick and thigh. Serve with the gravy.

Sicilian Roast Chicken: Finely grate the zest from 1 lemon and 1 orange (quarter the fruit and reserve). Place the zest in a cup with a teaspoon of ground ginger and stir in 1 tablespoon extra-virgin olive oil. Place the cleaned chicken in the roasting pan and rub the zest mixture all over the inside of the cavity. Squeeze the quartered lemon and orange over the same small bowl (and place the quarters in the cavity). Into the juice, whisk 2 tablespoons honey, 1 tablespoon olive oil, and 1 teaspoon ground ginger. Brush all over the chicken and season the chicken with salt and pepper. Roast and baste as directed, omitting the gravy.

Chicken Provençale: Season and roast the chicken as directed and transfer to a board. Pour the pan juices and peel an onion into a cup, skim and discard the fat, and reserve the juices. Add 2 garlic cloves (minced) to the roasting pan, place over medium heat, and cook, stirring for 1 minute. Return the pan juices to the pan, add the broth, and deglaze, and add the water and flour and cook as directed. Stir in 2 ripe plum tomatoes (finely diced) and 1/4 cup rinsed niçoise olives. Cook, stirring, for 1 minute, season to taste, and then stir in 1/4 cup chopped fresh basil.

Tracey's daughter, Margot, thirteen, called her from summer camp. When asked how the food was, Margot said, "Mommy, I really miss your spaghetti and your juicy chicken."

Chinese Roast Chicken: Omit the seasonings above and, before roasting, marinate the chicken for at least 30 minutes (or overnight) in the following: 4 garlic cloves (smashed), one 2-inch piece fresh ginger (peeled and finely chopped), 1/3 cup vegetable oil, 1/4 cup *each* soy sauce and honey, 2 tablespoons rice vinegar, and 1 teaspoon Chinese five-spice powder. Whisk all of the ingredients together in a large bowl and rub the chicken all over with the marinade. Cover with plastic wrap and chill until ready to cook. Roast and baste as directed but omit the gravy. Serve with the pan juices.

chicken little

No time for a big bird? Roast a 3- to 4-pound chicken the same way, but reduce the cooking time to about an hour or so. Use visual timing (insert the point of a small knife deep into the thigh—the juices will run clear if the bird is done) or use an ovenproof or an instant-read thermometer and look for an internal temperature of 160°F to ensure perfectly cooked, juicy chicken.

Chicken Fried Stuffing

Even though you are using leftover cooked chicken, these fun and tasty patties are a real treat (after Thanksgiving you can make them with turkey instead of chicken). For those who have vegetarians in the house, you can substitute diced tofu and vegetable broth for the chicken and chicken broth. Serve this with a green vegetable and a sauce like our Rockin' Ranch Dressing.

PREP: 10 minutes
COOKING: 12 minutes
SPEED LIMIT: 22 mpr

Makes 8 servings

PER 1-PATTY SERVING:
232 calories, 10g fat
(4g saturated),
22g carbohydrates,
3g fiber, 13g protein

3 tablespoons unsalted butter
1 large celery rib, finely chopped
1 bunch scallions, trimmed and finely chopped
3 (loosely packed) cups torn whole-wheat sandwich bread (about 6 ounces)
2 cups chopped cooked chicken (8 ounces)
1 small apple, peeled, cored, and finely diced
⅔ cup pitted prunes, chopped (optional)
1 large egg
½ cup canned low-sodium chicken broth
½ teaspoon kosher salt
½ teaspoon dried thyme
¼ teaspoon freshly ground black pepper
2 tablespoons extra-virgin olive oil
Lemon wedges or Rockin' Ranch Dressing (page 219), for serving

1. Melt 1 tablespoon of the butter in a small skillet over medium heat. Add the celery and scallions and cook, stirring until softened, about 4 minutes. Transfer to a large bowl, add the bread, chicken, apple, and prunes, if using, and stir to blend. Add the egg, broth, salt, thyme, and pepper and mix very well until thoroughly mixed. Take a handful of the mixture and form into a ½-inch-thick patty and place on a plate lined with waxed paper. Repeat with the remaining mixture to form 7 more patties.

2. Melt the remaining 2 tablespoons butter in the olive oil in a 12-inch skillet over medium heat, add the patties, and cook until golden underneath, about 4 minutes. Flip with a spatula and cook 4 minutes more. Serve with lemon wedges or dressing.

one-dish dinners: stews, casseroles, and souper meals

These one-pot dishes are all extremely satisfying. Just add a crisp green salad when serving. Two other great things about these dinners: There's less cleanup and these dishes taste even better the day after they are prepared, so you can enjoy leftovers—if there are any.

Country French Chicken Stew with Green Olives

Simply Saucy Beef Stew

Summertime Grilled Vegetable Lasagna

Nan's Shepherd's Pie

Sultan's Chicken-Couscous Bake

Lazy Lasagna

Get-Well-Soon Soup

Chicken Noodle Soup

Chicken Matzo Ball Soup

Asian Coconut–Chicken Noodle Soup

Bangers and Beans Quickie Soup

Mellow Yellow Split Pea Soup

Mellow Yellow Split Pea Soup with Ham

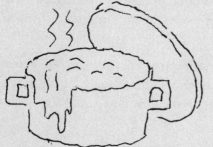

Country French Chicken Stew with Green Olives

This rustic stew features tender boneless chicken thighs in a velvety broth. Blanching the olives removes their saltiness and lets their subtle flavor come through. (Many varieties of green olives are sold pitted.) Serve with whole-wheat toast, noodles, or your favorite mash (pages 206–209).

PREP: 10 minutes
COOKING: 60 minutes

Makes 4 servings

PER SERVING:
482 calories, 27g fat
(5g saturated),
21g carbohydrates,
4g fiber, 35g protein

1 cup (about ¼ pound) green olives (preferably picholine), pitted and rinsed
1½ pounds boneless skinless chicken thighs
¼ teaspoon kosher salt
¼ teaspoon freshly ground black pepper
3 tablespoons unbleached all-purpose flour
2 tablespoons extra-virgin olive oil
2 medium onions, coarsely chopped
⅓ cup dry white wine or additional chicken broth
1 cup low-sodium canned chicken broth
½ cup filtered water
1 ripe medium tomato, finely diced

1. Bring about 2 cups of water to a boil in a small saucepan. Add the olives and simmer for 2 minutes; drain, rinse well with cold water, and repeat with fresh boiling water.

2. Meanwhile, place the chicken pieces in a large bowl, season with the salt and pepper, and sprinkle 2 tablespoons of the flour on top; toss well.

3. Heat the oil in a wide deep skillet or a 6-quart pot over medium heat. Add the chicken and cook until golden on both sides, about 8 minutes, turning once. Transfer the chicken to a plate.

4. Add the onions to the pan and cook, stirring often, until golden, about 6 minutes. Stir in the remaining tablespoon of flour and cook for 1 minute. Pour in the wine and stir until evaporated, about 2 minutes. Add the broth, water, and olives and bring to a boil.

5. Return the chicken pieces and any juices to the pan; reduce the heat, place the cover askew, and simmer gently until the chicken is tender and the sauce is thickened, about 40 minutes. Stir in the tomato, season to taste, and serve.

Two-year-old Zane S., of Amagansett, New York, says, "I like it. Me like it!"

Simply Saucy Beef Stew

Many kids dislike soft vegetables, the kind usually found in stew. This rendition is made without carrots or potatoes so you can serve it—with its thick, rich gravy—over your choice of perfectly cooked vegetables. Try adding a mash (pages 206–209), boiled spring potatoes, or Perfect Rice (page 196) and Blasted Winter Vegetables (page 199) or your favorite veg.

1/4 cup extra-virgin olive oil
5 pounds lean beef chuck, cut into 1- to 2-inch cubes
Kosher salt and freshly ground black pepper
3 extra-large onions, finely diced
5 garlic cloves, smashed and peeled
1/2 cup unbleached all-purpose flour
1 cup dry red or white wine
1 quart low-sodium beef broth
2 cups filtered water
1 tablespoon tomato paste
2 sprigs each fresh rosemary and thyme or 1 teaspoon each dried

PREP: 10 minutes
COOKING: About 2 1/2 hours

Makes 3 quarts

PER CUP:
286 calories, 15g fat
(4g saturated),
8.5g carbohydrates,
1g fiber, 25g protein

1. Heat 1 tablespoon of the oil in a 6- to 8-quart heavy Dutch oven over medium heat. Add a third of the beef, season lightly with salt and pepper, and cook, turning infrequently, until browned, about 8 minutes. Transfer to a plate and repeat with oil and the remaining beef and more salt in two batches.

2. Add the last tablespoon of oil, the onions, and garlic to the pot, and cook, stirring occasionally, until softened, about 6 minutes. Sprinkle the flour on top and cook, stirring constantly until thick and lightly browned, about 2 minutes. Whisk in the wine and bring to a boil, stirring, and then whisk in the broth, water, and tomato paste. Return the meat to the pot, add the rosemary and thyme, and bring to a boil, stirring occasionally. Reduce the heat to low, cover, and simmer gently, stirring occasionally, for 1 1/2 hours. Uncover the pot and continue simmering for up to 30 minutes more, until the meat is nicely tender but still holds its shape. Remove the sprigs and season to taste before serving.

Cooks' Note

❖ Buy concentrated tomato paste in tubes, which keeps well in the fridge after opening. This stew freezes well for up to six months.

Thirteen-year-old Margot, Tracey's daughter, said, "This is the only stew I really like because it doesn't have any mushy vegetables. I like my carrots crisp."

Summertime Grilled Vegetable Lasagna

This dish involves a few steps, but a lot of the work is done on the grill so there isn't too much mess. Prepare the Grilled Tomato Sauce first, and then soak the noodles and grill the vegetables.

PREP: 35 minutes
BAKING: 1 hour and
20 minutes

Makes 8 servings

PER SERVING:
*480 calories, 25g fat
(8g saturated),
42g carbohydrates,
6g fiber, 23g protein*

12 no-boil lasagna noodles
3 small eggplant (about 1¼ pounds total)
5 tablespoons extra-virgin olive oil
Kosher salt and freshly ground black pepper
3 medium zucchini (1½ pounds)
1 extra-large onion, sliced ¼ inch thick
One 15-ounce container reduced-fat ricotta cheese
2 large eggs
¼ cup finely grated Parmigiano-Reggiano
Grilled Tomato Sauce (page 212) or 1 quart jarred marinara sauce
½ pound mozzarella, preferably fresh, thinly sliced
½ cup lightly packed fresh basil leaves

1. Prepare a charcoal grill or preheat a gas grill at medium flame. Place the lasagna noodles in a large bowl of very hot water and let stand; turn the noodles occasionally while you prepare the fillings.

2. Trim the eggplant and slice lengthwise ⅛ to ¼ inch thick, discarding the first and last slices (with a lot of peel). Brush the slices lightly with about 3 tablespoons olive oil, season lightly with salt and pepper, and grill, covered, turning once or twice with tongs until lightly charred and tender, about 5 minutes.

3. Trim the zucchini and slice diagonally into ¼-inch-thick slices. Toss in a large bowl with another tablespoon of oil and ¼ teaspoon each of salt and pepper. Brush the onion with the remaining tablespoon of oil and grill the zucchini and onion until lightly charred and tender, about 5 minutes, turning occasionally.

4. Combine the ricotta, eggs, Parmesan, and ¼ teaspoon each of salt and pepper in a bowl and whisk until smooth.

5. Preheat the oven to 400°F. Lightly oil a 13- by 9-inch square glass baking dish. Add ½ cup of tomato sauce to the pan and tilt to coat. Place 3 noodles on top of the sauce, spacing evenly, and spoon on half of the ricotta, half of

the onion, and half of the eggplant. Add another ½ cup of sauce and 3 more noodles. Arrange all of the zucchini on top, spoon on ½ cup sauce, and add half of the mozzarella. Place 3 more noodles on top and spoon on the remaining ricotta, onion, and eggplant. Add ½ cup more sauce and arrange the remaining 3 noodles on top. Spoon on the remaining tomato sauce, cover snugly with foil, and bake for 1 hour.

6. Uncover the lasagna, arrange the basil leaves on top, and sprinkle on the remaining mozzarella; bake uncovered for about 20 minutes more, until golden on top. Let stand for 15 minutes before cutting and serving.

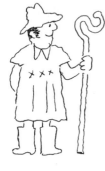

Nan's Shepherd's Pie

PREP: 35 minutes
BAKING: 10 minutes
SPEED LIMIT: 45 mpr

Makes 8 servings

PER SERVING:
414 calories, 17g fat
(7g saturated),
37g carbohydrates,
4g fiber, 30g protein

We've perfected Tanya's English grandmother's version of a succulent main-stay. Leftovers can be reheated in the microwave, and you can even prepare the casserole a day ahead and pop it in the oven for a stress-free weekend dinner with friends.

4 large russet potatoes (2½ pounds)
2 pounds (85%) lean ground sirloin
3 tablespoons extra-virgin olive oil
2 medium onions, chopped
1 large garlic clove, smashed, peeled, and finely chopped
One 15-ounce can tomato puree
¼ teaspoon cayenne pepper
1½ cups frozen petit peas (half of 1-pound bag), thawed
¾ cup half-and-half
1 teaspoon kosher salt
Freshly ground black pepper
*1 cup (packed) shredded reduced-fat extra-sharp Cheddar cheese
   (4 ounces)*

1. Peel the potatoes, cut in half lengthwise, and thinly slice; place in a large saucepan with cold water to cover by 1 inch. Bring to a boil over high heat, reduce the heat, and simmer until tender, about 10 minutes.

2. Right after you put the potatoes on to cook, begin the filling: Cook the ground beef in a 12-inch skillet over medium-high heat, breaking up the meat with a wooden spoon and turning frequently until the meat is nicely browned, about 7 minutes. Transfer the beef to a plate. Preheat the oven to 500°F.

3. Add 2 tablespoons of the oil to the same skillet. Add the onions and garlic and cook over medium heat, stirring often, until golden and tender, about 6 minutes. Return the browned meat to the pan and stir in the tomato puree and cayenne. Bring to a simmer and cook, stirring occasionally, until the mixture is thickened, about 10 minutes. Stir in the peas and cover to keep warm.

4. Drain the cooked potatoes well and return them to the pot. Mash well with a potato masher, and stir in the half-and-half and salt and pepper to taste. Spoon the warm meat mixture into a 2½- to 3-quart baking dish and

sprinkle the Cheddar on top. Spoon the potatoes on top of the cheese, spreading them over the meat, leaving a scant 1-inch border around the edge.

6. Drizzle the remaining tablespoon of olive oil over the top and bake until the potatoes are golden, about 10 minutes. Let cool for 5 minutes before serving.

"When my mom makes this, she always tells me about her grandma in England, and she gets happy," says Tanya's eight-year-old son William. "I get happy because I like how the potatoes are on top of the yummy meat."

Sultan's Chicken-Couscous Bake

This oven dish is inspired by the cuisine of Morocco. Brown boneless chicken breasts, nestle them in couscous, then cover and bake—the results are amazing, even as leftovers the next day. Buy whole pitted dates and chop them—they will be softer than packaged chopped dates—and look for unsulfured dried apricots; they are darker in color but have better flavor when cooked.

PREP: 10 minutes
BAKING: 24 minutes
SPEED LIMIT: 34 mpr

Makes 6 servings

PER SERVING:
560 calories, 21g fat
(3g saturated),
61g carbohydrates,
6g fiber, 36g protein

1 tablespoon plus ¼ cup extra-virgin olive oil
5 medium boneless skinless chicken breast halves (about 1¾ pounds),
   cut in half crosswise
Kosher salt and freshly ground black pepper
1½ cups water
One 10-ounce box instant couscous
½ cup pine nuts or slivered almonds
6 dried apricots, thinly sliced lengthwise
6 pitted dates, finely diced
1 tablespoon ground cumin
¼ teaspoon cinnamon
1 cup low-sodium canned chicken broth
3 tablespoons chopped flat-leaf parsley or cilantro
Orange wedges, for serving

1. Preheat the oven to 375°F.

2. Heat 1 tablespoon of the oil in a 12-inch skillet over medium-high heat. Add the chicken pieces smooth side down, season with salt and pepper, and cook until nicely browned underneath, about 2 minutes. Turn the chicken, season again with salt and pepper, and cook 2 minutes more. Transfer the chicken to a plate, pour 1 cup of the water into the skillet, and stir up any brown bits. Set aside.

3. Combine the dry couscous, pine nuts, sliced apricots, dried dates, cumin, and cinnamon in a 13- by 9-inch baking dish. Add the remaining ¼ cup oil, season with ¾ teaspoon salt and ¼ teaspoon pepper, and stir well to mix. Pour in the broth, the juices from the skillet, and the remaining ½ cup water and stir.

4. Arrange the chicken in the pan, spacing evenly in the couscous mixture. Cover the pan snugly with foil and bake for 20 minutes, until the couscous is tender and the chicken is just cooked through. Fluff up the couscous. Sprinkle the parsley on top and serve with orange wedges.

Lazy Lasagna

The hardest part about homemade lasagna is dealing with the noodles: Traditional noodles can stick and tear and add a lot of time to the process. Using egg noodles instead makes the dish doable even during the week.

2 teaspoons kosher salt

1 pound medium or wide egg noodles

1 pound lean ground beef

3 cups Quick Skillet Tomato Sauce (page 213) or jarred marinara

2 cups part-skim ricotta cheese (about 15 ounces)

¼ cup finely grated Parmigiano-Reggiano

1 large egg

¼ teaspoon freshly ground black pepper

3 cups (packed) shredded part-skim mozzarella (12 ounces)

PREP: 10 minutes
COOKING: 37 minutes
SPEED LIMIT: 40 mpr

Makes 8 servings

PER SERVING:
550 calories, 22g fat
(11g saturated),
52g carbohydrates,
3g fiber, 40g protein

1. Fill a 4-quart pot with water, add the salt, and bring to a boil. Add the noodles and cook according to the package directions, 5 to 7 minutes, and then drain in a colander. Do not rinse the noodles.

2. Meanwhile, cook the ground beef in a medium skillet over high heat, stirring occasionally with a wooden spoon and breaking up the meat, until the juices evaporate and the meat is browned, about 5 minutes. Remove from the heat and add 1 cup of tomato sauce.

3. Preheat the oven to 425°F. In a medium bowl, combine the ricotta, Parmesan, egg, and pepper and mix with a fork until blended.

4. Lightly grease a 13- by 9-inch baking dish, add ¾ cup of the remaining tomato sauce, and tilt to coat. Spoon half of the hot noodles evenly into the pan. Sprinkle 1 cup mozzarella on top and spoon on the ricotta mixture; spread as evenly as you can with a rubber spatula. Spoon on the remaining 1¼ cups of tomato sauce and then spoon on the remaining noodles. Sprinkle on 1 more cup of mozzarella and then spoon on the meat-sauce mixture. Sprinkle the remaining cup of mozzarella on top. Lightly grease a sheet of foil, place loosely on top of the casserole, and bake until piping hot, about 25 minutes. Let stand for 10 minutes before cutting and serving.

Cooks' Note

❖ Substitute Italian sausage meat, ground turkey, or soy crumbles for the beef. (Soy crumbles do not need browning.)

Get-Well-Soon Soup

Nothing cures the blahs (or any ailment) like homemade chicken soup with lots of meat, rich, flavorful broth, and some veggies. This is a simple soup to build upon (see the variations), and the recipe makes enough so you can freeze some for later.

PREP: 10 minutes
COOKING: 2 hours

Makes about 3 quarts

PER SERVING (1½ CUPS):
367 calories, 22g fat
(6g saturated),
8g carbohydrates,
1.5g fiber, 30g protein

1 quartered 4-pound chicken, rinsed
3 garlic cloves, peeled
1 medium onion, halved, with root end intact
1 medium parsnip, peeled and halved crosswise
1 large celery rib, halved crosswise
1 large carrot, peeled and halved crosswise
2 quarts low-sodium chicken broth
2 cups filtered water
3 sprigs fresh thyme or 1 teaspoon dried thyme
Kosher salt and freshly ground black pepper

1. Place the chicken pieces in a heavy 6- to 8-quart Dutch oven. Add the garlic, onion, parsnip, celery, and carrot; pour in the broth and water and add the thyme. Bring to a boil, reduce the heat to medium-low, cover, and simmer until the chicken is well cooked through, about 1½ hours.

2. Transfer the chicken pieces and vegetables with a slotted spoon to a platter. Remove the onion, garlic, and thyme sprigs and discard. Using a ladle, skim the fat off the broth and discard. Cut the chicken off the bones, discarding the skin and bones, and then cut into bite-sized pieces and add to the broth. Cut the carrot and parsnip into small dice and add to the broth. Season the soup with salt and pepper to taste.

Cooks' Note

❖ You can speed things up by cooking the soup in a pressure cooker, which keeps the maximum amount of nutrition and flavor in the soup. To do that, place all of the ingredients in a pressure cooker and add 6 cups of broth and 1 cup of water (instead of 10 cups liquid). Secure the lid according to the manufacturer's instructions. Bring to a boil, reduce the heat, and cook for 45 minutes. Release the pressure in the cooker and remove the lid. Proceed as directed above in step 2.

Chicken Noodle Soup: Add 2 cups of cooked egg noodles when you add the cut-up chicken to the broth. You can do the same with 2 cups of cooked brown rice, if desired.

Chicken Matzo Ball Soup: Make this recipe as instructed and then follow the recipe on the matzo box or can of matzo meal. However, use seltzer for the liquid instead of broth or water, and, for ease, use a 1- to 2-ounce-size ice-cream scoop to form the matzo balls.

Asian Coconut–Chicken Noodle Soup

This robust soup is a combination of Thai and Vietnamese flavors. We like to use large serving bowls and let the kids add their own garnishes. If you prefer, you can add thin egg noodles instead of rice noodles to the soup.

PREP: 20 minutes
plus cooling
COOKING: 1¼ hours

Makes 8 servings

PER SERVING:
477 calories, 15g fat
(10g saturated),
52g carbohydrates,
5g fiber, 35g protein

CHICKEN AND BROTH

1 quartered large broiler chicken (about 4 pounds), skin removed
2 quarts filtered water
2 onions, quartered
2 celery ribs, quartered crosswise
2 pieces fresh ginger (1 by 2 inches each), peeled
4 garlic cloves, smashed and peeled
1 teaspoon black peppercorns
1 pound medium or fine rice noodles or cooked egg noodles
1 teaspoon green or red Thai curry paste
One 13.5-ounce can unsweetened coconut milk, preferably light, shaken well
2 teaspoons Vietnamese or Thai fish sauce
2 teaspoons kosher salt

SOUP GARNISHES

1 to 2 bags (5 ounces each) baby spinach or other tender greens
2 cups mung bean sprouts
2 shallots, sliced
1 zucchini, very thinly sliced
½ cup fresh cilantro
1 lime, cut into wedges

1. Place the chicken parts, water, onions, and celery in a 5- to 6-quart pot. Thinly slice 1 piece of ginger and add to the pot with the garlic and peppercorns. Bring to a boil. Reduce the heat and simmer, partially covered with the lid, until the chicken is cooked through, 45 to 50 minutes.

2. Transfer the chicken pieces with tongs to a large bowl; pour the broth through a medium mesh strainer into a 4-quart saucepan, pressing on the solids in the strainer. Let the broth stand for 5 minutes and then skim the fat from the surface with a ladle. Let the chicken cool for 20 minutes.

3. Meanwhile, submerge the rice noodles in a bowl of warm water and let soak for 10 minutes. Clean out the original soup pot, fill with water, and bring to a boil.

4. Remove and discard the chicken skin. Remove the chicken meat, tear into small pieces, and place in a large bowl.

5. Place the broth over medium-high heat in a medium saucepan, add the curry paste, coconut milk, fish sauce, and salt and bring to a boil.

6. Finely chop the remaining piece of ginger and place a little into each soup bowl. Next, add a handful each of chicken, spinach leaves, and bean sprouts to each bowl. Sprinkle some shallots and zucchini on top.

7. Place a strainer into the pot of boiling water and add a handful of soaked noodles for 1 serving of soup. Cook until tender, about 1 minute, and then strain out of the water and add to one of the bowls. Ladle in about 1½ cups of broth. Garnish with cilantro and lime. Repeat with the remaining servings.

Cooks' Notes

* You can prepare the chicken and broth ahead: Let cool separately; degrease the broth and pull apart the chicken. Combine the chicken and broth and pack in containers. Freeze for up to 3 months. Thaw in the refrigerator overnight.

* Adorable, kid-friendly connected chopsticks are available at Sur La Table and other specialty stores. Hand them out along with large spoons for enjoying the soup.

Bangers and Beans Quickie Soup

If you don't want to add spicy sausage, use any type of mild, fully cooked sausage, chopped smoked ham, diced and thinly sliced prosciutto, or chopped cooked bacon in the soup. You can garnish the soup with Basil Oil (page 221), fresh Parmesan cheese, or a dab of plain yogurt with a bit of chopped fresh flat-leaf parsley.

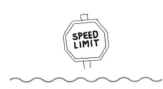

PREP: 5 minutes
COOKING: 25 minutes
SPEED LIMIT: 30 mpr

Makes 2 quarts

PER CUP:
212 calories, 9g fat
(2g saturated),
22g carbohydrates,
5g fiber, 9g protein

2 tablespoons extra-virgin olive oil
1 onion, finely diced
8 ounces (about 2 large) chicken andouille sausages (or any other fully cooked sausage), thinly sliced or finely diced
1 medium potato (about 5 ounces), peeled and finely diced
Two 15-ounce cans cannellini beans or small white beans
One 14-ounce can low-sodium chicken broth
1½ cups filtered water
1 cup Quick Skillet Tomato Sauce (page 213) or other marinara sauce
2 teaspoons finely chopped fresh rosemary or 1 teaspoon dried rosemary, crumbled
Freshly ground black pepper

1. Heat the oil in a large, deep saucepan over medium heat. Add the onion and cook, stirring, until softened, about 5 minutes. Add the sausage and potato and cook over medium-high heat, stirring often, until lightly browned, about 4 minutes. Stir in the beans, broth, water, marinara, and rosemary and bring to a boil. Reduce the heat and simmer until the soup is thickened slightly, about 15 minutes.

2. Transfer 1½ cups of the soup to a blender and puree until smooth (or use an immersion blender to partially puree to thicken). Stir back into the soup in the pot. Season to taste with pepper and serve.

Mellow Yellow Split Pea Soup

This golden soup is warm, thick, and inviting—your kiddies will gobble it up. Make the soup with or without ham (see the variation).

1 tablespoon extra-virgin olive oil
1 large onion, finely diced
2 large garlic cloves, smashed, peeled, and minced
1 pound (about 2½ cups) yellow split peas, picked over and rinsed
2 quarts (8 cups) filtered water
2 cups clear vegetable broth or additional water
2 carrots, peeled and chopped
1 large celery rib, halved lengthwise and thinly sliced
Kosher salt and freshly ground black pepper

PREP: 5 minutes
COOKING: 1¾ hours

Makes a generous 2 quarts

PER 1-CUP SERVING:
255 calories, 2g fat
(0g saturated),
43g carbohydrates,
1g fiber, 16g protein

1. Heat the oil in a large 4-quart saucepan over medium heat. Add the onion and garlic and cook, stirring often, until softened, about 4 minutes. Add the split peas, water, and broth and bring to a boil. Reduce the heat and simmer uncovered, stirring occasionally, for 30 minutes.

2. Add the carrots and celery, cover, and continue simmering, stirring occasionally, until the peas are broken down, 45 minutes to 1 hour longer. Add additional water as desired if the soup becomes too thick. (Be sure to watch and stir often toward the end of cooking to prevent the soup from sticking to the pan and burning.) Season with about 1 teaspoon each salt and pepper.

Mellow Yellow Split Pea Soup with Ham: Finely dice 4 ounces of boneless smoked, baked, or boiled ham and stir into the finished soup before adding any salt. Let the flavors blend off the heat for about 20 minutes before reheating and then season to taste.

get fresh!

If you have any chives or sprigs of fresh thyme on hand, add them to the finished soup: Add whole sprigs of thyme and thinly slice the chives and stir them in.

blue plate specials: classic dishes you and your kids crave

This group of recipes comprises classic American dishes—something you might like to order at a diner. We've updated these dishes, lightening and simplifying them. Many will undoubtedly become your kids' favorites and staples in your repertoire.

Spaghetti and Meatballs

Mega Mac 'n' Cheese

Crunchy Mega Mac 'n' Cheese

Lemon Turkey London Broil

Pantry-Style Grilled Butterflied Lamb

Peerless Pot Roast with Brown Gravy

Southern Semifried Chicken

Slow-Simmered Chili con Carne

Spaghetti and Meatballs

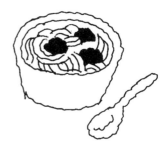

There are certain dishes that can make everything "all better" and this is one of them. To streamline this recipe, we begin with one of those great big cans of Italian tomatoes. The finished sauce of tomatoes, garlic, and olive oil is just thick enough to lightly coat the pasta and highlight the tender, moist meatballs, which are not fried or roasted but gently poached in the sauce. This makes about 4 quarts of meatballs and sauce, enough to serve with 2 pounds of cooked dried pasta, but it's worth making in such a large quantity, as the meatballs and sauce freeze beautifully.

For Sauce

10 garlic cloves, in their peels

3 tablespoons extra-virgin olive oil

One 6-pound, 10-ounce can Italian peeled tomatoes
   or four 28-ounce cans

1¾ teaspoons kosher salt

½ teaspoon freshly ground black pepper

For Meatballs

1¾ cups plain dried bread crumbs

8 large eggs

¾ cup freshly grated Parmigiano-Reggiano

2 teaspoons kosher salt

1 teaspoon freshly ground black pepper

2 pounds lean ground round

2 pounds whole-wheat spaghetti, such as Da Vinci brand

Chopped fresh basil or Italian parsley, for serving

PREP: 30 minutes

COOKING: About 2½ hours

Makes about 16 servings

PER SERVING:
428 calories, 10g fat
(3g saturated),
61g carbohydrates,
10g fiber, 29g protein

1. Make the sauce: Cut the ends off of the garlic, crush the cloves with the side of a large knife, and discard the peels and any green stems in the centers of the cloves. Heat the oil in a large pot over medium heat until hot. Add the garlic and stir until golden and fragrant, about 1 minute. In the can, using kitchen shears or scissors, cut the tomatoes in half. Then add the tomatoes and their liquid, the salt, and pepper to the pot.

2. Bring the mixture to a full boil over medium-high heat, reduce the heat to medium-low, cover, and cook, adjusting the heat as necessary to maintain a lively simmer and stirring often, until the pieces of tomato are very tender, about 1 hour and 45 minutes.

3. While the sauce is simmering, prepare the meatballs: Line a large baking sheet with waxed or parchment paper.

4. Combine the bread crumbs, eggs, Parmesan, salt, and pepper in a large bowl, whisking to blend. Crumble the ground beef into the bowl and stir with a wooden spoon or mix with your hands until well blended. Scoop up a rounded tablespoon of the meat mixture and roll with your hands into a 1½-inch ball; place on the baking sheet. Repeat with the remaining meat mixture. You should have about 4 dozen meatballs.

5. When the sauce is ready, put the water on to boil for the pasta and add the meatballs into the tomato sauce, carefully placing them in the pot one at a time; without stirring, cover the pot and let cook for 15 minutes. When the pasta water boils, add the pasta and stir frequently, to prevent clumping.

6. Meanwhile, uncover the sauce and simmer, stirring occasionally, until the meatballs are tender and cooked through and the sauce is thickened slightly, about 15 minutes more. Season the sauce to taste and serve over the pasta. Sprinkle with basil.

Cooks' Note

❖ Freeze cooked meatballs and sauce in quart containers. Let thaw in the refrigerator overnight and then reheat in a medium saucepan, covered, over medium heat.

"Yuuuu-mmmm-yyyyy," says Tanya's eight-year-old son Sanger whenever he has this for dinner.

Mega Mac 'n' Cheese

There are two bad things about prepared macaroni and cheese: the artificial ingredients and excess salt, which should be enough to sway you from buying it. For best results, use organic milk and a fine, small whole-wheat macaroni, such as Da Vinci brand, which is thin and cooks up nicely tender and not mealy.

One 12-ounce box whole-wheat elbow macaroni
2 tablespoons unsalted butter
1 large shallot, finely chopped
2 tablespoons unbleached all-purpose flour
2¼ cups reduced-fat (2%) milk
2 tablespoons cornstarch
10 ounces extra-sharp Cheddar cheese, shredded (2½ cups)
½ cup heavy cream
1½ teaspoons kosher salt
Freshly ground black pepper

PREP: 10 minutes
COOKING: 25 minutes
SPEED LIMIT: 35 mpr

Makes 10 cups

PER CUP:
332 calories, 18g fat
(12g saturated),
31g carbohydrates,
3g fiber, 14g protein

1. Bring a large saucepan of water to a boil; add the macaroni and cook, stirring often, until al dente, about 8 minutes. Drain in a colander and rinse with cool water until cool. Reserve.

2. Melt the butter in the same saucepan over medium heat. Add the shallot and cook, stirring, until tender, about 5 minutes. Stir in the flour and cook for 1 minute. Whisk in 1 cup of the milk and cook, whisking, until thickened, about 2 minutes. Whisk the cornstarch into the remaining 1¼ cups milk and then whisk into the sauce in the pan. Bring to a boil, reduce the heat, and simmer, whisking, for 1 minute longer. Add the cheese and stir until melted. Stir in the cream and salt.

3. Stir the cooked macaroni into the cheese sauce and cook over medium heat, stirring, until hot, about 3 minutes. Season to taste with salt and pepper.

Crunchy Mega Mac 'n' Cheese: Transfer the mac and cheese to a buttered baking dish. Combine ½ cup plain dried bread crumbs and ½ cup more shredded Cheddar, sprinkle on top of the macaroni mixture, and broil until golden.

Lemon Turkey London Broil

This recipe is great for a simple dinner or a party. You can easily double or even triple the recipe as needed. Use leftovers for Turkey Hash (page 137). Serve with one of our potato recipes and a green salad.

PREP: About 1 hour (includes marinating)
COOKING: 45 minutes

Makes 8 servings

PER SERVING:
*203 calories, 3g fat
(1g saturated),
0g carbohydrates,
0g fiber, 40g protein*

*1 lemon
1 medium shallot, thinly sliced
2 garlic cloves, smashed and peeled
1/3 cup extra-virgin olive oil
1 boneless turkey breast half (about 3 pounds)
1 teaspoon kosher salt
1/2 teaspoon coarsely ground black pepper*

1. Finely grate the lemon peel into a large nonreactive bowl (or a gallon resealable plastic bag), taking care to grate only the bright yellow part, not the bitter white pith underneath. Cut the lemon in half and squeeze the juice into the bowl. Add the shallot, garlic, and oil. Rinse the turkey breast, pat dry, and add to the marinade, turning to coat well. Cover and chill for 1 hour or overnight.

2. Prepare the grill: Preheat a gas grill at medium flame or arrange hot charcoal in a circular fashion for indirect heat.

3. Remove the turkey from the marinade, season with the salt and pepper, and place skin side down on the grill rack. Cover and cook, turning once or twice and rotating the breast as necessary, until an instant-read thermometer inserted horizontally into the center of the thickest part of the breast reaches 155°F, about 45 minutes.

4. Transfer the turkey breast to a board with grooves and let stand for 5 minutes before thinly slicing against the grain.

Ruby S., five years old and living in Amagansett, New York, said, "I really liked the way the turkey tasted grilled. I couldn't taste the garlic much but it was delicious."

Pantry-Style Grilled Butterflied Lamb

Remember Grandma's way of overcooking leg of lamb? If it made you think you didn't like lamb, this dish will convince you otherwise. The marinade can be made in a snap, and the longer you marinate the lamb, the better. Serve with one of our salads.

1/4 cup plus 2 tablespoons pure maple syrup
1/4 cup whole-grain mustard
1/4 cup vegetable oil
3 tablespoons soy sauce
2 tablespoons red wine vinegar
4 garlic cloves, smashed and peeled
2 teaspoons dried thyme
One 4 1/2-pound boneless butterflied leg of lamb
Freshly ground black pepper
1/2 teaspoon kosher salt

PREP: About 1 hour
(includes marinating)
GRILLING: 33 minutes

Makes 8 servings

PER SERVING:
355 calories, 16g fat
(6g saturated),
3g carbohydrates,
0g fiber, 47g protein

1. Combine the maple syrup, mustard, oil, soy sauce, vinegar, garlic, and thyme in a container or bowl just large enough to hold the lamb; whisk to blend. Add the lamb, turning to coat, cover, and chill for 1 hour and up to 2 days, turning the lamb a couple of times.

2. Prepare the grill. Preheat a gas grill at medium flame or arrange hot charcoal in a circular fashion for indirect heat.

3. Remove the lamb from the marinade and let any excess drip off. Place the lamb on the grill and season with pepper. Cover and cook for 15 minutes, rotating the meat once during cooking. Turn the lamb, cover, and cook about 18 minutes more, until the internal temperature in the thinnest part of the lamb reaches 145°F on an instant-read thermometer and the thickest part reaches 130°F. Transfer the lamb to a board, cover loosely with foil, and let stand for 10 minutes. Thinly slice the lamb, sprinkle with the salt, and serve with any collected juices.

"This dish gets Max's seal of approval!" says fifteen-year-old Max D., of Tavernier, Florida. "We should have this more often."

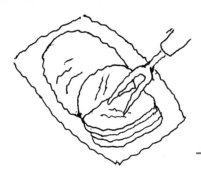

Peerless Pot Roast with Brown Gravy

This classic has a rich, meaty sauce that is thickened with tender braised onion pureed in the blender. Serve with any mash (pages 206–209) and a steamed green vegetable.

PREP: 20 minutes
BRAISING: 3 hours

Makes 8 servings

PER SERVING:
277 calories, 10g fat
(3g saturated),
7.5g carbohydrates,
1g fiber, 38g protein

One 3½-pound boneless chuck or rump roast
Kosher salt and freshly ground black pepper
1 tablespoon extra-virgin olive oil
3 pounds yellow onions (8 medium), quartered
1 (dried) ancho chile, seeded and torn into pieces (optional)
2 cups canned low-sodium beef broth
1 cup water

1. Preheat the oven to 325°F. Pat the beef dry with paper towels and season lightly on both sides with the salt and pepper.

2. Heat the oil in a 6- to 8-quart heavy pot over medium heat until hot, add the beef, and cook until nicely browned on both sides, about 14 minutes total, turning once.

3. Add the onion, chile, if using, broth, and water and bring to a simmer over medium-high heat. Cover the pot with the lid and transfer to the oven. Let braise for 2½ to 3 hours, turning the meat every 45 minutes or so, until very tender. Transfer the beef to a plate and let the sauce cool for at least 15 minutes.

4. Skim any excess fat from the surface and then puree the sauce in a blender in batches until smooth. Transfer the sauce to a 4-quart pot or a deep skillet, bring to a simmer, and season to taste with salt and pepper. Slice the beef about ½ inch thick and reheat gently in the sauce.

Southern Semifried Chicken

Everyone loves fried chicken, but many never make it because of the fat and the mess. Our version solves both problems: The chicken is marinated in a buttermilklike mixture and coated with whole-wheat flour, bread crumbs, and spices. We briefly pan-fry the chicken in olive oil and finish the cooking in the oven, so the chicken comes out crispy outside, tender inside, and not greasy. If you want to reduce even more fat and calories, remove and discard the skin before marinating.

2 cups reduced-fat (2%) milk
1 tablespoon distilled white vinegar
One 4-pound broiler chicken, cut into eighths, 4 chicken breast halves
*   on the bone, or 8 drumsticks*
¾ cup whole-wheat flour
½ cup plain dried bread crumbs
1 tablespoon kosher salt
1 teaspoon dried thyme, crumbled
¼ teaspoon freshly ground black pepper
½ cup extra-virgin olive oil

1. Combine the milk and vinegar in a large nonreactive bowl; add the chicken pieces, turning to coat, and chill for 1 hour or overnight.

2. Preheat the oven to 400°F. Line a large shallow baking sheet with heavy-duty foil, lightly grease the foil, and set aside.

3. Combine the flour, bread crumbs, salt, thyme, and pepper in a medium bowl; whisk to blend. Coat the chicken pieces one at a time in the crumb mixture and place on a plate. Repeat with the remaining chicken pieces.

4. Heat the oil in a 10-inch cast-iron or other heavy skillet over medium heat until hot. Add half of the chicken pieces to the pan skin side down, and cook until golden underneath, 3 to 4 minutes. Turn and cook 2 minutes more. Transfer the chicken pieces to the prepared baking sheet. Repeat browning with the remaining chicken.

5. Transfer the baking sheet to the oven and bake until the chicken is browned and sizzling and the juices run clear when the thickest part of a thigh or breast is pierced with the tip of a knife, about 30 minutes.

PREP: About 1 hour (includes marinating)
COOKING: 36 minutes

Makes 4 servings

PER SERVING (1 PIECE LIGHT MEAT, 1 PIECE DARK MEAT):
580 calories, 27g fat (8g saturated), 16g carbohydrates, 1g fiber, 62g protein

"I don't like this chicken—I love it!" says Caroline C., age ten, from Weston, Connecticut. "This chicken is out of this world!"

Slow-Simmered Chili Con Carne

This luscious chili—a shredded beef bonanza—is great to make ahead for a party and also freezes well. We make use of the food processor to cut the time it takes to chop the veggies, and also simmer the chili in the oven to prevent the burning that can occur when chili is made on top of the stove. Although it takes several hours to cook, it needs only minimal maintenance. Serve with brown rice, shredded Cheddar or Monterey Jack cheese, thinly sliced scallions, Chunky Guacamole (page 104), and plain whole milk yogurt.

PREP: 20 minutes
COOKING: About 4 hours

Makes about 4½ quarts (18 servings)

PER SERVING
(1 CUP CHILI):
309 calories, 13g fat
(4g saturated),
16g carbohydrates,
4g fiber, 31g protein

3 tablespoons vegetable oil
5 pounds trimmed beef chuck stew meat, cut into 2-inch pieces
Kosher salt and freshly ground black pepper
3 medium onions, trimmed and halved
3 Anaheim chiles or green bell peppers, trimmed, halved, and seeded
6 garlic cloves, smashed and peeled
4 teaspoons chili powder
2 teaspoons dried oregano
½ teaspoon ground cumin
½ teaspoon ground coriander
½ teaspoon cayenne pepper
Two 28-ounce cans crushed tomatoes
2 cups canned low-sodium beef broth
Three 15.5-ounce cans small red beans, pinto beans, or black beans, drained and rinsed
1 ounce Ibarra Mexican or bittersweet chocolate, chopped (optional)

1. Heat ½ tablespoon of the oil in an ovenproof 7- to 8-quart pot with a lid over medium heat. Add one-third of the beef and season lightly with salt and pepper. Cook, turning the meat on all sides, until nicely browned, about 5 minutes. Transfer the meat with tongs or a slotted spoon to a large bowl. Repeat browning in two more batches with the remaining beef and ½ tablespoon more oil for each batch. Reserve the pot.

2. While the meat is searing, arrange a rack in the lower third of the oven and preheat the oven to 325°F. Cut the onion and fresh chile halves into 1-inch chunks. Add the garlic to a food processor and process until the garlic is chopped and sticks to the side of the work bowl. Add the onion and

chili (in batches if necessary) and pulse (using 3-second pulses) until chopped; reserve.

3. Add the remaining 1½ tablespoons of oil to the same pot; add the chili powder, oregano, cumin, coriander, and cayenne and stir for 1 minute over medium-low heat. Add the contents of the food processor to the pot and cook, stirring, until the vegetables are slightly softened, about 3 minutes. Stir in the tomatoes and broth, increase the heat to medium, and bring to a boil. Return the meat to the pot, cover with a lid, and bring to a simmer over medium heat.

4. Transfer the pot to the oven and set the timer for 3½ hours. Every 45 minutes, carefully remove the pot from the oven and place on the stovetop; stir and then return to the oven. After 3½ hours the meat should be tender enough to shred when pushed against the side of the pot with a wooden spoon.

5. Stir in the beans and chocolate, if using, and let stand for 10 minutes before seasoning to taste.

Cooks' Notes

* To make the chili hotter, stir in minced fresh jalapeño just before serving.

* Although you can eat the chili right away, the flavor improves if you make it a day or two ahead: Just let cool and chill for up to 4 days, or freeze in covered containers for up to 4 months.

"I've never tried chili before, but this was good! Not too spicy—it was perfect," said Gabriel C., age seven, from the Bronx, New York.

meat-free mains: entrees without meat but with plenty of flavor

These creative, hearty main courses contain vegetables, grains, dairy, and eggs. They are not for a vegan diet, but they will prove to your kids that anyone can have a great, satisfying dinner without meat.

Bean and Green Enchiladas

Penne Primavera

Pop's Spinach Pie

Mushroom-Spinach Pie

Harvest Tomato Tart

Mamma Mia Manicotti

Indian-Spiced Spinach

Middle Eastern Couscous with Tofu and Vegetables

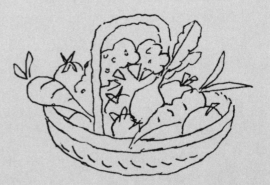

Bean and Green Enchiladas

This twist on a Mexican classic is a fantastic way to make a meal of veggies. Serve the enchiladas with reduced-fat sour cream and extra salsa.

1½ pounds fresh baby spinach leaves or 3 boxes (10 ounces each) frozen
    leaf spinach (see Cooks' Notes), thawed
¼ cup canola oil
1 large onion, chopped
One 15-ounce can pinto beans, drained and rinsed
¼ teaspoon kosher salt
¼ teaspoon freshly ground black pepper
2 cups (packed) shredded Monterey Jack or Swiss cheese (8 ounces)
Eight 5- to 6-inch soft corn tortillas
1½ cups green salsa (salsa verde), such as Herdez brand

PREP: 10 minutes
COOKING: 34 minutes
SPEED LIMIT: 44 mpr

**Makes 8 enchiladas
to serve 4 to 8**

PER ENCHILADA:
329 calories, 16g fat
(7g saturated),
35g carbohydrates,
8g fiber, 13g protein

1. Lightly oil a 13- by 9-inch baking dish and set aside.

2. Bring 2 inches of water to boil in a 6-quart pot. Add the spinach and stir until wilted, about 2 minutes. Drain the spinach in a colander; rinse with cold running water until cool, and then squeeze the leaves in batches to remove as much liquid as possible; reserve.

3. Add 1 tablespoon of the oil and the onion to the same pot and cook over medium heat, stirring often until softened, about 5 minutes. Remove from the heat and stir in the spinach, beans, salt, pepper, and half of the shredded cheese.

4. Heat 1 tablespoon of the remaining oil in a cast-iron skillet over medium heat. Add a tortilla, cook for 30 seconds, turn, and cook 30 seconds more. Drain and pat dry on paper towels. Repeat with the remaining tortillas, adding more oil when the skillet seems dry.

5. Fill the tortillas: Add about ½ cup of the spinach mixture in a row down the center of each tortilla, then roll up snugly. Repeat with the remaining tortillas and spinach mixture, and then arrange the enchiladas in 2 crosswise rows in the baking dish.

6. Just before baking, preheat the oven to 400°F. Pour the salsa down the center of both rows of enchiladas. Bake for about 10 minutes, remove from the oven, and sprinkle the remaining cup of cheese on top, and then bake 10 minutes more until the cheese is melted and golden.

Cooks' Notes

❖ If using thawed frozen spinach, coarsely chop and then squeeze out as much moisture as possible. Skip step 2 and prepare as directed.

❖ To do ahead: You can assemble the enchiladas through step 4 the day before and chill. Let stand at room temperature for 1 hour, cover with sauce, and bake as directed. You can also freeze the assembled enchiladas for up to 1 month. Wrap well in plastic. Let thaw in the fridge overnight before baking as directed.

Lila E., age fifteen, from Westport, Connecticut, liked the spinach/cheese part of this dish while her brother, Jacob, twelve, really liked the beans.

Penne Primavera

With this colorful dish, the whole family can get almost all of their daily veggies in one sitting. Look for whole-wheat pasta that is lighter in color; kids prefer it because it has a better texture than dark, grainy pasta.

2 teaspoons kosher salt

8 ounces whole-wheat penne (2 rounded cups)

2 cups snow peas, trimmed

1 tablespoon extra-virgin olive oil

1 tablespoon unsalted butter

1 medium onion, coarsely chopped

1 small yellow bell pepper, trimmed, seeded, and sliced into $\frac{1}{4}$-inch-thick strips

1 broccoli stalk, cut into tiny florets (about 2 cups)

$\frac{1}{4}$ cup filtered water

2 small zucchini, trimmed, halved lengthwise, and sliced into $\frac{1}{4}$-inch-thick half-moons

1 cup heavy cream

2 cups grape tomatoes, halved

$\frac{1}{2}$ cup finely grated Parmigiano-Reggiano, plus more for serving

Freshly ground black pepper

SPEED LIMIT

PREP: 15 minutes
COOKING: 20 minutes
SPEED LIMIT: 35 mpr

Makes 4 servings

PER SERVING:
513 calories, 24g fat (12g saturated), 57g carbohydrates, 9g fiber, 18g protein

1. Fill a 6-quart pot with 3 quarts of water, add the salt, and bring to a boil. Add the pasta and cook according to the package directions, stirring often, until al dente, about 8 minutes.

2. Place the snow peas in a colander in the sink and pour the pasta over the snow peas to drain well and warm the peas; do not rinse.

3. Heat the oil and butter in the same pot over medium heat. Add the onion and cook, stirring occasionally, for 3 minutes. Add the bell pepper, broccoli, and filtered water; cover and cook for 3 minutes. Add the zucchini and cook uncovered until the vegetables are nearly tender, about 3 minutes more.

4. Pour in the cream and bring to a boil. Cook, stirring occasionally, for 1 minute. Add the tomatoes, pasta, and snow peas, toss well, and cook, stirring occasionally, until the pasta is hot and saucy, about 2 minutes. Stir in the Parmesan, season to taste with salt and plenty of pepper, and serve extra cheese on the side.

Wow! We are impressed by Kobey W., age seven, from Potter, Maine, who said, "I love the pasta and sauce and I would like even more vegetables in it!"

Pop's Spinach Pie

Both of our households are obsessed with spinach pie. Almost every Sunday Tanya whips up one big enough to serve eight, so that on a busy weeknight, the second half of the pie can be cut into portions and heated up quickly. If using frozen leaf spinach, choose a quality brand like Cascadian Farm, which is organic. You can find phyllo dough in the supermarket freezer—we like Kronos and Fillo Factory brands.

PREP: 20 minutes

COOKING: 1 hour and 10 minutes

Makes 8 servings

PER SERVING:
259 calories, 13g fat (4g saturated), 26g carbohydrates, 7g fiber, 12g protein

1/4 cup extra-virgin olive oil
One 2 1/2-pound bag fresh baby spinach or two 1-pound bags frozen leaf spinach
1 large onion, chopped
2 garlic cloves: smashed, peeled, and finely chopped
1 cup reduced-fat ricotta cheese
2 large eggs
1/2 cup finely grated Parmigiano-Reggiano
3/4 teaspoon kosher salt
1/2 teaspoon cinnamon (optional)
1/4 teaspoon crushed red pepper flakes
1/4 teaspoon freshly ground black pepper
Six 17- by 11-inch sheets frozen phyllo dough, thawed according to package directions

1. Preheat the oven to 350°F. Lightly brush a 13- by 9-inch baking dish with a little olive oil and set aside.

2. Bring 2 inches of water to boil in a 6-quart pot. Add half of the spinach leaves and stir until wilted, about 2 minutes. Add the remaining spinach a few handfuls at a time, stirring until wilted. Once all of the spinach is wilted, drain in a colander. Rinse with cold running water until cool. Squeeze the spinach in batches by hand or through a fine-mesh sieve to remove as much liquid as possible, and place in a large bowl. (If using frozen spinach, add the contents of both bags to the boiling water; cover and cook until tender, about 4 minutes. Drain, rinse, and squeeze as directed.)

3. Wipe out the pot, add 1 tablespoon of the olive oil, and heat over medium heat. Add the onion and garlic and cook, stirring occasionally, until soft, about 5 minutes. Transfer to the bowl with the cooled spinach. Add the ricotta, eggs, Parmesan, salt, cinnamon, if using, crushed red pepper flakes, and black pepper. Stir with a fork until well blended.

4. Lay the phyllo sheets on top of one another on a work surface. Brush one-half of the top sheet lightly with some oil and fold the plain side over on top of the oiled side. Carefully transfer the sheet to the prepared baking dish and lightly brush with oil. Repeat the process with 2 more sheets of phyllo. Spoon the spinach mixture on top of the phyllo and spread evenly. Repeat layering on top of the spinach filling with the remaining 3 sheets of dough and olive oil, brushing the top of the pie with the last of the oil. Bake for about 1 hour, until the top of the pie is crispy and golden brown.

Cooks' Notes

- ❖ Reheat chilled leftovers in a 350°F oven or toaster oven for about 10 minutes.

- ❖ Use leftover ricotta to make tender Protein Power Pancakes (page 47) or serve the ricotta with fresh berries, drizzled with honey for breakfast or dessert.

Mushroom-Spinach Pie: Add a 6-ounce package of medium white mushrooms, thinly sliced, and cook them along with the onion and garlic. Tanya sometimes adds ½ cup of raisins or currants to the mushroom-spinach filling.

"I really love eating this because it gives me big muscles,"
says Tanya's eight-year-old son William.

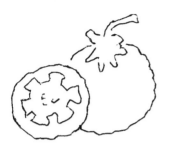

Harvest Tomato Tart

Look for colorful heirloom tomatoes, such as Brandywine, Black Kirm, and Rainbow, for layering in this tart, which celebrates summer's bounty. Everyone will love the Parmesan-flavored crust. For those who love gooey, melted mozzarella, the assembled tart can be heated in a 375°F oven for 10 minutes.

Prep: 20 minutes plus chilling and cooling
Baking: 33 minutes

Makes one 9-inch savory tart to serve 6 as a main dish

per ⅙ tart:
385 calories, 24g fat
(12g saturated),
25g carbohydrates,
3g fiber, 18g protein

Tart Shell
¾ cup unbleached all-purpose flour
½ cup whole-wheat flour, preferably white whole-wheat
¼ cup finely grated Parmesan cheese, preferably Parmigiano-Reggiano
¼ teaspoon freshly ground black pepper
1 stick cold unsalted butter, cut up
3 to 4 tablespoons cold water

Filling
1½ pounds assorted tomatoes, sliced ¼ inch thick
Kosher salt and freshly ground black pepper
8 ounces lightly salted fresh mozzarella cheese, thinly sliced and patted dry
3 tablespoons Basil Oil (page 221)

1. Prepare the pastry dough: Combine the flours, Parmesan, and pepper in the food processor. Add the butter and pulse until crumbly. Add 3 tablespoons cold water and pulse just until the dough begins to gather into a ball on the blade. (If necessary, add up to 1 tablespoon more cold water.)

2. Turn the dough out onto a work surface, gather up any crumbs, and knead briefly to make a barely smooth dough. Form into a disk; wrap in plastic and chill for 30 minutes.

3. Bake the pastry shell: Roll out the dough on a lightly floured surface to a 12-inch round. Carefully fit the dough into a 9-inch tart pan with a removable bottom or a 9-inch pie pan. Prick the flat surface of the dough all over at 1-inch intervals with a fork; chill for 15 minutes. Preheat the oven to 375°F.

4. Place a sheet of aluminum foil over the chilled pastry shell and press into the bottom edge of the dough. Fill with about a cup of dry beans or pie weights. Bake the shell for 18 minutes, remove the foil and weights, and bake 15 minutes more, until the crust is golden. Let cool completely on a rack.

5. Assemble the tart: When ready to serve, transfer the tart shell to a serving plate (keep the pie shell in the pie pan). Arrange one-third of the tomato slices in the bottom of the crust; season lightly with salt and pepper, top with half of the mozzarella slices, and drizzle 1½ tablespoons basil oil on top. Repeat layering with half of the remaining tomato slices, salt and pepper, the remaining mozzarella, and 1½ tablespoons basil oil. Arrange the last of the tomato slices on top of the tart. Serve at room temperature.

Cooks' Notes

❖ You can use raw rice or dried beans for pie weights. Once they have cooled, store them in a bag and keep with your baking supplies for future use.

❖ The tart shell can be baked up to 2 days ahead; let cool, cover with foil, and keep at room temperature.

Megan L., age six, from LaGrange, Kentucky, who made this with her mom, Pamela, said, "Delicious! I can't stop eating this!"

Mamma Mia Manicotti

Tracey's friend Gina Marie Miraglia at *Gourmet* magazine puts a stick of mozzarella inside her manicotti, but we like Fontina even better. Don't forget to butter the baking dish for easy cleanup.

PREP: 20 minutes
BAKING: 30 minutes
SPEED LIMIT: 50 mpr

Makes 8 large manicotti

PER MANICOTTO:
302 calories, 20g fat
(10g saturated),
13g carbohydrates,
1g fiber, 19g protein

Eight 9-inch store-bought crepes or homemade crepes (see our website, www.realfoodforhealthykids.com)
1½ cups marinara sauce, preferably Quick Skillet Tomato Sauce (page 213)
2 cups part-skim ricotta cheese (1 pound)
1 large egg
¼ cup finely grated Parmigiano-Reggiano, plus more for serving
¼ teaspoon kosher salt
¼ teaspoon freshly ground black pepper
Pinch of nutmeg
12 ounces Italian Fontina cheese, 1 cup grated, the remainder cut into 8 chunky horizontal slices

1. If using homemade crepes, prepare them and reserve.

2. Arrange a rack in the upper third of the oven and preheat the oven to 400°F. Lightly butter a 13- by 9-inch glass baking dish. Pour 1 cup of the marinara sauce into the baking dish and tilt to coat the bottom with the sauce; set aside.

3. Combine the ricotta, egg, Parmesan, salt, pepper, and nutmeg and stir until well blended. Lay a crepe on a work surface. Mound about ⅓ cup of the grated cheese mixture in the center and press a horizontal slice of Fontina into the cheese. Pick up the rounded edge closest to you (the bottom) and fold over the cheese. Fold in the right and left sides and roll the crepe away from you to make a packet. Place in the baking dish. (You will have 2 lengthwise rows of 4 manicotti arranged crosswise.) Repeat with the remaining crepes and filling.

4. Spoon the remaining sauce over the manicotti, cover snugly with foil, and bake for 30 minutes. The crepes should be puffed and the filling bubbly. Remove the foil and sprinkle the remaining 1 cup grated cheese on top. Bake about 5 minutes more to melt the cheese. Serve with more Parmesan.

"These are almost as good as dessert!" said Kelly M., of Middletown, New Jersey.

Indian-Spiced Spinach

Does your family love creamed spinach? If so, try this Indian version of it, a popular vegetarian dish known as *Palak Paneer*. It's a great way to introduce anyone to wonderfully fragrant Indian cuisine. Traditionally, it is made with *sag*, fresh farmer's cheese (available at most supermarkets), which you can substitute for the tofu. Make sure that the tofu or cheese is well drained so it keeps its shape during browning.

PREP: 10 minutes
COOKING: 15 minutes
SPEED LIMIT: 25 mpr

Makes 4 servings (or 8 side-dish servings)

PER 1/2-CUP SERVING
(BASED ON 4 SERVINGS):
*391 calories, 27g fat
(16g saturated),
33g carbohydrates,
14g fiber, 11g protein*

One 2 1/2-pound bag fresh baby spinach or two 1-pound bags frozen
    leaf spinach (see Cooks' Notes)
Two 1/4-inch-thick slices peeled fresh ginger
1 serrano chile, trimmed (seeded, if desired)
1/4 cup water
1 teaspoon ground coriander
1/2 teaspoon sweet paprika
1/2 teaspoon turmeric
1/4 teaspoon ground cumin
1/4 cup ghee (clarified butter) or vegetable oil (see Cooks' Notes)
One 7-ounce piece medium-firm drained tofu, cut into bite-sized pieces
1/2 cup heavy cream
1 teaspoon kosher salt
1/2 teaspoon ground garam masala (see Cooks' Notes)

1. Bring 2 inches of water to boil in a 6-quart pot. Add half of the spinach and stir until wilted, about 2 minutes. Add the remaining spinach a few handfuls at a time, stirring until wilted and then adding more. Drain the spinach in a colander. Rinse with cold running water until cool and squeeze the leaves in batches to remove as much liquid as possible.

2. Pulse the spinach in a food processor until coarsely chopped; transfer to a bowl. Combine the ginger and chile in the food processor and process to finely chop. Add the water, coriander, paprika, turmeric, and cumin and process to blend; reserve.

3. Heat the ghee or oil in a large nonstick skillet over medium heat. Add the tofu and cook, turning occasionally with a spatula, until light golden, about 5 minutes. Add the ginger-spice mixture to the skillet and boil, stirring, until reduced by half, about 3 minutes. Add the spinach and cook, turning, until heated through. Add the cream, salt, and garam masala and cook, stirring until hot, about 2 minutes, and serve.

Cooks' Notes

❖ If using frozen spinach, add the contents of both bags to the boiling water; cover and cook until wilted, about 4 minutes. Drain, rinse, and squeeze as directed.

❖ Ghee is available at many grocery stores in the international foods aisle. Garam masala is a spice mixture of cinnamon, cardamom, bay leaf, dried chiles, fennel, and black pepper. You can purchase it and the other spices at Indian shops and some specialty stores or from Kalustyan's in New York City (www.kalustyans.com).

Middle Eastern Couscous with Tofu and Vegetables

Tracey's vegan friend Lena Pfeffer makes a dish like this regularly for quick weekday dinners and casual entertaining. Pearl-shaped Israeli couscous is tender and velvety and a delightful change from pasta and rice. For substituting instant couscous, see the Cooks' Note.

PREP: 10 minutes
COOKING: 25 minutes
SPEED LIMIT: 35 mpr

Makes 2 quarts (about 8 servings)

PER CUP:
245 calories, 7g fat
(1g saturated),
36g carbohydrates,
2g fiber, 10g protein

2 cups canned low-sodium vegetable broth
1/2 cup filtered water
3 tablespoons extra-virgin olive oil
One 10-ounce package white mushrooms, quartered
One 14-ounce container firm tofu, drained, patted dry, and cut into
    1/3-inch dice
1 onion, finely chopped
3 garlic cloves, smashed, peeled, and minced
One 10-ounce container Israeli (Middle Eastern) couscous, about
    1 3/4 cups
2 medium zucchini and/or summer squash, trimmed and finely diced
1/4 cup drained sun-dried tomatoes (packed in oil), finely diced
1 teaspoon kosher salt
Freshly ground black pepper
1 to 2 teaspoons finely grated fresh lemon peel
2 tablespoons finely chopped fresh basil or flat-leaf parsley (optional)

1. Bring the broth and water to a boil in a small saucepan, remove from the heat, and cover to keep warm. (Alternatively, heat the broth and water in the microwave.)

2. Meanwhile, heat 1½ tablespoons of the oil in a large 4-quart saucepan over medium-high heat. Add the mushrooms and cook, stirring occasionally, until nicely browned, about 6 minutes. Add the tofu and cook, stirring occasionally, until golden, about 3 minutes. Transfer the tofu mixture to a bowl.

3. Add the remaining 1½ tablespoons oil, the onion, and garlic to the same pot and cook over medium-high heat, stirring, until golden, about 3 minutes. Add the couscous and stir until lightly toasted, about 2 minutes. Add the hot broth, the tofu mixture, zucchini, and sun-dried tomatoes and bring to a boil. Reduce the heat, cover, and simmer gently, stirring occasionally to prevent

sticking, until the couscous is tender, about 8 minutes. Stir in the salt, pepper, lemon peel, and basil, if using. Serve hot.

Cooks' Note

❖ If you can't find Israeli couscous you can substitute $1\frac{1}{2}$ cups of instant couscous. Add the couscous (without toasting) along with the hot broth, tofu, and vegetables; cover the pot, remove from the heat, and let stand until the couscous is tender, about 5 minutes.

"I really like the green and white bits, Mommy," says two-year-old Kaylen M., of Port Chester, New York.

sidekicks: vegetables and more to round out a meal

Hasty Hash Browns

   Cheddar-Potato Cake

   Swiss Cheese Potato Cake

   Goat Cheese Potato Cake

Cheddar Scalloped Potatoes

Grasshopper Potato Salad

Perfect Rice

Grilled Spudniks

   Loaded Spudniks

Creamed Spinach

Blasted Winter Vegetables

Zucchini-Parmesan Pancakes

Harvest Ratatouille

Totem Poles (Roasted Asparagus)

   Asparagus in a Blanket

Turkish Green Beans

Cowboy Beans

Rainbow Slaw

Super-Mash!

Tater-Brocky

   Tater-Cali

Squish Squash

   Butternut Squash Soup

Yummy Yammy-Parsnip Mash

Blender Hollandaise

Thick 'n' Spicy Barbecue Sauce

Grilled Tomato Sauce

Quick Skillet Tomato Sauce

Eat-Yer-Veggies Cheese Sauce

ABC Vinaigrette

   ABC Salad

Teriyaki Vinaigrette

Mexican Adobo Dressing

Blue on Blue Dressing

Rockin' Ranch Dressing

Tzatziki

Basil Oil

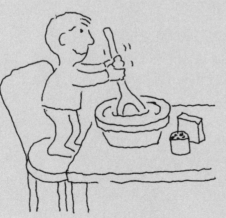

This section has a reliable roundup of satisfying starches and vegetable side dishes, as well as recipes for salad dressings and sauces. You may like our sides so much they could become the center of your dinner plate—and you need only to add a simple lean protein to make a meal. The mashes are terrific any time of the year and are a great way to get kids to enjoy eating their veggies.

The sauces and dressings are a great foundation for your repertoire. They are extremely versatile, easy to make, and have a nutritional makeover so they are as good as they can be. There are also some dressings and sauces in other sections of the cookbook, including Sesame Sauce (page 95) and Horseradish Dunk (page 103).

~ VEGGIES AND GRAINS ~
Hasty Hash Browns

Using high-quality frozen shredded potatoes makes for fast potato dishes like this one. Serve the hash browns with eggs, grilled meats, or fish. Kids love the addition of a layer of cheese (see variations). Look for organic frozen potatoes, such as Cascadian Farm brand.

3 tablespoons extra-virgin olive oil
1 medium onion, finely chopped
One 1-pound bag frozen shredded potatoes, thawed
1 teaspoon kosher salt
¼ teaspoon freshly ground black pepper

PREP: 5 minutes
COOKING: 25 minutes
SPEED LIMIT: 30 mpr

Makes 4 servings

PER SERVING:
197 calories, 10g fat
(1g saturated),
23g carbohydrates,
3g fiber, 3g protein

1. Place the oven rack in the upper third of the oven and preheat the oven to 500°F. Heat 2 tablespoons of the oil in a 9-inch ovenproof skillet over medium-low heat.

2. Add the onion and cook, stirring occasionally, until softened, about 5 minutes. Add the remaining tablespoon of oil and add the potatoes, salt, and pepper, stirring to mix. Increase the heat to medium-high, spread the potatoes out in the skillet, and let cook for 5 minutes undisturbed.

3. Turn the potato mixture with a spatula, roughly smooth the top, and transfer to the oven. Bake for 10 minutes, turn the potatoes again, and bake 5 to 10 minutes more, until golden brown on the top and bottom. Serve hot.

Cheddar-Potato Cake: Sprinkle ¾ cup (3 ounces) shredded sharp Cheddar on one-half of the hash browns, and then, with a spatula, turn the other half on top. Let stand for a few minutes to melt the cheese.

Swiss Cheese Potato Cake or Goat Cheese Potato Cake: Use ¾ cup shredded Swiss cheese or crumbled fresh goat cheese instead of the Cheddar.

Cheddar Scalloped Potatoes

This rendition is lighter in calories and fat than most versions. For easy potato slicing, use a food processor or an inexpensive mandoline.

PREP: 10 minutes
BAKING: 1 hour and
5 minutes

Makes 8 servings

PER SERVING:
203 calories, 6.5g fat
(4g saturated),
29g carbohydrates,
2g fiber, 8g protein

2 medium leeks
2 tablespoons unsalted butter, plus more for greasing the pan
1 garlic clove, smashed, peeled, and minced
¾ cup canned low-sodium chicken broth
1 tablespoon cornstarch
1 tablespoon unbleached all-purpose flour
¾ teaspoon kosher salt
¼ teaspoon freshly ground black pepper
1¼ cups whole milk
2 pounds russet (baking) potatoes (4 medium-large)
1 cup (packed) shredded extra-sharp Cheddar cheese (4 ounces)

1. Cut the dark green portion off the leeks and discard. Quarter the leeks lengthwise, leaving the roots intact, and rinse any grit from in between the layers. Trim and discard the roots from the leeks and then thinly slice.

2. Arrange the rack in the upper third of the oven and preheat the oven to 425°F. Lightly butter a 2-quart shallow casserole (such as a 12-inch oval) and set aside.

3. Melt the butter in a medium saucepan over medium heat. Add the leeks and garlic and cook, stirring often, until softened, about 6 minutes.

4. Meanwhile, in a 2-cup glass measuring cup, whisk together the broth, cornstarch, flour, salt, and pepper. Add the broth mixture to the leeks and whisk until simmering, thickened, and smooth. Cook, whisking, 1 minute more. Whisk in the milk and bring to a boil. Remove from the heat.

5. Peel the potatoes (if desired) and then thinly slice. Immediately layer half of the potato slices in the casserole (to prevent discoloration), sprinkle half of the Cheddar evenly on top, and then top with the remaining potato slices. Pour the sauce evenly over the potatoes and sprinkle the remaining Cheddar on top.

6. Cover the casserole snugly with foil and bake for 45 minutes. Remove the foil and continue cooking for about 20 minutes, until the potatoes are very tender and the top is lightly golden. Let cool slightly before serving.

Grasshopper Potato Salad

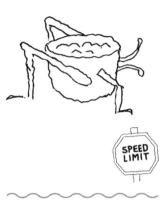

There aren't any bugs in this salad, but you can let your kid think it's chock-full. Canned green chiles and chopped scallions add zip, and yogurt adds tang. Serve warm or at room temperature with meat, poultry, or fish. You can peel the potatoes before cutting them up, but it isn't necessary.

1½ pounds thin-skinned white potatoes (3 medium), cut into 1-inch chunks
¾ cup plain reduced-fat yogurt
¼ cup reduced-fat mayonnaise
One 4.25-ounce can chopped mild green chiles
½ tablespoon rice vinegar or distilled white vinegar
1½ teaspoons kosher salt
¼ teaspoon freshly ground black pepper
4 scallion greens, thinly sliced (white portions reserved for another use)
1 large celery rib, finely diced
½ cup finely diced peeled Granny Smith (or any other crisp) apple

PREP: 10 minutes
COOKING: 15 minutes
SPEED LIMIT: 25 mpr

Makes 6 servings

PER SERVING:
164 calories, 4g fat
(1g saturated),
30g carbohydrates,
2.5g fiber, 4g protein

1. Place the potatoes in a large saucepan with cold water to cover. Bring to a boil, reduce the heat, and simmer until tender, about 15 minutes. Drain well in a colander.

2. In a large bowl, whisk together the yogurt, mayonnaise, chiles, vinegar, salt, and pepper. Add the warm potatoes and toss well. Add the scallion greens, celery, and apple and toss again.

Perfect Rice

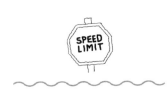

We like rice that is fluffy, chewy, and sticks together slightly—like the kind you can get at a great Chinese restaurant. This recipe is for long-grain or short-grain rice, but not sweet rice or sticky rice, which needs to be soaked before cooking. Your rice will come out consistently reliable to serve with anything. If you want to season the rice or add butter, do so after cooking.

PREP: 5 minutes
COOKING: 20 minutes
SPEED LIMIT: 25 mpr

Makes about 8 cups

PER ½ CUP:
*113 calories, 1g fat
(0g saturated),
24g carbohydrates,
1g fiber, 2g protein*

3 cups long-grain brown rice, brown basmati, or jasmine rice
3 cups cold filtered water

1. Place the rice in a heavy 2- to 3-quart saucepan with a lid. Add enough cold water to fill the pot, swish the rice and water around with your hand for a minute, and then drain well, catching the rice in a strainer. Repeat this process twice, until the poured-off water is clear.

2. Return the rice to the pot and add the measured water. Place over high heat and bring to a boil without disturbing, then (as soon as possible) cover with a lid and reduce the heat to the lowest setting. Let steam for 20 minutes without removing the lid or until tender.

3. Fluff the rice with a fork, remove from the heat, and cover with the lid to keep warm for up to 30 minutes.

Cooks' Note

❖ If you want to make a half batch of rice, use a 1-quart pot. (We do not recommend treated rice, such as rice mixes and converted or "quick" rice.)

Grilled Spudniks

These potatoes will send the kids into orbit! They are great to make—whatever else you're cooking on the grill. Because the spuds are sliced thin they cook quickly.

3 medium baking potatoes (1½ pounds)
3 tablespoons extra-virgin olive oil
Kosher salt and freshly ground black pepper

1. Prepare the grill: Arrange coals for indirect heat, or set a gas grill at medium flame.

2. Slice the unpeeled potatoes lengthwise into ¼-inch-thick slices. Brush on both sides with the oil and sprinkle lightly with salt and pepper.

3. Place the potato slices on the grill, cover, and cook for 5 minutes. Turn the potato slices with tongs, cover, and cook 5 minutes more, until golden and crisp on the outside and tender inside.

Loaded Spudniks: For a snack or an appetizer, simply top the grilled potato slices with shredded cheese and heat until melted. Add sliced scallions, chopped tomatoes, and chopped green chiles and serve with plain yogurt or reduced-fat sour cream.

PREP: 5 minutes
GRILLING: 10 minutes
SPEED LIMIT: 15 mpr

Makes 6 servings

PER SERVING:
*155 calories, 7g fat
(1g saturated),
21g carbohydrates,
2g fiber, 2g protein*

Creamed Spinach

Who doesn't love a deliciously naughty dish of creamy spinach? Ours is slimmed down yet still retains a lusciousness that is addictive.

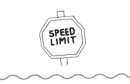

PREP: 10 minutes
COOKING: 10 minutes
SPEED LIMIT: 20 mpr

Makes 6 servings

PER SERVING:
*240 calories, 13g fat
(8g saturated),
29g carbohydrates,
9g fiber, 7g protein*

*One 2½-pound bag baby leaf spinach
2 tablespoons unsalted butter
1 large onion, finely chopped
2 tablespoons unbleached all-purpose flour
1½ cups whole milk
1 tablespoon cornstarch
½ cup heavy cream
1½ teaspoons kosher salt
¼ teaspoon freshly ground black pepper*

1. Bring 2 inches of water to boil in a 6-quart pot. Add half of the spinach leaves and stir until wilted, about 2 minutes. Add the remaining spinach a few handfuls at a time, stirring until wilted and then adding more spinach. Drain the spinach in a colander. Rinse with cold running water until cool.

2. Melt the butter in the same pot over medium heat. Add the onion and cook, stirring occasionally, until golden, about 5 minutes. Add the flour and stir for 1 minute. Gradually whisk in the milk and bring to a boil. In a measuring cup, stir the cornstarch into the cream and then whisk that mixture into the milk mixture along with the salt and pepper. Whisk while simmering for 2 minutes and then reduce the heat to low.

3. Squeeze the spinach in batches by hand or in a fine-mesh sieve to remove as much liquid as possible. Stir the spinach into the sauce and serve.

Cooks' Note

❖ You can make the spinach a day ahead and reheat in a saucepan, stirring over medium heat until hot, or reheat in a bowl in the microwave.

*"This is the best green food I ever had!" says Christina H.,
nine years old, of Atlanta, Georgia.*

Blasted Winter Vegetables

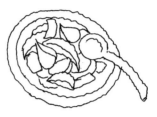

The kids will curse veggies no more after trying these tasty flash-roasted vegetables. Serve them warm as a side dish or cool as a salad.

1 pound parsnips, peeled and cut into 2-inch-long sticks $\frac{1}{2}$ inch thick
1 pound carrots, peeled and cut crosswise into 2-inch-long sticks
   $\frac{1}{2}$ inch thick
1 bunch scallions, trimmed and cut into 1-inch pieces
2 tablespoons extra-virgin olive oil
2 teaspoons fresh rosemary leaves or 1 teaspoon dried
$\frac{1}{2}$ teaspoon kosher salt
Freshly ground black pepper
3 cups medium-size broccoli florets (from large bunch)
4 garlic cloves, smashed, peeled, and thinly sliced
3 sprigs fresh thyme

PREP: 5 minutes
ROASTING: 20 minutes
SPEED LIMIT: 25 mpr

Makes 8 servings

PER SERVING:
100 calories,
4g fat (.5g saturated),
16g carbohydrates,
5g fiber, 2g protein

1. Arrange the oven rack in the upper third of the oven and preheat the oven to 500°F. Line a large shallow baking sheet with parchment or foil. Combine the parsnips, carrots, and scallions on the sheet; drizzle the oil on top, toss well, and then spread the vegetables out in an even layer. Sprinkle the rosemary, salt, and pepper on top.

2. Roast the vegetables for 10 minutes. Add the broccoli and garlic, stir to mix, and spread the vegetables out again in an even layer. Scatter the thyme on top and bake about 10 minutes longer, until the vegetables are tender and golden brown on the edges.

Zucchini-Parmesan Pancakes

In September, when zucchini is abundant, the versatile veggie is inexpensive and the prime ingredient in these little green pancakes, which are tender and flavorful.

PREP: 25 minutes
COOKING: 15 minutes
SPEED LIMIT: 40 mpr

Makes 6 servings (about a dozen 3-inch pancakes)

PER SERVING
(2 PANCAKES):
175 calories,
10g fat (5g saturated),
10g carbohydrates,
1.5g fiber, 10g protein

1 pound zucchini (3 to 4 small)
1 tablespoon kosher salt
1 large egg
¾ cup finely grated Parmesan cheese, preferably Parmigiano-Reggiano
¼ cup whole-wheat flour
¼ cup unbleached all-purpose flour
2 tablespoons minced fresh chives or scallion greens
1 teaspoon baking powder
½ teaspoon baking soda
¼ teaspoon freshly ground black pepper
1 tablespoon extra-virgin olive oil
1 tablespoon unsalted butter, softened

1. Trim the zucchini and coarsely shred in a food processor or with a box grater; place in a colander, sprinkle the salt on top, and toss well. Let stand for 15 minutes to draw out moisture from the zucchini.

2. Squeeze the zucchini one handful at a time to remove as much liquid as possible and then transfer to a medium bowl. Add the egg, Parmesan, flours, chives, baking powder, baking soda, and pepper. Mix well with a rubber spatula until blended.

3. Lightly oil a griddle or a nonstick large skillet with the olive oil and heat over medium heat until hot. Add a heaping tablespoon of batter for each pancake to the skillet, spreading each mound lightly into a 3-inch circle. Let cook until golden brown underneath, about 4 minutes. Flip with a spatula and cook until golden on the other side, about 3 minutes more. Transfer the pancakes to a platter and immediately spread with a little butter. Repeat with the remaining batter.

"They are so yummy, Mommy!" says six-year-old Ruby S., of Amagansett, New York. Mom Juliana now makes them all the time for her.

Harvest Ratatouille

This vegetable stew, a Provençal classic, is slow-cooked, so it melts in your mouth. See the Cooks' Note for ideas on how to make it a main course.

2 medium eggplant (10 to 12 ounces each), quartered and cut
    into ½-inch dice (not necessary to peel)
½ teaspoon kosher salt, plus more to taste
One 28-ounce can Italian peeled tomatoes
5 tablespoons extra-virgin olive oil
5 small zucchini (about 1¼ pounds), trimmed, halved lengthwise, and
    sliced ¼ inch thick crosswise
1 yellow bell pepper, trimmed, seeded,
    and cut into thin strips
1 large onion, coarsely chopped
3 garlic cloves, smashed, peeled, and minced
Freshly ground black pepper

PREP: 20 minutes
COOKING: 45 minutes

**Makes 9 cups (8 to
10 side-dish servings)**

PER CUP:
135 calories,
8g fat (1g saturated),
14g carbohydrates,
5g fiber, 3g protein

1. Place the eggplant in a colander, sprinkle with the salt, and toss; let stand in the sink for 15 minutes. Rinse the eggplant and pat dry with a towel.

2. Meanwhile, drain the tomatoes in a sieve set over a bowl, reserving the juice. Halve and seed the tomatoes, scraping the seeds into the sieve. Coarsely dice the tomato flesh and add to the bowl with the juice and reserve.

3. Heat 1½ tablespoons of the oil in a nonstick 12-inch skillet over medium-heat, add the zucchini, and cook, stirring often, until golden, about 4 minutes. Transfer to a 4- to 6-quart pot. Add 2 tablespoons of oil and the eggplant to the skillet and cook, stirring, until soft and golden, about 4 minutes. Transfer to the pot.

4. Add the remaining 1½ tablespoons oil to the skillet. Add the bell pepper, onion, and garlic and cook, stirring, over medium heat until softened, about 6 minutes. Transfer to the pot. Add the tomatoes and juice and bring to a boil. Reduce the heat to medium-low, partially cover with a lid, and simmer, stirring occasionally, until the vegetables are tender and the mixture is thickened, about 30 minutes. Season with salt and pepper to taste.

Cooks' Note

❖ For a main course, serve the ratatouille over whole-wheat pasta or Perfect Rice (page 196) or sandwich between split focaccia (page 66) or use in an omelet (page 42).

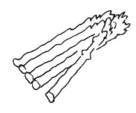

Totem Poles
(Roasted Asparagus)

Even the finicky will enjoy the intense flavor of toasty roasted spears of thick asparagus.

PREP: 5 minutes
ROASTING: 10 minutes
SPEED LIMIT: 15 mpr

Makes 8 servings

PER SERVING:
*30 calories, 1g fat
(0g saturated),
2g carbohydrates,
1g fiber, 1g protein*

2 pounds thick asparagus
1 tablespoon extra-virgin olive oil
Kosher salt and freshly ground black pepper

1. Arrange a rack in the upper third of the oven and preheat the oven to 500°F. Line a large shallow baking sheet with foil or parchment paper.

2. Snap the bottom ends off the asparagus. Rinse the spears and place in a pile on the sheet. Drizzle the oil on top and toss to coat; arrange in an even layer and season lightly with salt and pepper.

3. Roast the asparagus for 8 to 10 minutes, just until fork-tender.

Asparagus in a Blanket: Let the asparagus cool and then wrap in very thin slices of imported prosciutto de Parma. You can then dip the spears into Horseradish Dunk (page 103).

Fifteen-year-old Hayley K., of Rhinebeck, New York, is tall, lean, and strong and has always loved her veggies. "Roasted asparagus is awesome—hot or cold."

all steamed up!

Steaming is a healthy, fast method for cooking vegetables like asparagus. The natural flavor of the veggies is retained, and if done properly, their color will be bright and their texture crisp-tender. Here are a few tricks to steaming:

You can use a metal steaming insert or a bamboo steamer. Fill a large saucepan or a wok with an inch or two of water and bring to a boil. Meanwhile, cut up the vegetables—try to cut various vegetables uniformly, so they will cook evenly. (Carrots and potatoes take a little longer to cook, so cut them smaller and place in the steamer first, before any green vegetables.) Insert the steamer into the pan, place the veggies inside the steamer, and cover with the pan lid. Let cook until the vegetables are just fork-tender, checking after about 3 minutes. Serve immediately.

Turkish Green Beans

This is a delicious take on green bean casserole. We especially like to make this recipe with haricots verts, thin French green beans.

12 ounces green beans, stem ends trimmed
2 tablespoons unsalted butter
1 medium onion, finely chopped
1 garlic clove, smashed, peeled, and minced
½ teaspoon dried marjoram
¾ cup plain whole milk yogurt
¼ teaspoon kosher salt
Freshly ground black pepper

PREP: 4 minutes
COOKING: 6 minutes
SPEED LIMIT: 10 mpr

Makes 6 servings

PER SERVING:
*75 calories, 5g fat
(3g saturated),
7g carbohydrates,
2.5g fiber, 2g protein*

1. Bring 1 inch of water to a boil in a medium skillet. Add the beans, reduce the heat slightly, and simmer until crisp-tender, 2 to 3 minutes. Drain in a colander and rinse with cold water to cool. Cut the beans into 1-inch pieces and reserve.

2. Wipe out the skillet. Add the butter and melt over medium heat. Add the onion, garlic, and marjoram and cook, stirring often, until golden, about 5 minutes. Stir in the beans and cook, stirring, until just tender, 2 to 3 minutes (add ¼ cup water during cooking if the mixture seems dry).

3. Add the yogurt, salt, and pepper and stir until saucy, and then transfer the bean mixture to a serving dish.

Cowboy Beans

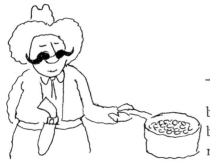

These rootin' tootin' beans have a kick yet are not far from typical baked beans. We prefer to cook the dried variety from scratch because canned beans contain so much sodium. To save some time, follow the quick-soak method described on the bag of beans.

1 pound dried small red beans, picked over and rinsed
8 cups filtered water
3 thick strips bacon, diced
2 medium onions, chopped
2 large garlic cloves, smashed, peeled, and finely chopped
One 14-ounce can crushed tomatoes
1 cup Thick 'n' Spicy Barbecue Sauce (page 211) or prepared
   barbecue sauce

PREP: 5 minutes plus soaking
SIMMERING: About 1½ hours

Makes 8 servings

PER SERVING:
310 calories, 7g fat (2g saturated), 45g carbohydrates, 5g fiber, 17g protein

1. Soak the beans according to the package directions.

2. Rinse the beans and place in a 4-quart pot with 7 cups of water. Bring to a boil, reduce the heat, and simmer, partially covered with a lid, until the beans are tender, about 45 minutes. Let cool and then drain. Wipe out the pot.

3. Cook the bacon in the same pot over medium heat, stirring occasionally, until crisp, about 5 minutes. Add the onions and garlic and cook over medium-low heat, stirring occasionally. Stir in the beans, crushed tomatoes, barbecue sauce, and the remaining cup of water. Bring to a boil, reduce the heat to medium-low, cover, and simmer for 45 minutes, stirring occasionally.

Cooks' Notes

❖ Dried beans, like any vegetable, need to be washed before cooking. Pick the beans over to remove any bits of debris before rinsing.

❖ If you're really short on time, you can substitute three 19-ounce cans of red beans or pinto beans (drained and rinsed) and go straight to step 3.

Six-year-old Rosey M., of Studio City, California, said,
"These beans are like a tornado in my mouth.
Is that why cowboys like them?
I like them, too."

Rainbow Slaw

Making this festive slaw is a snap with a food processor, but you can also chop it by hand with a large sharp knife. Serve it with Oven-Barbecued Beef (page 145), sandwiches, or grilled or roasted meats.

1/2 cup mayonnaise
1/3 cup plain whole milk yogurt or sour cream
1/3 unsweetened pineapple juice
1 1/4 teaspoons kosher salt
1/2 teaspoon freshly ground black pepper
1 medium red or green cabbage (about 1 3/4 pounds)
4 medium carrots, peeled
1 red bell pepper, finely diced
1 cup fresh corn kernels (from 2 ears) or thawed frozen corn (optional)
1/4 cup minced fresh chives
1 cup fresh baby spinach leaves

1. Combine the mayonnaise, yogurt, pineapple juice, salt, and pepper in an extra-large salad bowl and whisk to blend.

2. Fit a food processor with a slicing disk. Cut the cabbage in quarters and cut out the core of each section. Cut each quarter in half. Add the cabbage pieces to the feed tube of the processor and process to slice. Add to the bowl with the dressing. Repeat until all of the cabbage is sliced.

3. Switch to the shredding disk. Trim the carrots and cut into lengths that will fit into the feed tube. Shred the carrots in the processor. Add to the cabbage along with the bell pepper, corn, if using, and chives. Toss well to mix.

4. Just before serving, add the spinach and toss again.

PREP: 20 minutes
SPEED LIMIT: 20 mpr

**Makes about 2 quarts
to serve 8**

PER CUP:
177 calories,
12g fat (1g saturated),
17g carbohydrates,
4g fiber, 3g protein

Super-Mash!

The most important mash of all is the mighty spud. You can use baking potatoes or white potatoes with their skins, but we like peeled Yukon golds best. We needn't tell you what to serve these with—they go with everything. Feel free to do what you want to dress them up, including adding a drizzle of Basil Oil (page 221). You can add a bit of butter, but mashers without butter reheat better in the microwave.

PREP: 5 minutes
COOKING: 20 minutes
SPEED LIMIT: 25 mpr

Makes about 6 cups

PER 3/4 CUP:
100 calories,
5g fat (0g saturated),
22g carbohydrates,
2g fiber, 2.5g protein

2 pounds Yukon gold potatoes (about 5 medium potatoes)
1 teaspoon kosher salt
1/4 teaspoon freshly ground black pepper
1/2 cup plus 2 tablespoons reduced-fat (2%) milk

1. Peel the potatoes and cut into 1-inch chunks. Place in a large saucepan and add cold water to cover and a teaspoon of salt. Bring to a boil, reduce the heat to medium, and simmer until the potatoes are fork-tender, about 18 minutes.

2. Drain the potatoes well in a colander and then return to the pot. Add salt and pepper and mash well with a potato masher. Gradually beat in the milk using a wooden spoon. Season with more salt to taste and serve hot.

Cooks' Note

❖ You can substitute whole milk or half-and-half in the mash, but 2% milk is plenty rich. For a special treat, stir in a spoonful of sour cream or plain whole milk yogurt just before serving.

Tater-Brocky

Do your kids love mashed potatoes but have a fear of broccoli? Here is a good way to get them to have their taters and broccoli, too. We love Yukon golds here because they mash up fluffy. The broccoli, garlic, and Parmesan add a zesty Italian twist. Serve these green-speckled spuds with plain or highly seasoned meat or fish from our "Double Plays" (pages 135–152).

1½ pounds Yukon gold potatoes (4 medium), peeled
2 garlic cloves, smashed, peeled, and sliced
2 cups coarsely chopped broccoli
½ cup half-and-half
¼ cup finely grated Parmigiano-Reggiano
½ teaspoon kosher salt
¼ teaspoon freshly ground black pepper

1. Slice the potatoes in half and then cut into ½-inch-thick slices. Place in a medium saucepan with the garlic and cold water to cover. Bring to a boil, reduce the heat, and simmer until nearly tender, about 10 minutes. Add the broccoli and cook until barely tender, about 5 minutes more.

2. Drain the vegetables in a colander, return to the pot, and coarsely mash. Stir in the half-and-half, Parmesan, salt, and pepper. Serve warm.

Tater-Cali: Substitute cauliflower for the broccoli and add ½ cup shredded Swiss cheese instead of the Parmesan.

PREP: 10 minutes
COOKING: 20 minutes
SPEED LIMIT: 30 mpr

Makes 6 servings (about 4½ cups)

PER SERVING (¾ CUP):
162 calories,
4g fat (2.5g saturated),
26g carbohydrates,
4g fiber, 6g protein

Squish Squash

This mash works with both butternut and acorn squash, but most kids prefer the sweetness of butternut. Roast extra squash to make a batch of luscious Butternut Squash Soup (see below), which you can freeze.

1 medium butternut squash (about 1½ pounds)
2 tablespoons unsalted butter
Pinch of nutmeg
Kosher salt and freshly ground black pepper

1. Preheat the oven to 400°F and line a baking sheet with foil.

2. Trim the top off the squash with a large sharp knife. Cut the squash in quarters. Arrange the pieces skin side up on the baking sheet and bake for about 45 minutes, until the skin is beginning to brown and the squash is fork-tender.

3. Let the squash cool for about 10 minutes (until cool enough to handle), scoop out the seeds and discard, and then scoop the flesh into a bowl. Add the butter and nutmeg and mash coarsely with a potato masher. Add salt and pepper to taste.

Butternut Squash Soup: Combine 2 cups cooked squash flesh, 2 cups vegetable broth, ½ teaspoon kosher salt, ¼ teaspoon freshly ground black pepper, and a pinch of nutmeg. Puree in a blender in batches and transfer to a medium saucepan. Cook over medium heat, stirring, until hot. Season to taste. Makes 1 quart. Garnish each serving with a small dollop of plain yogurt or reduced-fat sour cream, or a spoonful of soft blue cheese, such as Gorgonzola Dolce.

PREP: 10 minutes
ROASTING: 1 hour and 15 minutes

Makes 6 servings

PER ½ CUP:
72 calories,
4g fat (2g saturated),
10g carbohydrates,
3g fiber, 1g protein

Yummy Yammy-Parsnip Mash

Kids love the subtle sweetness of parsnips and sweet potatoes smashed together. For a smoother finish, you can puree in the food processor.

1 pound parsnips (4 medium), peeled, halved lengthwise, and cut into
  ½-inch pieces
1 pound orange sweet potatoes (2 medium), peeled, halved lengthwise,
  and cut into 1-inch pieces
2 tablespoons light brown sugar
1 tablespoon unsalted butter
¼ cup low-sodium canned vegetable broth or chicken broth
2 tablespoons heavy cream
¾ teaspoon kosher salt
½ teaspoon pumpkin pie spice or ground ginger
2 pinches of freshly ground black pepper

PREP: 5 minutes
COOKING: 21 minutes
SPEED LIMIT: 26 mpr

Makes 8 servings

PER ½ CUP:
106 calories, 3g fat
(2g saturated),
19g carbohydrates,
3.5g fiber, 1.5g protein

1. Fill a medium saucepan half full of water and bring to a boil. Add the parsnips and sweet potatoes, reduce the heat, and simmer until the vegetables are tender, about 18 minutes. Drain well in a colander and return the vegetables to the pan.

2. Add the brown sugar and butter and mash coarsely with a potato masher. Stir in the broth, cream, salt, pie spice, and pepper and cook, stirring occasionally, until warm, about 3 minutes.

Blender Hollandaise

Hollandaise is a natural paired with poached eggs, steak, salmon, roasted vegetables, and steamed broccoli and asparagus.

PREP: 5 minutes
COOKING: 3 minutes
SPEED LIMIT: 8 mpr

Makes about 1¼ cups (about 10 servings)

PER 2-TABLESPOON SERVING:
179 calories, 20g fat (12g saturated), 0g carbohydrates, 0g fiber, 1g protein

2 sticks unsalted butter
3 large egg yolks
1½ tablespoons fresh lemon juice
½ cup boiling filtered water
Kosher salt and freshly ground black pepper

1. Bring an inch of water to a simmer in a medium saucepan over medium heat.

2. Meanwhile, place the butter in a small saucepan and melt over low heat.

3. Combine the yolks and lemon juice in a blender. Turn on to medium speed and add the boiling water, pouring in a fine stream. Slowly drizzle in the hot melted butter and blend at high speed for 1 minute.

4. Transfer the sauce to a stainless-steel bowl. Place over the saucepan of simmering water and stir constantly with a whisk until the sauce is as thick as whipped cream, about 3 minutes. Season to taste with salt and pepper and serve warm.

Cooks' Note

❖ You can keep the sauce warm over a hot (not simmering) water bath for up to an hour.

Thick 'n' Spicy Barbecue Sauce

This very thick delicious sauce will keep, refrigerated, for up to 2 months. You can add more honey or vinegar according to your preference.

1/4 cup vegetable oil

2 medium onions, finely chopped

2 garlic cloves, smashed, peeled, and minced

1 cup medium salsa, such as Sunny Summer Salsa (page 107)
or store-bought, such as Green Mountain Gringo

1 cup tomato sauce, such as Quick Skillet Tomato Sauce (page 213)

1/2 cup cider vinegar

1/2 cup honey

1. Heat the oil in a medium saucepan over medium heat. Add the onion and garlic and cook, stirring often, until softened, about 6 minutes. Stir in the remaining ingredients and bring to a boil. Reduce the heat and simmer, stirring often, until thickened, about 15 minutes.

2. Carefully puree the sauce in 2 or 3 batches in a blender or food processor and let cool. Transfer to a jar, cover, and chill until ready to use.

PREP: 10 minutes
COOKING: 21 minutes
SPEED LIMIT: 31 mpr

Makes 1 quart

PER 1/4 CUP:
82 calories,
3.5g fat (.5g saturated),
12g carbohydrates,
1g fiber, 1g protein

Grilled Tomato Sauce

This sauce is delicious tossed with pasta and you can use it for any recipe in this book that calls for tomato sauce. We like the intensity of the tomato flavor that is achieved through grilling over charcoal—this is a great way to make use of red-hot coals that you've just finished cooking on. If you don't have a grill, you can cook the tomatoes on the stove in a grill pan over medium heat or under the broiler with great results.

PREP: 5 minutes
COOKING: 15 minutes
SPEED LIMIT: 20 mpr

Makes 4 cups, enough for 1 pound pasta

PER ½ CUP:
100 calories, 8g fat
(3.5g saturated),
4g carbohydrates,
1g fiber, 2.5g protein

12 large ripe plum tomatoes (1¾ pounds)
2 tablespoons extra-virgin olive oil
⅓ cup heavy cream
1 teaspoon kosher salt
¼ teaspoon freshly ground black pepper
2 tablespoons chopped fresh parsley
¼ cup finely grated Parmigiano-Reggiano

1. Prepare a grill.

2. With a small sharp knife, carefully cut out the core of each tomato and discard. Toss the tomatoes in the oil in a large bowl. Add the tomatoes to the grill, reserving the bowl with the oil. Cover the tomatoes and cook, turning occasionally with tongs, until the skins are charred and the flesh is softened, about 15 minutes. Place the tomatoes on a plate, let cool slightly, and carefully remove the blackened skins using the tongs.

3. Transfer the tomatoes back to the bowl with the oil and mash with a potato masher (or place in a food processor and pulse the tomatoes and the reserved oil) until chunky. Add the cream, salt, pepper, parsley, and Parmesan and stir to combine.

Cooks' Note

❖ While the tomatoes are grilling, cook 1 pound of your favorite pasta in boiling salted water, stirring often, until al dente, and drain. When the sauce is ready, add it to the pasta, along with more chopped fresh parsley or basil. Season to taste with salt and pepper and serve with more Parmesan.

Quick Skillet Tomato Sauce

When it seems like there is nothing around the house to eat, head for the pantry. Hopefully, you have a couple of cans of tomatoes and some pasta on hand. Because this sauce is cooked quickly, you must be careful not to get splattered with the bubbling tomatoes when stirring. For safety, use an oven mitt and stand back!

3 tablespoons extra-virgin olive oil
6 garlic cloves
Two 28-ounce cans crushed tomatoes
Kosher salt and freshly ground black pepper

PREP: 5 minutes
COOKING: 30 minutes
SPEED LIMIT: 35 mpr

Makes about 6 cups

1. Heat the oil in a 10-inch skillet with a lid over medium heat.

2. Meanwhile, trim the stem ends off the garlic, crush each clove with the side of a large knife, and discard the peel. Add the garlic to the oil and cook, stirring, until golden, 1 to 2 minutes. Pour in the tomatoes, cover, and bring to a boil. Reduce the heat to low, cover with the lid, and simmer, stirring occasionally, until the sauce is smooth and thick, about 25 minutes. Season to taste with salt and pepper.

PER ½ CUP:
77 calories, 3.5g fat
(.5g saturated),
9g carbohydrates,
2g fiber, 2g protein

Cooks' Note

❖ If you like a chunkier, slightly thinner sauce, use 2 cans of Italian peeled tomatoes; drain them (discarding the juice) and chop the tomatoes by hand or pulse in the food processor until coarsely chopped. Proceed as directed to make a generous 3 cups.

Eat-Yer-Veggies Cheese Sauce

Cheese, like bacon, makes almost everything taste better. Serve this simple sauce on steamed or roasted vegetables, Perfect Poached Eggs (page 43), plain grilled chicken, hamburgers, sausages, or even whole-wheat toast. You'll never eat processed cheese again!

COOKING: 6 minutes

SPEED LIMIT: 6 mpr

Makes about 1 cup

PER 2-TABLESPOON SERVING:
95 calories, 7g fat (4g saturated), 3g carbohydrates, 0g fiber, 5g protein

1 cup whole milk
1 tablespoon cornstarch
1 tablespoon unsalted butter
1 tablespoon unbleached all-purpose flour
1 cup (packed) shredded sharp Cheddar cheese (4 ounces)
½ teaspoon kosher salt
¼ teaspoon freshly ground black pepper

1. Stir together the milk and cornstarch in a small bowl.

2. Melt the butter in a medium saucepan over medium heat, add the flour, and stir for 1 minute. Gradually whisk the milk into the pan. Cook, stirring with the whisk, until the mixture boils. Reduce the heat and simmer, whisking, for 2 minutes. Stir in the cheese, salt, and pepper.

ABC Vinaigrette

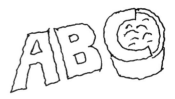

Freshly made salad dressing is as easy as 1–2–3 and better than going to the store to buy the bottled stuff. If you want to make a big batch to keep in the fridge for a few days, quadruple the recipe, adding the ingredients to a glass jar with a lid. Let stand at room temperature for about 10 minutes before using.

> 1½ teaspoons red wine vinegar
> ½ teaspoon Dijon mustard
> 2 tablespoons extra-virgin olive oil
> Kosher salt and freshly ground black pepper

Whisk together the vinegar and mustard in a medium bowl. Gradually whisk in the oil and season with 3 pinches of salt and several grindings of black pepper.

ABC Salad: To make a perfect light lunch or side, just combine the dressing in a large salad bowl—wooden if you have one—add 6 cups lightly packed prewashed organic baby greens, and toss. You can top the salad with roasted meat or poultry, hard-cooked eggs, or grilled shrimp or vegetables.

PREP: 5 minutes
SPEED LIMIT: 5 mpr

Makes 4 servings

PER SERVING:
77 calories, 7g fat
(1g saturated),
2.5g carbohydrates,
2g fiber, 1g protein

Teriyaki Vinaigrette

This dressing with an Asian twist is great when you want to serve a side salad with a stir-fry or another Asian dish. Try drizzling the dressing over steamed or roasted vegetables.

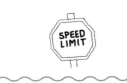

PREP: 5 minutes
SPEED LIMIT: 5 mpr

Makes about ½ cup

PER ½ TABLESPOON:
44 calories, 5g fat
(.5g saturated),
0g carbohydrates,
0g fiber, 0g protein

1 tablespoon soy sauce
2 tablespoons rice wine vinegar
⅓ cup mild olive oil
Kosher salt and freshly ground black pepper

Combine the soy sauce and vinegar in a small jar. Add the oil and shake well until blended. Season to taste with salt and pepper and shake again.

Mexican Adobo Dressing

You may think "Russian dressing" when you look at this, but the smoky slightly spicy flavor is more "south of the border" thanks to chipotle chile in adobo. Try drizzling on a green salad, smear it on Mini-Cuban Sandos (page 92), or dip crudités into it. You can go from little spice to quite a bit, depending on how much chile you put in.

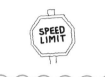

½ cup mayonnaise
3 tablespoons ketchup
1 teaspoon distilled white vinegar
1 teaspoon yellow mustard or Dijon mustard
1 teaspoon chopped chipotle chile in adobo, or more to taste

PREP: 5 minutes
SPEED LIMIT: 5 mpr

Makes about ³/₄ cup

PER TABLESPOON:
*70 calories, 7g fat
(1g saturated),
1g carbohydrates,
0g fiber, 0g protein*

Combine all of the ingredients in a small bowl and stir to blend. Add more chipotle, up to 1 tablespoon, as desired. Store the unused portion in a small glass jar with a tight-fitting lid and chill for up to 1 month.

Cooks' Note

❖ Canned chipotles in adobo are available at most supermarkets in the Latino section. It's a good idea to coarsely chop up the whole can (by hand or in the food processor) and store in a covered jar in the refrigerator for up to 4 months. A little goes a long way!

Blue on Blue Dressing

No blue cheese dressing can beat this. Use Greek yogurt or organic whole milk or low-fat yogurt, such as Stonyfield.

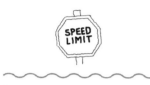

PREP: 5 minutes
STANDING: 20 minutes
SPEED LIMIT: 25 mpr

Makes about 3 cups

PER TABLESPOON:
35 calories,
3g fat (1g saturated),
.5g carbohydrates,
og fiber, 1g protein

> *One 6-ounce piece firm blue cheese, preferably Maytag or Danish blue*
> *1 cup plain whole milk yogurt*
> *½ cup reduced-fat mayonnaise*
> *3 tablespoons rice vinegar*
> *¾ cup reduced-fat (2%) milk*

Place the blue cheese in a medium bowl and coarsely crumble with a fork. Stir in the yogurt, mayonnaise, and vinegar, mixing well. Stir in the milk and let stand, stirring occasionally, for 20 minutes. Transfer the dressing to a large jar and chill for up to 1 month.

Cooks' Note

❖ The dressing tends to thicken over time. Stir in a little water if you want to thin the dressing, and shake to blend.

Rockin' Ranch Dressing

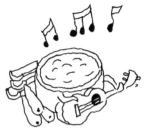

We keep a batch of this delicious dressing in our fridges at all times for quick salads, as a dip for veggies, and for drizzling on burgers, sandwiches, and more. Store the dressing in a glass jar with a lid.

1 cup reduced-fat mayonnaise
1 cup plain low-fat yogurt, such as Stonyfield
1 large garlic clove, smashed, peeled, and minced
Kosher salt and freshly ground black pepper
2 tablespoons minced fresh chives

Place the mayonnaise in a medium bowl. Whisk in the yogurt and garlic and season to taste with salt and pepper. Stir in the chives and serve.

PREP: 5 minutes
SPEED LIMIT: 5 mpr

Makes about 2 cups

PER TABLESPOON:
30 calories, 2.5g fat
(.5g saturated),
1g carbohydrates,
0g fiber, .5g protein

"The ranch dressing was so, so, so good. It really made my carrots smile," said Julia B., five years old and living in Rye, New York.

Tzatziki

This Greek yogurt and cucumber sauce is great served with seafood and spicy meat dishes. It's a nice fresh change from tartar sauce.

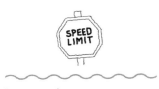

PREP: 5 minutes
SPEED LIMIT: 5 mpr

Makes about 1½ cups

PER 2-TABLESPOON
SERVING:
*29 calories, 2g fat
(.5g saturated),
2g carbohydrates,
0g fiber, 1g protein*

2 small Kirby cucumbers, peeled, seeded, and finely chopped
1 small garlic clove, smashed, peeled, and minced
⅔ cup whole milk yogurt
¼ cup light mayonnaise
¾ teaspoon kosher salt
Freshly ground black pepper

Combine all of the ingredients in a small bowl and stir well with a fork to blend. Keep covered in the refrigerator until ready to use.

Cooks' Note

❧ The best yogurts are those whole milk ones from Greece, which are available in many supermarkets. They are very rich with a deep satisfying flavor. Another great option is to buy yogurt from your local organic dairy farmer.

Basil Oil

Make a big batch of this in late summer, when delicious basil is so abundant. Transfer the basil oil to a jar, add a layer of extra-virgin olive oil on top to seal it, and cover tightly with a lid and refrigerate (or freeze). It will stay fresh for several weeks if you keep the top covered with oil. Drizzle the oil over eggs, pasta, potatoes, soup, meats, or poultry.

2 cups lightly packed fresh basil leaves
1 cup extra-virgin olive oil
1 tablespoon red wine vinegar
½ teaspoon kosher salt

Wash the basil leaves thoroughly and spin dry. Transfer to the blender with ½ cup of the oil. Add the vinegar and salt and blend at medium speed until the basil is finely chopped. With the blender running, drizzle in the remaining ½ cup oil and blend at high speed until smooth.

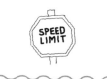

PREP: 5 minutes
SPEED LIMIT: 5 mpr

Makes 1 cup

PER TABLESPOON:
*127 calories, 14g fat
(2g saturated),
0g carbohydrates,
0g fiber, 0g protein*

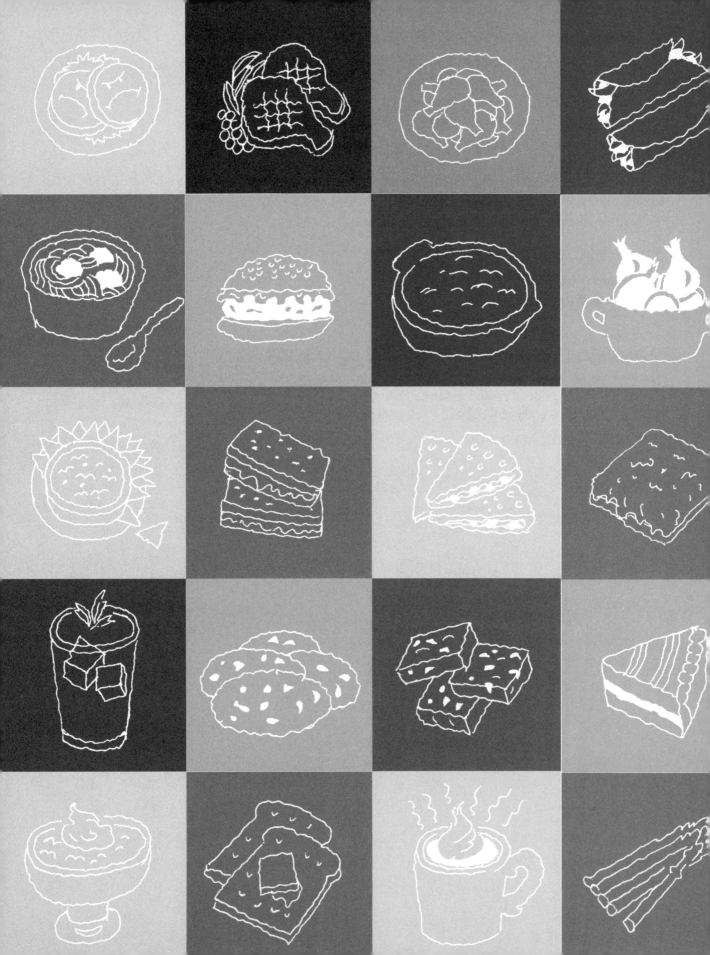

chapter seven

Quality Quenchers
Cold and Warm Drinks
for Thirsty Kids

Nutritionists will tell you there are few dietary evils greater than soft drinks. These should be exiled from most households and be an item that children can have only on rare occasions. If, from the beginning, soda is accurately described to kids as artificially colored, calorie-rich, carbonated chemicals, perhaps fewer will opt to drink it.

A regular Coca-Cola packs about 155 empty calories in a 12-ounce can, so if a child has one at lunch and dinner, that adds 310 excess calories a day, nearly a quarter of his daily calorie intake. And he won't necessarily eat less later to compensate, which means he might have too many calories for a given day. Then there is the caffeine, which, according to the National Sleep Foundation, robs our children of sleep—just one caffeinated beverage each day could add up to $3\frac{1}{2}$ hours of lost sleep a week.

Beverages like Snapple aren't a much better deal—one 12-ounce can has about 170 calories and 40 grams of sugar in some form or another, which would take an hour of exercise to burn off. There is also high-fructose corn syrup, which is added to so many beverages because it is cheaper than sugar. Avoid everything that contains it. (It's even in salad dressings and other foods you wouldn't think of.) In addition, some children may be sensitive to the artificial coloring used, which can contribute to hyperactivity.

Nutritionists are not crazy about sugary fruit juices either. We know one could argue that at least with juice kids are getting some vitamins and minerals, but they would get more nutrition and fiber from whole fruit, at one-third the calories.

Diet sodas that contain artificial sweeteners claim to be safe, yet no one knows for sure. More testing is needed on sugar substitutes such as aspartame (NutraSweet) and sucralose (Splenda), and although they may not seem harmful in the short term, we don't know their long-term effects.

But just as we need to watch for empty calories in drinks and foods, some mothers have justified concern about children who are slight, who often don't eat much. These children need to have beverages that are more caloric and nutritious to help with their growth. It is important to add protein and vitamins, whenever possible, to the diets of these children—through fresh ingredients and supplementation (protein powder or other), if necessary. Likewise, drinking fresh juices (with the aid of a juicer) enables some kids to get added vitamins they won't get if they are picky eaters. Drinks can be a fantastic way to add real nutrition.

So, what is a parent to offer kids, besides our top two beverage choices of water and skim milk? Here are some nutritious options when something a little more interesting is desired. What follows are refreshing creative beverages, both cool and hot, that are light on sugar and caffeine—perfect for any day and any age.

creative coolers: cold and refreshing quaffers

From lemonade to smoothies, these quenching quaffers will go down cold and fast. They are a breeze to whip up, and you can teach your kids how to make them. You will notice that some of these recipes specify filtered water. As we explained in our Introduction, we prefer filtered water, water that comes out of a filtered tap, from a Brita or Pur filtered pitcher, or from a bottle, to water straight from the tap.

Boardwalk Fresh Lemonade

Berry Delicious Iced Tea

Island-Style Smoothie

Blueberry Cheesecake Smoothie

Strawberry Cheesecake Smoothie

Mango Lassi

Fresh Iced Tea

Minted Iced Green Tea

Boardwalk Fresh Lemonade

We love getting freshly squeezed lemonade at the boardwalk or from road-side stands helmed by little ones. For a different taste, try adding a little sprig of fresh mint to the finished drink.

¼ cup fresh lemon juice (from 2 medium lemons)
¾ cup water
2 tablespoons sugar
1 tablespoon honey
Ice, for serving

Combine the lemon juice and water in a tall glass. Add the sugar and honey and stir for about a minute to dissolve. Add ice to fill the glass, and serve.

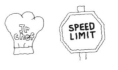

PREP: 2 minutes
SPEED LIMIT: 2 mpr

Makes 1 serving

PER SERVING:
140 calories, 0g fat,
40g carbohydrates,
0g fiber, 0g protein

"It's good!" says six-year-old Rosey M., of Studio City, Los Angeles.
"It's almost spicy and it's sweet. Daddy, I think
you could work at a lemonade store."

Berry Delicious Iced Tea

There is very little caffeine here, as the tea gets steeped for only a minute, but if it makes you concerned, substitute decaffeinated tea bags. This refreshing cooler is definitely one that the kids will love.

PREP: 20 minutes
SPEED LIMIT: 20 mpr

Makes ½ gallon (about 8 servings)

PER 8-OUNCE SERVING:
53 calories, 0g fat, 15g carbohydrates, 1g fiber, 0g protein

2 cups fresh raspberries or blackberries (12 ounces), plus more for garnish
1 cup plus 1 quart filtered water
¼ cup honey
¼ cup sugar
5 bags black tea bags or orange pekoe tea bags, tied together, tags removed
1 quart iced filtered water
Ice, for serving

1. Combine the berries, 1 cup of water, the honey, and sugar in a small saucepan and bring to a boil. Reduce the heat and simmer gently until the berries begin to break down, about 6 minutes. Strain the mixture through a fine sieve set over a heatproof bowl, pressing on the solids; set aside to cool.

2. Bring the remaining quart of water almost to a boil in a large saucepan. Remove from the heat and immediately add the tea bags. Let steep for 1 minute, then remove and discard the bags. Stir in the iced water. When the tea mixture is cool, transfer to a pitcher and stir in the berry syrup. Pour the finished tea over ice in tall glasses and garnish with more fresh berries.

*"I love this tea! I would definitely drink it on a hot day," says
Brittany R., age thirteen and living in Porter, Maine.*

Island-Style Smoothie

This fruit smoothie can be packed with protein if you add a scoop of soy protein powder, or for more fiber add a teaspoon of wheat germ.

1 cup vanilla low-fat yogurt
1 cup canned tropical fruit salad in natural juice, such as Dole
1 generous cup ice cubes
1 ripe medium banana
¾ cup reduced-fat unsweetened canned coconut milk (stir before adding)

Combine all of the ingredients in a blender. Blend on low speed and then increase to high speed, blending until smooth.

PREP: 5 minutes
SPEED LIMIT: 5 mpr

Makes 1 quart to serve 4

PER CUP:
135 calories, 3.5g fat
(3g saturated),
23g carbohydrates,
1g fiber, 3.5g protein

Blueberry Cheesecake Smoothie

PREP: 5 minutes
SPEED LIMIT: 5 mpr

**Makes about 3 cups
to serve 2**

PER SERVING:
205 calories, 6.5g fat
(3g saturated),
36g carbohydrates,
4g fiber, 4g protein

This tastes like a tangy blueberry milk shake. For a surprise treat, add a peeled fresh peach (or some drained canned peaches in light syrup) to the mixture before blending.

2 cups fresh or thawed frozen blueberries
1 graham cracker square
1 cup ice cubes
½ cup prepared lemonade or limeade
4 tablespoons Neufchâtel (reduced-fat) cream cheese
1 tablespoon honey

Combine all of the ingredients in order in a blender. Blend at medium and then high speed until smooth, about 2 minutes.

Strawberry Cheesecake Smoothie: Substitute fresh or frozen strawberries for the blueberries.

Mango Lassi

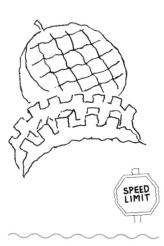

A *lassi* is an Indian drink, and traditionally a few drops of rosewater are added to the mango mixture before blending. This cooler is a cross between a fruit smoothie and a sherbet. Serve with mint sprigs, if desired.

1 ripe medium mango (about 12 ounces)
1 cup plain reduced-fat or whole milk yogurt
1 heaping cup ice cubes
½ cup pure mango nectar, apricot nectar, or unsweetened apple juice or orange juice
1 tablespoon honey

1. Cut up the mango: Place the fruit flat on a cutting board. Place your hand flat on top. Slice into the mango horizontally just above the center with a thin sharp knife and cut all the way across the top of the pit, which is flat but rather thick. Set the peel with the flesh aside, turn the fruit over, and repeat cutting over the pit. Score the flesh in the peel lengthwise, cutting several times, and then cut crosswise. Cut the scored pieces of mango away from the peel, cutting as close to the peel as possible. Place the fruit in the blender. Repeat with the remaining half.

2. Add the yogurt, ice, nectar, and honey and blend until smooth. Pour into two 10-ounce glasses and serve with straws.

Cooks' Notes

❖ We especially like this drink made with creamy 2% milk–fat Greek-style yogurt, such as Fage brand, which comes in 7-ounce containers.

❖ Frozen unsweetened cut-up mango is available in some supermarkets; measure out a generous cup and let thaw before using to make the drink.

Allaire M., a four-year-old living in Port Chester, New York, says she likes it because "it's not too sweet and it's kinda thick and tasty. Is this a milk shake?"

PREP: 10 minutes
SPEED LIMIT: 10 mpr

Makes 2 servings

PER 10-OUNCE SERVING:
144 calories, 1.3g fat
(1g saturated),
28g carbohydrates,
2g fiber, 6g protein

Fresh Iced Tea

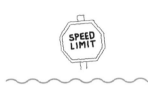

Iced tea is a favorite beverage, especially in the South, where you get a choice of "sweet" or "unsweet" tea. Our recipe makes lightly sweetened iced tea. In summer, add sprigs of fresh lemon verbena when you add the iced water and then strain.

PREP: 10 minutes
SPEED LIMIT: 10 mpr

Makes 2 quarts to serve 8

PER 8-OUNCE SERVING:
*72 calories, 0g fat,
22g carbohydrates,
0g fiber, 0g protein*

1 quart filtered water
7 black tea bags or orange pekoe tea bags
½ cup sugar
1 quart iced filtered water
Ice, for serving
Orange or lemon slices

Bring 1 quart water almost to a boil in a large saucepan. Remove from the heat, add the tea bags, and let steep for 2 minutes. Remove the bags and discard. Stir in the sugar and iced water. When the ice has melted, pour the tea over ice in tall glasses and serve with orange or lemon slices.

cute cubes

If you have ice-cube trays, try filling some with pure fruit juice, fruit puree, or melted chocolate whisked together with light cream. Freeze the cubes and add to a glass and fill with milk, seltzer, or fruit-accented seltzer.

Minted Iced Green Tea

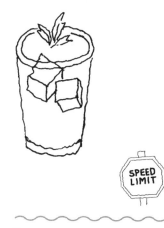

This is a great twist on regular iced tea and is especially good with spicy food. Removing the water from the heat just before boiling prevents iced tea from clouding.

> 1 quart filtered water
> 12 green tea bags
> ¾ cup sugar
> ¼ cup honey
> 1 quart iced filtered water
> 4 large sprigs fresh mint, preferably spearmint
> Ice, for serving

1. Bring 1 quart water almost to a boil in a large saucepan. Tie the tea bags together, add to the pot, and let steep for 10 minutes. Remove the bags and stir in the sugar and honey. Let cool.

2. Stir in the iced water and transfer to a large pitcher. Add the mint sprigs and let stand for at least 15 minutes. Pour the finished tea over ice in tall glasses. Garnish with more fresh mint if desired.

PREP: 25 minutes
SPEED LIMIT: 25 mpr

Makes ½ gallon (8 servings)

PER 8-OUNCE SERVING:
77 calories, 0g fat,
22g carbohydrates,
0g fiber, 0g protein

juicy-fizzy

A combination of juice and club soda or seltzer is a great way to quench the thirst of even a die-hard cola drinker. And there are so many great flavors of unsweetened juices to use these days—even crazy combos such as Mango-Passion, Pineapple-Banana, and Carrot-Orange-Apple.

Fill any size glass halfway with ice. Add bubbly water to fill two-thirds up. Top off the remaining third with a pure juice of choice or with a splash of juice concentrate, which you can buy at natural food stores. You can add fresh berries or fresh fruit slices. The kids will love making their own homemade "soda" and you can feel good about them drinking it.

hot stuff: warming and wonderful

Warm drinks go with winter like a new pair of mittens and snuggling by a fire. But these days the popularity of coffee bars is at an all-time high, and teenagers (and even younger kids) are drinking more coffee than ever, with plenty of sugar to go with the caffeine. (A Starbucks 16-ounce Toffee Nut Latte tallies up at 420 calories, and the same size White Chocolate Mocha is a whopping 510!) Introduce your young ones to these better choices for warming up on a frosty day.

Chai Latte

Mexican Hot Coco-lot

Lightly Spiced Mulled Cider

The Great Pumpkin Toddy

Happy Apple Toddy

Hot Strawberry Soothie

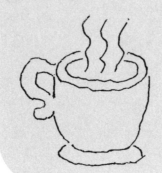

Chai Latte

Chai simply means tea in India, and milky Indian tea infused with sweet and peppery spices is soothing and delicious. The kids will love a cup of this tea after school with a couple of Chocolate Snaps (page 272). It is fun to use a teapot and pour the tea into cups through a small tea strainer.

1½ teaspoons (decorticated) cardamom seeds (out of the pods)
1 teaspoon coriander seeds
½ teaspoon whole cloves
¼ teaspoon cumin seeds
3 black peppercorns
One 2- to 3-inch cinnamon stick, lightly crushed
1 slice (quarter-sized) peeled fresh ginger
1½ cups filtered water
1 tablespoon loose decaffeinated Darjeeling or 2 decaffeinated black
    tea bags
½ cup hot milk
1 tablespoon honey
1 tablespoon sugar

PREP: 10 minutes
SPEED LIMIT: 10 mpr

Makes 2 large cups of tea

PER 1-CUP SERVING:
89 calories, 1.5g fat
(1g saturated),
18g carbohydrates,
1g fiber, 2.5g protein

1. Place the cardamom, coriander, cloves, cumin, and peppercorns in a small saucepan over medium heat and toast, stirring, until fragrant and lightly colored, about 3 minutes. Add the cinnamon, ginger, and water and bring to a boil.

2. Meanwhile, place the tea or tea bags in a warmed teapot or add it to the saucepan. Pour the milk into a 2-cup glass measuring cup and microwave at full power for 1 minute. Add the hot milk, honey, and sugar to the tea mixture and let steep for 2 minutes. Strain into cups and serve warm.

Mexican Hot Coco-lot

This cocoa has a cinnamon twist. Kids will love it with a hearty winter breakfast or in the afternoon as a warming after-school treat. If you can find it, Mexican chocolate has cinnamon already in it and is a great substitute for the regular chocolate.

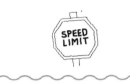

PREP: 2 minutes
COOKING: 3 minutes
SPEED LIMIT: 5 mpr

Makes 1 serving

PER 1-CUP SERVING
(WITHOUT WHIPPED
CREAM):
*279 calories, 14g fat
(8g saturated),
33g carbohydrates,
.5g fiber, 10g protein*

1 cup reduced-fat (2%) milk
1 ounce good-quality milk chocolate or semisweet chocolate, finely chopped (about 1½ tablespoons)
1 teaspoon unsweetened cocoa powder
1 teaspoon sugar
Prepared lightly sweetened whipped cream (optional)
Pinch of ground cinnamon

1. Place ¾ cup of the milk in a small saucepan. Add the chocolate, cocoa, and sugar and stir over medium heat until the mixture is steaming hot and the chocolate is melted, about 3 minutes.

2. Transfer the hot chocolate mixture to a mug and stir in the remaining ¼ cup of the cold milk to cool the mixture. Top with whipped cream, if using, and a dash of cinnamon.

Cooks' Note

❖ Canned organic whipped cream is now available in some markets.

Lightly Spiced Mulled Cider

This is the perfect warm drink to imbibe after an active day playing outside in fall or winter.

One 3-inch cinnamon stick, lightly crushed
3 whole cloves
3 whole allspice berries
1 quart fresh unpasteurized apple cider

Combine the spices in a small saucepan. Pour in the cider and then warm gently over medium-low heat until hot, about 10 minutes. Pour the finished cider through a fine-mesh tea strainer into 4 mugs.

PREP: 10 minutes
SPEED LIMIT: 10 mpr

Makes 4 servings

PER SERVING:
125 calories, 0g fat,
31g carbohydrates,
0g fiber, 0g protein

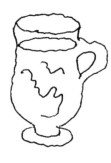

The Great Pumpkin Toddy

PREP: 5 minutes
COOKING: 5 minutes
SPEED LIMIT: 10 mpr

Makes 1 serving

PER SERVING:
128 calories, 3.7g fat
(2.3g saturated),
18g carbohydrates,
1g fiber, 6.5g protein

We both love warm milk with honey—even did so when we were kids. Adding a little pumpkin puree and maple syrup makes a warm cup of milk even better, plus it adds a nutritious boost.

> ¾ cup reduced-fat (2%) milk
> 2 tablespoons solid pack pumpkin puree
> ½ tablespoon pure maple syrup
> 2 pinches of pumpkin pie spice (optional)

Combine all of the ingredients in a small saucepan; place over medium heat and cook, stirring with a whisk, until steaming hot, about 5 minutes. Pour into a mug and let cool slightly before serving.

Happy Apple Toddy: Substitute 2 tablespoons apple butter for the pumpkin puree.

Hot Strawberry Soothie

This is a very delicious unusual warm drink. Look for good-quality organic white chocolate without artificial flavors and sweeteners. You can use fresh or thawed frozen berries for this pretty pink, warming drink.

1¼ cups reduced-fat (2%) milk
½ cup sliced strawberries
2 ounces white chocolate, finely chopped (scant ⅓ cup)

1. Pour the milk into a small saucepan and heat over medium heat until steaming hot.

2. Place the strawberries in the blender, add half of the hot milk, and blend at medium speed for 30 seconds. Add the white chocolate and, with the motor running, carefully pour in the remaining hot milk. Put on the lid and increase the speed to high and blend for 1 minute. Pour the frothy drink into 2 mugs.

PREP: 1 minute
COOKING: 1 minute
SPEED LIMIT: 2 mpr

Makes 2 servings

PER SERVING:
246 calories, 13g fat (7.5g saturated), 28g carbohydrates, 1g fiber, 7g protein

store-bought drinks we like

Think outside the juice box with these drinks. For more recommendations, go to www.realfoodforhealthykids.com.

Whole Kids organic juices
Whole Kids lemonades
365 Organic Lemonade
R. W. Knudsen concentrates
Millborne Farm's Probiotic Yogurt Drinks
The Switch Carbonated 100% Juice
Martinelli's Organic Sparkling Cider
Honest Tea Tazo
Inkos Sweetheart Iced Tea
Kristall Lemon-Lime

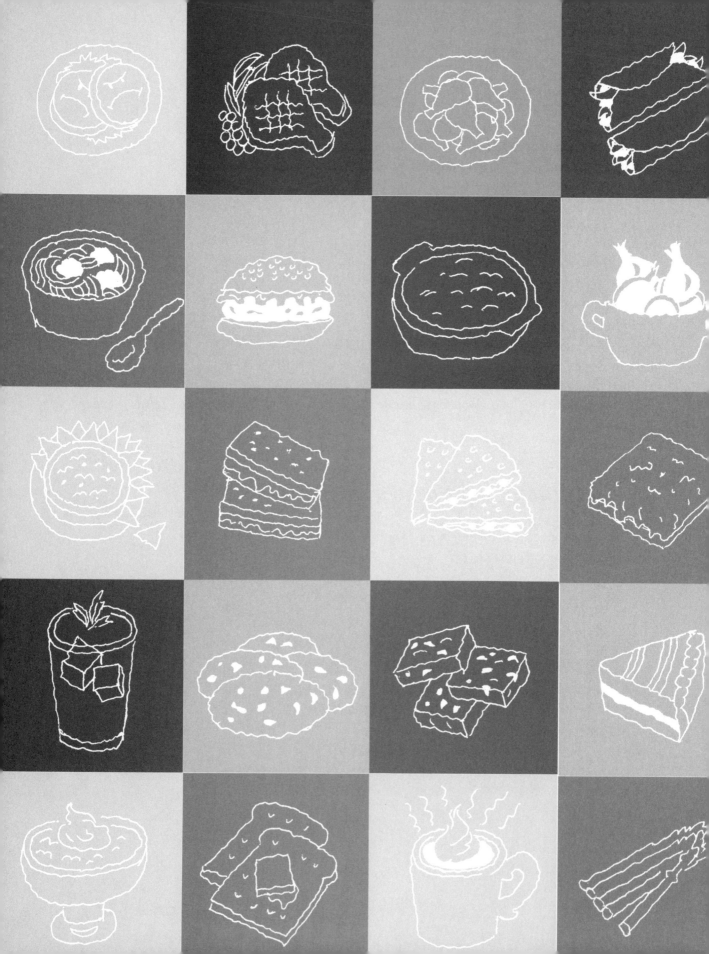

chapter eight

Divine Desserts
From Birthday Cake to Tangy Granita

Despite Mae West's adage that too much of a good thing is a good thing, dessert should be served when desired but always in moderation. Serving up sweet endings is a powerful and tangible way to teach lessons of moderation, to learn how to know when to stop. Dessert should never be used as a bribe; that could instill a lifetime of using food as reward and punishment. That said, if subtly broadcast, sweets can be a powerful motivator to getting children to dine at the table in a polite manner. But we parents know all about walking a tightrope, don't we?

We've divided our dessert chapter into cakes with complementary frostings that are perfect for birthday parties and special occasions; cakes that are perfect for every day but taste anything but ordinary; and cool and creamy desserts that are especially good when it's hot.

special occasion cakes and frostings

14-Karat Gold Cake

Black Bottom Cupcakes

Strawberry-Freckled Cake

Secret Agent Chocolate Cake

Bunny Bliss Carrot Cake

Honey-Fudge Frosting

Cream Cheese Frosting

Old-Fashioned Vanilla Frosting

Party On!

Parties are the stuff of memories, but throwing one, which includes cleaning, shopping, and cooking (and that's not including stuffing goody bags and creating activities, etc.), can be exhausting and strenuous. So, we've given you some simple but sophisticated birthday cake recipes—one vanilla, one chocolate, and one carrot—that are easy to make, plus a few variations, versatile frostings, and some tips on how to make and decorate the cakes.

14-Karat Gold Cake

This is the ultimate yellow cake. Make it special with frosting (see Honey-Fudge Frosting, page 247) for a birthday, or serve it plain for an everyday treat. It is moist, lightly sweet, and slightly tangy. (See Cooks' Notes for different pans and baking times.)

3 cups all-purpose unbleached flour

1 tablespoon baking powder

1 teaspoon fine salt

½ teaspoon baking soda

1 cup sour cream

1 cup reduced-fat (2%) milk, at room temperature

2 sticks unsalted butter, softened

2 cups sugar

4 large eggs, at room temperature

2 teaspoons pure vanilla extract

PREP: 15 minutes plus cooling and frosting
BAKING: 45 minutes

Makes one 9-inch 2-layer cake (about 12 servings)

PER SERVING:
395 calories, 21g fat (13g saturated), 49g carbohydrates, .5g fiber, 6.5g protein

1. Preheat the oven to 350°F. Lightly butter two 9- by 2-inch round cake pans, line with parchment or waxed paper, and then lightly butter the paper.

2. Whisk together the flour, baking powder, salt, and baking soda in a bowl and set aside. In a separate bowl, stir together the sour cream and milk.

3. Cream the butter and sugar in the bowl of an electric mixer at high speed until fluffy, about 5 minutes. Beat in the eggs, one at a time, beating well at medium speed after each addition. Mix in the vanilla.

4. Add half of the flour mixture to the batter and mix at low speed until incorporated. Add the sour cream mixture and the remaining flour mixture and mix at low until smooth (do not overbeat). Scrape the batter evenly into the prepared pans, smoothing the tops.

5. Bake the cake layers 40 to 45 minutes, until the tops are springy to the touch and a tester inserted into the center of the layers comes out clean. Let cool for 10 minutes in the pans on racks, cut around the sides with a small knife, turn the layers out of the pans onto racks and let cool completely.

Cooks' Notes

❖ You can also use two 9-inch springform pans to make the cake.

❖ To make a **13- by 9-inch single layer cake**, bake for 50 to 55 minutes. Place the cake on a tray and frost the top and sides with icing.

- For a **rectangular three-layer cake**, spread the batter in a 17- by 11- by 1-inch shallow baking sheet and bake for 25 to 28 minutes; let the cake cool in the pan for 20 minutes and then invert onto the rack to cool completely. Cut the cake crosswise into thirds. Spread about ¾ cup icing in between the layers and frost the top and sides with the remaining icing.

- For **3 dozen cupcakes**, spoon the batter into 3 dozen paper-lined ½-cup capacity muffin cups, filling about halfway. Place a pan in the upper and lower thirds of the oven and bake for 20 to 25 minutes. (Bake the third cupcake pan after the first two are done.)

Black Bottom Cupcakes: Melt 4 ounces chopped semisweet chocolate and let cool slightly. Transfer 2 cups yellow batter to a bowl, add the melted chocolate, and stir with a rubber spatula to blend. Spoon about 2 tablespoons of the chocolate batter into each of 36 lined muffin cups. Spoon the yellow batter on top and bake as directed. Frost with Old-Fashioned Vanilla Frosting (page 249) and top with real chocolate sprinkles (available from King Arthur Flour, the Bakers Catalogue).

Strawberry-Freckled Cake: This is a yellow cake with flecks of fresh strawberry, which are folded into the batter just before adding to the pan. Wash, pat dry, and hull a pint of fresh strawberries—look for firm small berries with deep color. Cut the berries in half, cut into small dice, and gently fold into the finished batter. Bake as directed as a cake or cupcakes, and frost.

"Mom, this is like the most delicious cake,
even without the chocolate covering it,"
says Tanya's eight-year-old son Sanger.

Secret Agent Chocolate Cake

This cake is deceptive: It contains whole-wheat flour and has no butter. Also, the cake is mixed in one pot. It is so moist you can serve it with a simple dusting of confectioners' sugar, but feel free to smear it with Old-Fashioned Vanilla Frosting (page 249) or Honey-Fudge Frosting (page 247). It's the only chocolate cake recipe you'll ever need.

PREP: 15 minutes
BAKING: 20 minutes
SPEED LIMIT: 35 mpr

Makes one 9-inch 2-layer cake (about 12 servings)

PER SERVING:
251 calories, 9.5g fat
(3.5g saturated),
48g carbohydrates,
3g fiber, 5.5g protein

> 2 cups filtered water
> 1 cup granulated sugar
> 1 cup (packed) dark brown sugar
> 4 ounces unsweetened chocolate, coarsely chopped
> 3 large eggs
> ½ cup unsweetened Dutch-process cocoa powder
> 2 teaspoons pure vanilla extract
> 1 cup unbleached all-purpose flour
> ¾ cup white whole-wheat flour
> 2 teaspoons baking powder
> 1 teaspoon baking soda
> ¼ teaspoon fine salt

1. Preheat the oven to 350°F. Lightly butter two 9- by 2-inch round cake pans, line with waxed or parchment paper, and then lightly butter the paper.

2. Combine the water, granulated sugar, and brown sugar in a 4-quart saucepan. Bring to a boil, whisking occasionally. Remove from the heat and add the chocolate; whisk occasionally until melted, about 2 minutes.

3. In a small bowl, whisk the eggs. Add all at once into the warm chocolate mixture, whisking briskly. Whisk in the cocoa powder and vanilla. Add the flours, baking powder, baking soda, and salt, and stir with the whisk until well blended.

4. Scrape the batter into the prepared pans. Bake for about 20 minutes, until a cake tester inserted into the center comes out clean. Let the layers cool in the pans on racks for 20 minutes, and turn out onto racks to cool completely.

Cooks' Notes

❖ To make a **13- by 9-inch single layer cake**, bake for 35 to 40 minutes. Place the cake on a tray and frost the top and sides with icing.

- For a **rectangular three-layer cake**, spread the batter in a 17- by 11- by 1-inch shallow baking sheet and bake for 15 to 20 minutes; let the cake cool in the pan for 20 minutes and then invert onto a rack to cool completely. Cut the cake crosswise into thirds. Spread about ¾ cup icing in between the layers and frost the top and sides with the remaining icing.

- For **3 dozen cupcakes**, spoon the batter into 3 dozen paper-lined ½-cup capacity muffin cups, filling about halfway. Place a pan in the upper and lower thirds of the oven, and bake for about 18 minutes. (Bake the third cupcake pan after the first two are done.)

Bunny Bliss Carrot Cake

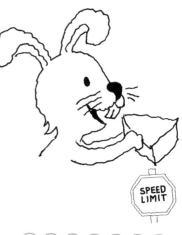

The roots of this recipe are from Teresa Ouellette, who worked with Tracey in Hartford, Connecticut, during her college days. Although the cake wasn't for sale, lucky customers sometimes got a slice for free. This cake is lighter than most carrot cakes.

3 large eggs
½ cup granulated sugar
½ cup (packed) light brown sugar
2 teaspoons baking powder
1 teaspoon baking soda
1 teaspoon cinnamon
¼ teaspoon fine salt
¾ cup safflower or other vegetable oil
1⅓ cups unbleached all-purpose flour
⅔ cup white whole-wheat flour
1 pound carrots, peeled and shredded
Cream Cheese Frosting (page 248)
1 cup chopped toasted walnuts, for garnish (optional)

PREP: 10 minutes plus cooling
BAKING: 30 minutes
SPEED LIMIT: 40 mpr

Makes one 9-inch 2-layer cake, 12 servings

PER SERVING (WITHOUT FROSTING):
276 calories, 15.5g fat (2.5g saturated),
33g carbohydrates,
2g fiber, 4g protein

1. Preheat the oven to 350°F. Lightly oil two 9-inch round cake pans. Line with parchment or waxed paper and then lightly oil the paper.

2. Combine the eggs and sugars in the bowl of an electric mixer and then beat at medium-high speed until fluffy, about 3 minutes. Add the baking powder, baking soda, cinnamon, and salt and mix at low speed until blended. With the mixer running, gradually add the oil, mixing until incorporated. Add the flours and stir until blended. Stir in the carrot.

3. Scrape the batter into the prepared pans. Bake two 9-inch layers for 30 to 35 minutes (bake two 8-inch layers for 35 to 40 minutes) until a tester inserted into the center of a cake layer comes out clean. Let cool for ten minutes in the pans on racks. Cut around the sides with a small knife, turn out onto racks, and let cool completely.

4. Place a cake layer on a platter, spread half of the frosting on top, and sprinkle half of the nuts on top, if using. Add the second cake layer, spread the remaining frosting on top, and sprinkle with the remaining nuts.

Cooks' Notes

❖ Shred the carrots on a box grater or in a food processor.

❖ For one 13- by 9-inch single layer cake, bake for about 1 hour.

❖ Bake two dozen cupcakes in paper liners for 25 minutes.

*Max M., seven years old and living in Bethel, Connecticut,
called these "the most extreme cupcakes,"
and really liked them, although he would opt to
add more sugar to the cream cheese frosting.*

Honey-Fudge Frosting

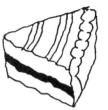

This creamy chocolaty frosting, which has less sugar than most frostings, is sublime for the 14-Karat Gold Cake (page 241) and the Secret Agent Chocolate Cake (page 243). Make sure your cake is cool before you begin making the frosting and follow the instructions carefully. When the frosting is ready, use it at once, when it is most spreadable.

1¼ cups heavy cream
¾ cup sugar
½ cup honey
¼ teaspoon fine salt
5 ounces unsweetened chocolate, coarsely chopped
1 stick cold unsalted butter, sliced into tablespoons
1½ teaspoons pure vanilla extract

PREP: 10 minutes
COOKING: 6 minutes
SPEED LIMIT: 16 mpr

Makes 3⅓ cups (12 servings)

PER SERVING:
*287 calories, 23g fat
(14g saturated),
25g carbohydrates,
2g fiber, 2g protein*

1. Combine the cream, sugar, honey, and salt in a heavy medium saucepan, whisking to blend. Bring to a boil over medium-high heat, reduce the heat, and simmer over medium-low heat, whisking occasionally, for 5 minutes (the mixture will thicken slightly).

2. Remove the saucepan from the heat, add the chocolate, and whisk until smooth. Add the butter and whisk until melted, about 1 minute. Stir in the vanilla. Transfer the chocolate mixture to a medium-large stainless-steel bowl.

3. Prepare an ice water bath: Fill a bowl or a pot, larger than the bowl with the chocolate mixture, halfway with ice and cold water. Insert the bowl of chocolate into the ice water. Beat the chocolate mixture with a handheld mixer at high speed until cool and fluffy and thick enough to spread, about 5 minutes.

Cream Cheese Frosting

This tangy frosting is great for our Bunny Bliss Carrot Cake (page 245) and Secret Agent Chocolate Cake (page 243). It's perfect for those kids who like things a little less sweet.

PREP: 5 minutes
SPEED LIMIT: 5 mpr

Makes about 1½ cups

PER SERVING:
114 calories, 8g fat
(5g saturated),
9g carbohydrates,
0g fiber, 1.4g protein

> 6 tablespoons unsalted butter, softened
> 6 ounces Neufchâtel (reduced fat) cream cheese (three-quarters of an 8-ounce package)
> ⅔ cup confectioners' sugar
> 1½ tablespoons granulated sugar
> 1 teaspoon pure vanilla extract
> ¼ teaspoon fine salt

Combine all of the ingredients in a large bowl, mix with an electric mixer on low to blend, and beat at medium-high speed until fluffy, about 5 minutes in all.

Old-Fashioned Vanilla Frosting

This old standby icing, perfect for cakes or cupcakes, remains a favorite with kids from six to sixty! It's important to use the best pure vanilla you can find.

2 sticks (½ pound) unsalted butter, softened

3 cups confectioners' sugar

4 tablespoons heavy cream

2 teaspoons pure vanilla extract

¼ teaspoon fine salt

Beat the butter with an electric mixer at high speed until light and fluffy, about 4 minutes. Gradually add the confectioners' sugar and mix at low speed until combined and then beat at high speed 2 minutes more. Add the cream, vanilla, and salt and beat at high speed until fluffy, about 3 minutes more.

PREP: 9 minutes

SPEED LIMIT: 9 mpr

Makes enough to fill and frost a 9-inch 2-layer cake (about 3 cups)

PER SERVING (BASED ON 12 SERVINGS): 271 calories, 17g fat (11g saturated), 30g carbohydrates, 0g fiber, .5g protein

decorating birthday cakes

Decorating a birthday cake can be easy and fun, and there are many ways to decorate without a pastry bag or any special techniques.

- ❖ Begin with a delicious cake made of fresh, pure ingredients. Place the cake on an attractive plate, or cover a piece of cardboard at least 4 inches larger than the diameter of the cake with festive wrapping paper to use as the base.

- ❖ Take your time spreading the icing on a little at a time; a small offset spatula is perfect for this. As you ice the cake, rotate it in front of you (instead of rotating yourself around the cake). You can choose a smooth finish or a swirly one—flowing waves of icing typically require more frosting.

- ❖ Wrap ribbon all around the bottom edge of the cake and secure with a pin that you will remove as soon as the candles are blown out.

- ❖ We avoid artificial colors and flavors in all of our cooking. Many children are sensitive to these additives. There are, however, some companies that make natural food colors. India Tree makes natural food coloring paste and decorating sugar sprinkles, which are available at Whole Foods and other markets. You can buy pure chocolate sprinkles from King Arthur Flour.

- ❖ What's in a name? Spell out the birthday child's name with little candy-coated chocolates, raspberries or blueberries, naturally flavored gumdrops, mini-nonpareils, or small homemade or store-bought alphabet cookies (Newman's Own Organics has little arrowroot letter cookies).

- ❖ You can also decorate around the cake platter with organic edible flowers and other small seasonal items, such as tiny pumpkins and nuts.

- ❖ Some stores that sell cakes will print a photograph on edible rice paper, which can be transferred on top of a cake.

- ❖ Keep a supply of candles in different colors and shapes on hand.

better baking

If you're a nervous baker, follow these helpful tips when making these cakes:

Quality is the name of the game: When baking, always choose quality ingredients, including unsalted butter, pure vanilla extract, and fine salt. It is best to buy large eggs for all of your cooking; whole-wheat flour should be among your refrigerated staples. Gold Medal sells finely ground whole-grain whole-wheat flour, and King Arthur Flour sells white whole-wheat flour, which is even softer. They are interchangeable, but sometimes we have listed our preferences within certain recipes.

Tools of the trade: If you like to bake, it makes sense to invest in a standing electric mixer for easy mixing, and an internal oven thermometer for temperature regulation and perfect results. Purchase some heavy baking sheets and pans and a good rack or two. We like to purchase items from King Arthur Flour Baker's Catalogue, Sur La Table, Williams-Sonoma, and Zabar's.

Temper-temper: For best results, bake with room-temperature ingredients. You can warm butter, milk, and water in the microwave (don't overheat!) and warm eggs in their shells in a bowl of hot water. Eggs are easier to separate when cold; to get the best volume when whipping egg whites, whip them at room temperature. Also be sure that absolutely no traces of yolk get into the whites, or they will not whip properly.

Old-fashioned Cakes and Baked Fruit Treats

This section is filled with new recipes as well as tried-and-true family favorites that have stood the test of time. As with all of our recipes, we have tried to use sugar and butter in moderation and have included whole-wheat flour whenever possible.

Nana Elizabeth's Sour Cream Cake

Lemon Sour Cream Cake

Anita's True Sponge Cake

Vanilla Angel Food Cake

Chocolate-Flecked Angel Cake

Easy-Does-It Applesauce Cake

Big Peach and Blackberry Cobbler

Peach Cobbler

Plum Cobbler

Cheery Cherry Plank

Plum Plank

Pear and Hazelnut Tart

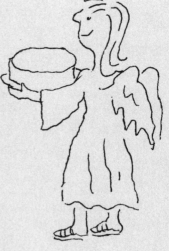

Nana Elizabeth's Sour Cream Cake

This subtle Bundt cake comes from Tracey's paternal great-grandmother. It is a timeless cake that is a family favorite, and now it can be for your family.

2 ½ cups unbleached all-purpose flour
½ teaspoon baking soda
½ teaspoon fine salt
2 sticks (½ pound) unsalted butter, softened
2 cups plus ¼ cup sugar
3 large eggs, at room temperature
1 cup full-fat sour cream or plain whole milk yogurt
1 teaspoon vanilla extract
2 teaspoons ground cinnamon
Confectioners' sugar, for dusting (optional)

PREP: 15 minutes plus cooling
BAKING: 1 hour

Makes 10 servings

PER SERVING:
442 calories, 24g fat (15g saturated), 55g carbohydrates, .5g fiber, 6g protein

1. Adjust an oven rack in the lower third of the oven and preheat the oven to 325°F. Lightly butter a 10-cup Bundt pan or tube pan; dust with flour and tap out the excess.

2. Combine the flour, baking soda, and salt in a bowl and whisk to blend; reserve.

3. Cream the butter and 2 cups of the sugar in the bowl of an electric mixer, beating at high speed and scraping down the bowl as necessary until fluffy, about 5 minutes. Add the eggs one at a time, beating well after each addition. Add half of the flour mixture and mix at low speed until just blended. Add the sour cream and vanilla and the remaining dry mixture; mix at low speed just until smooth.

4. Spoon half of the batter into the prepared pan. Mix the remaining ¼ cup sugar with the cinnamon in a cup and sprinkle on top of the batter in the pan. Spoon the remaining batter on top of the cinnamon layer and carefully smooth the top. Bake until a cake tester inserted into the center of the cake comes out clean, about 1 hour.

5. Let the cake cool for 15 minutes in the pan, turn out onto a rack, and let cool completely. Dust the cake with confectioners' sugar, if using, before cutting.

Lemon Sour Cream Cake: Add 2 teaspoons finely grated fresh lemon peel to the batter along with the sour cream. Omit the cinnamon-sugar layer in the batter; spoon all of the lemon batter into the pan and bake as directed. While the cake is baking, make a glaze: Increase the additional sugar from $1/4$ cup to $1/2$ cup and place in a small bowl with $1/2$ cup fresh lemon juice; whisk until the sugar is dissolved. Unmold the warm cake as directed on a rack and place the rack over a shallow baking pan. Prick the cake top at $3/4$-inch intervals with a toothpick. Brush one-quarter of the glaze on top of the cake and let stand for 5 minutes. Repeat until all of the glaze has soaked into the cake, and let cool completely.

Elijah S., age five, from Booneville, Indiana, found this cake
to be "delicious" and now asks his mom,
Missy, to make it often.

Anita's True Sponge Cake

This golden few-ingredient cake comes from Tracey's maternal grand-mother. The girls in Tracey's extended family relish the handwritten recipes from this special woman, including this tall moist cake, which is as light as air and a great vehicle for summer fruit and whipped cream.

8 large eggs, at room temperature
¾ cup granulated sugar
1 teaspoon vanilla extract
½ cup unbleached all-purpose flour
Pinch of fine salt

FOR SERVING
4 cups mixed berries, such as blueberries, raspberries, and quartered
   strawberries
1 tablespoon granulated sugar
1 tablespoon confectioners' sugar, for dusting
Lightly sweetened freshly whipped cream

1. Arrange a rack in the lower third of the oven and preheat the oven to 325°F.

2. Separate the eggs one at a time, placing the egg whites in a bowl and the yolks in the bowl of a standing electric mixer. Add the sugar and vanilla to the bowl of yolks. Mix at low speed to blend for a few seconds and then beat at high speed until the mixture becomes pale in color and very thick, about 8 minutes; the mixture will blister on the surface when you stop beating. Add the flour and mix at low speed until just incorporated.

3. In a clean bowl with a clean, dry whisk attachment, beat the egg whites and salt at medium speed until soft peaks form, 1 to 2 minutes. Increase the speed to high and beat until the mixture holds stiff peaks but is not dry, 1 minute or less. Fold one-third of the whites into the yolk mixture, and then fold in the remaining whites until no streaks remain.

4. Scrape the batter into a 10-inch tube pan and smooth the top. Bake for about 35 minutes, until a tester inserted into the center comes out clean. Carefully invert the cake pan onto a glass bottle (wine or other) with a neck that is narrow enough to fit inside the center tube of the pan, place in a safe place, and let cool completely, about 1½ hours.

PREP: 20 minutes plus cooling
BAKING: 35 minutes
SPEED LIMIT: 55 mpr

Makes one 10-inch cake to serve about 10

PER SERVING (WITHOUT WHIPPED CREAM):
155 calories, 4g fat
(1g saturated),
26g carbohydrates,
1.5g fiber, 6g protein

5. When ready to serve, toss the berries with granulated sugar and let stand. Run a long thin straight-edged knife around the center tube and the outside edge of the cake and remove the tube insert from the pan. Cut around the bottom of the cake to release it from the tube bottom and then invert the cake onto a serving platter. Just before serving, dust the cake with confectioners' sugar and cut with a serrated knife in a sawing motion. Serve the berries and whipped cream along the side.

Cooks' Note

❖ When separating eggs it is important not to get any yolk into the whites, because the fat from the yolk will prevent the whites from whipping to their full volume. If you're not good at separating eggs, use a small bowl and a large bowl for the whites; add 1 white to the small bowl and then pour that white into the larger bowl. Repeat with each egg. This way, if some yolk gets into a single white, you can discard that egg white and it will not harm the total amount.

Vanilla Angel Food Cake

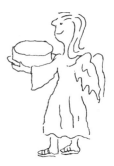

This cake is fluffy, sweet, and light—and fat-free. A standing mixer is preferable to use because you want the volume of the egg whites to be as big as possible. Drizzle the cake with warm Honey-Fudge Frosting (page 247) before beating and completely cooling or serve with sliced peeled peaches and whipped cream.

> 1 cup plain cake flour (not self-rising)
> 1½ cups sugar
> 13 large egg whites
> 1 teaspoon cream of tartar
> ¼ teaspoon fine salt
> 2 teaspoons vanilla extract

PREP: 10 minutes
BAKING: 45 minutes
SPEED LIMIT: 55 mpr

Makes 10 servings

PER SERVING:
147 calories, 0g fat,
33g carbohydrates,
0g fiber, 6g protein

1. Arrange a rack in the lower third of the oven and preheat the oven to 375°F.

2. Place the flour and ¾ cup of the sugar in a bowl and stir well with a whisk for 1 minute to combine and aerate; reserve.

3. Place the egg whites, cream of tartar, and salt in the bowl of an electric mixer; mix at low speed until frothy, about 1 minute. Increase the speed to medium and beat until the mixture holds soft peaks when the beater is lifted, about 2 minutes. Then, with the mixer running at low speed, gradually sprinkle in the remaining ¾ cup sugar, 1 tablespoon at a time. Once all of the sugar has been added, beat at medium speed until stiff, about 3 minutes.

4. Sift one-third of the flour mixture on top of the whites; fold in gently with a rubber spatula until just blended. Repeat with the remaining flour in two batches. Fold in the vanilla and then scrape into a 10-inch tube pan, smoothing the top. Bake for about 45 minutes, until a tester inserted into the center of the cake comes out clean, and the top is light brown. Invert the pan onto a glass bottle (wine or other) with a neck that is narrow enough to fit inside the center tube of the pan and let cool completely before unmolding the cake.

5. To unmold the cake, run a long thin knife around the inside and outside edges of the cake to release it from the pan and then invert onto a serving platter.

Chocolate-Flecked Angel Cake: Coarsely chop 4 ounces of quality bittersweet or semisweet chocolate, place in a food processor, and pulse until finely ground. Fold into the batter after the vanilla and bake as directed.

Four-year-old angel Sarah C., from Rye Brook, New York, made this cake with her mom, Wendi: "Who was the angel in the angel food cake? Is it me?"

Easy-Does-It Applesauce Cake

This moist cake keeps well for several days, covered, in the refrigerator. You can serve it for breakfast or stow a piece in a lunch box.

PREP: 15 minutes plus cooling

BAKING: 40 minutes

Makes 8 servings

PER SERVING:
319 calories, 12.5g fat
(8g saturated),
53g carbohydrates,
2g fiber, 3.5g protein

½ cup white whole-wheat flour
½ cup unbleached all-purpose flour
1 teaspoon apple pie spice or pumpkin pie spice
1 teaspoon baking soda
¼ teaspoon fine salt
1 stick unsalted butter, softened
½ cup (packed) light brown sugar
½ cup granulated sugar
1 large egg, at room temperature
1 cup unsweetened applesauce, at room temperature
1 cup dark raisins or currants
Cream Cheese Frosting (page 248), optional

1. Place a rack in the lower third of the oven and preheat the oven to 350°F. Lightly butter an 8-inch square metal baking pan or a 9- by 2-inch round pan and then dust the inside with a little flour, tilting to coat; shake out the excess flour.

2. In a bowl, whisk together the flours, apple pie spice, baking soda, and salt and reserve.

3. Beat the butter and sugars in a bowl with an electric mixer at high speed until fluffy, about 3 minutes. Add the egg and beat at high speed until well blended. Add the applesauce and mix at low speed until blended and then add the flour mixture, mixing at low speed until incorporated. Stir in the raisins.

4. Scrape the batter into the prepared pan and bake for 35 to 40 minutes, until a cake tester inserted into the center comes out clean. Let cool completely in the pan on a rack and then frost with Cream Cheese Frosting, if using.

Big Peach and Blackberry Cobbler

When ripe golden or white peaches are in season, there is no better way to showcase them than in this whole-wheat enriched fruity dessert.

FILLING

4 pounds ripe fresh peaches, peeled, pitted, and sliced, or 3 pounds
   frozen sliced peaches, thawed
¾ cup (packed) light brown sugar
2 tablespoons unbleached all-purpose flour
¼ teaspoon fine salt
2 half-pints fresh blackberries

TOPPING

1½ cups unbleached all-purpose flour
¾ cup white whole-wheat flour
½ cup granulated sugar
2 teaspoons baking powder
¼ teaspoon fine salt
1 stick cold unsalted butter, cut up
1¼ cups low-fat buttermilk
1 large egg

PREP: 20 minutes
BAKING: 45 minutes

Makes 10 servings

PER SERVING:
360 calories, 11g fat
(6g saturated),
64g carbohydrates,
5g fiber, 7g protein

1. Preheat the oven to 400°F. Butter a 13- by 9-inch or other 3-quart shallow casserole. Place the peach slices in the casserole. Sprinkle the light brown sugar, flour, and salt on top. Stir gently to mix. Sprinkle the blackberries on top. Bake for 20 minutes; the mixture should begin to boil.

2. While the peaches are cooking, make the topping: In a bowl, toss together the flours, sugar, baking powder, and salt. Add the butter pieces and cut into the dry mixture with your fingertips, a pastry blender, or two knives until crumbly. With a fork, beat together the buttermilk and egg in a small bowl, and then stir into the dry mixture until the dough comes together into a ball.

3. Remove the fruit from the oven after 20 minutes. Using a soup spoon or a tablespoon, drop about 20 dollops of the dough on top of the hot fruit, spacing evenly in a single layer. Bake for 20 to 25 minutes more, until the topping is golden and springy to the touch.

Peach Cobbler: Omit the berries.

Plum Cobbler: Substitute halved and pitted plums for the peaches.

"Can I have some more please?" said Aidan C., fourteen, who lives in the Bronx, New York, and loved how the "light and spongy topping complemented the peaches."

Cheery Cherry Plank

Y ou can make this tart with fresh or frozen fruit. Because the crust is flat, the pastry is easy to make, even for the novice. Serve the tart with vanilla frozen yogurt or lightly sweetened whipped cream and watch the mutineers get in line.

PREP: 20 minutes plus
10 minutes cooling
BAKING: 25 minutes
SPEED LIMIT: 45 mpr

Makes 5 servings

PER SERVING:
*339 calories, 17g fat
(10.5g saturated),
45g carbohydrates,
3.5g fiber, 6g protein*

1 cup unbleached all-purpose flour
½ cup white whole-wheat flour
2 tablespoons sugar
1½ teaspoons baking powder
¼ teaspoon baking soda
¼ teaspoon fine salt
4 tablespoons plus 2 tablespoons cold unsalted butter
½ cup half-and-half
50 sweet dark cherries, stemmed and pitted (4 cups, about 1 pound)

1. Combine the flours, 1 tablespoon of the sugar, the baking powder, baking soda, and salt in a food processor and pulse to blend. Cut 4 tablespoons of the butter into 8 slices, add to the flour mixture, and pulse until the mixture is crumbly. Add the half-and-half and process just until a dough comes together. Form the dough into a small brick shape, wrap in plastic, and chill while you prepare the topping.

2. Melt the remaining 2 tablespoons butter in a small saucepan or in the microwave and reserve.

3. Preheat the oven to 425°F. Roll the dough out on a 14-inch-long sheet of parchment paper to a rough 12- by 6-inch rectangle. Trim the edges with a knife to neaten, and discard the trimmings. Transfer the dough base on the parchment to a baking sheet and brush the dough with half of the melted butter. Arrange the cherries in 5 lengthwise rows of 10 on top of the dough, leaving a ¾-inch border all around. Dab with the remaining butter and sprinkle the remaining tablespoon of sugar on top.

4. Bake for about 25 minutes, until the crust is golden. Let cool for 10 minutes on the baking sheet. Cut crosswise into 5 slices.

Cooks' Notes

❖ A spring-release cherry pitter can be purchased at a specialty store for about $12.

❖ When working with fresh cherries, it's best to wear plastic gloves, as the juice stains your hands.

❖ You can make the tart up to 1 day ahead: Completely cool the tart, cover with foil, and keep at room temperature overnight. Rewarm in a 325°F oven for 5 minutes.

Plum Plank: Substitute 5 large ripe plums, quartered, pitted, and sliced for the cherries. Bake as directed.

Pear and Hazelnut Tart

Frozen puff pastry is the base for this quick but impressive dessert. Try to find an all-butter brand, such as Dufour, and roll it out just enough to smooth out the creases. Serve the tart for brunch or dessert.

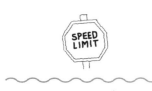

PREP: 20 minutes plus cooling
BAKING: 20 minutes
SPEED LIMIT: 40 mpr

Makes one 10-inch tart to serve 6 to 8

PER WEDGE:
*90 calories, 4g fat
(.5g saturated),
11g carbohydrates,
2g fiber, 1g protein*

*¹⁄₃ cup hazelnuts
1 sheet (10 by 9 inches) frozen puff pastry, thawed according to package
    directions
2 tablespoons sugar
2 firm ripe pears, such as Bartlett*

1. Preheat the oven to 400°F.

2. Spread the nuts on a large shallow baking sheet and roast in the oven for about 8 minutes, until fragrant and lightly toasted. Lay a clean kitchen towel on a work surface, transfer the nuts to the center, and fold up in the towel. Let cool for 5 minutes and then rub the nuts in the towel to remove most of the skin. Reserve the nuts and wipe off the baking sheet.

3. Roll the pastry out on a lightly floured surface to a 12-inch square. Use a plate as your guide and cut a 10-inch round out of the pastry. Transfer the pastry round to the same baking sheet. Prick the pastry all over with a fork, leaving a ¹⁄₂-inch border all around.

4. Transfer the peeled roasted nuts to the food processor, leaving the skins on the towel. Add the sugar to the nuts and process until finely ground. Sprinkle two-thirds of the nut mixture on top of the pastry. Chill while you prepare the pears.

5. Cut each of the pears into quarters (with or without peel), cut out the core and discard, and thinly slice the pear pieces. Starting just inside the border, arrange the pear slices in overlapping concentric circles, using the larger slices first and then the smaller. Continue until all of the pear is used. Sprinkle the remaining nut mixture on top and bake for about 25 minutes, until the pastry is puffed and golden. Let cool slightly before serving.

cool and creamy: cheesecake and more

These luscious chilled treats are particularly great to make in summer, but you can enjoy them all year long.

Brown Mouse

Peanut Butter–Chocolate Mouse

Dreamy Creamy Cheesecake

Watermelon Gell-ee

Lively Lemon Granita

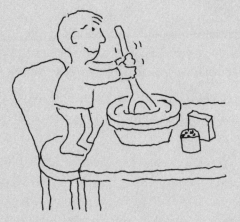

Brown Mouse

A mouse is quicker than a mousse but just as chocolaty. You can make it anytime, but it is definitely special enough for a celebration. Although we worship the egg, which ordinarily gives mousse its velvety texture, we've taken it out and use marshmallow cream instead. Be sure to buy good-quality chocolate chips for your mouse!

PREP: 15 minutes
CHILLING: 1 hour

Makes 5 cups (ten ½-cup servings)

PER ½-CUP SERVING:
397 calories, 27g fat
(17g saturated),
38g carbohydrates,
2g fiber, 3.5g protein

1 cup semisweet chocolate chips, such as Ghirardelli (6 ounces)
½ cup milk chocolate chips, such as Ghirardelli (2 ounces)
2 cups heavy cream
1 teaspoon vanilla extract
Pinch of fine salt
1 container (about 7 ounces) marshmallow cream (see Cooks' Notes)

1. Place the semisweet and milk chocolate chips and ¼ cup of the cream in a small microwavable bowl. Cook at medium (50%) power for 3 minutes and stir until smooth. Transfer to a medium bowl (this will help the chocolate cool).

2. Combine the remaining 1¾ cups cream, the vanilla, and salt in the bowl of an electric mixer. Beat at medium-high speed until stiff enough to hold its shape when you lift the beater but not too dry.

3. Scoop half of the marshmallow cream into the chocolate and fold with a rubber spatula until half blended. Add the remaining marshmallow cream and fold in until almost no streaks remain. Add ⅓ of the whipped cream and fold in until half blended. Add the remaining whipped cream and fold until no streaks remain.

4. Scrape the mouse into a 6- to 8-cup serving bowl or spoon into individual cups or dessert glasses. Cover with plastic and chill until cold, at least 1 hour.

Cooks' Notes

❖ You can use bar chocolate instead of chips; simply chop it to about the size of chips.

❖ We like Tiny Trapeze brand marshmallow cream; it is made with rice syrup instead of high-fructose corn syrup.

"This brown mouse was soo, sooo delicious," says eight-year-old Maeve D., of Valencia, California.

Peanut Butter–Chocolate Mouse: Reduce the semisweet chocolate to 4 ounces; after melting, stir in ¼ cup natural peanut butter and then proceed with the recipe.

Dreamy Creamy Cheesecake

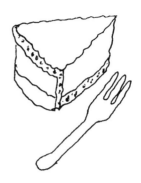

This is the only cheesecake recipe you will ever need. It produces a rich cheesecake, about 2 inches high, with plenty of graham cracker crust. Serve with a little fresh fruit.

CRUST

    9 whole graham crackers (or 1½ cups packaged graham cracker crumbs)
    ¼ cup sugar
    6 tablespoons unsalted butter, melted

FILLING

    Two 8-ounce packages Neufchâtel (reduced-fat) cream cheese, at room temperature
    ¾ cup sugar
    3 large eggs, at room temperature
    1 teaspoon vanilla extract
    ½ teaspoon finely grated fresh lemon peel (about ¼ lemon)

TOPPING

    1 cup sour cream
    2 tablespoons sugar
    1 teaspoon vanilla extract

PREP: 20 minutes plus cooling and chilling
BAKING: 1 hour and 15 minutes

Makes a 9-inch cheesecake to serve 8 to 10

PER SERVING:
345 calories, 22g fat (13g saturated), 30g carbohydrates, .5g fiber, 8.5g protein

1. Preheat the oven to 350°F. Lightly butter the bottom and sides of a 9- by 2½-inch springform pan.

2. Prepare the crust: If using whole graham crackers, pulse the crackers in a food processor to make fine crumbs. Add the sugar and process to mix. Remove the blade and stir in the melted butter. (Alternatively, mix together the crumbs and sugar in a bowl and stir in the butter.) Press the crumbs mixture over the bottom and three-quarters of the way up the side of the pan. Freeze the pan for 10 minutes and then bake for 10 minutes to set. Let cool on a rack.

3. Make the filling: Beat the cream cheese and sugar with an electric mixer at high speed until fluffy, about 5 minutes. Beat in the eggs one at a time, beating well after each addition. Add the vanilla and lemon peel and mix at medium speed until incorporated. Scrape the batter on top of the crust and bake for about 55 minutes, until set but wobbly in the center. Transfer the cake to the stovetop and increase the oven temperature to 450°F.

4. Prepare the topping: Whisk together the sour cream, sugar, and vanilla. Spoon on top of the hot cake, spreading evenly. Return the cake to the oven and bake for 8 to 10 minutes, until just set. Let cool completely on a rack and then refrigerate until cold, at least 3 hours and up to 24 hours. To serve, cut around the edge of the cake with a thin knife and remove the side of the pan. Serve cold.

"This is the best cheesecake I've ever eaten," says ten-year-old Ceri D., of Valencia, California.

Watermelon Gell-ee

Here is a cooling dessert made with fresh watermelon. If desired, add sliced strawberries or raspberries before chilling. If you prefer, chill the gelatin in a single large bowl or a mold, but allow for extra chilling to set.

> One 4½-pound wedge seedless watermelon, cut up, at room
> temperature (see Cooks' Note)
> 2 packets (¼ ounce each) unflavored gelatin
> ¼ cup sugar
> 2 tablespoons fresh lemon juice

PREP: 1 hour including chilling

Makes 8 servings

PER ¾ CUP:
62 calories, og fat,
15g carbohydrates,
.5g fiber, 2g protein

1. Extract the juice from the watermelon with a juicer or puree in a food processor and strain through a fine sieve. (You should have about 4 cups of juice.)

2. Place 1 cup of watermelon juice in a heatproof bowl. Sprinkle the gelatin on top and let stand and soften for 5 minutes, and then microwave for 45 seconds to melt the gelatin. Stir in the sugar and lemon juice; stir the gelatin mixture into the remaining watermelon juice. Spoon the mixture into eight 6-ounce custard cups or ramekins and chill until set, about 30 minutes.

Cooks' Note

❖ If your watermelon is cold, you may need to microwave the juice 30 seconds longer to melt the gelatin. For ease, you can buy watermelon already cut up at the market.

Lively Lemon Granita

Serve this cooling lemony treat for a snack or dessert. The kids can take turns stirring the mixture. It is fun to serve the granita in frozen hollowed-out lemon halves.

4 large lemons
1⅓ cups filtered water
½ cup sugar
⅓ cup honey

PREP: 10 minutes
FREEZING: About 4 hours

Makes 6 servings

PER SERVING:
*105 calories, 0g fat,
29g carbohydrates,
0g fiber, 0g protein*

1. Finely grate the zest from 1 lemon or remove the peel in strips with a vegetable peeler (avoiding any bitter white pith) and place in a small saucepan. Add the water and sugar and cook over moderate heat until the sugar is dissolved, 2 to 3 minutes. Remove from the heat, stir in the honey, and let cool to room temperature.

2. Trim a little off both ends of the remaining 3 lemons (so they will stand upright on either end). Halve the lemons and squeeze out the juice, with a citrus juicer or reamer, keeping the halves intact. Place the hollowed-out lemon cups in a shallow container large enough to hold them and freeze until ready to use.

3. Stir ½ cup lemon juice into the cooled syrup. (Cover and chill any additional juice for another use.) Pour the lemon-syrup mixture through a fine-mesh strainer into a 1-quart (8- or 9-inch square) metal baking dish and then place flat in the freezer. After 30 minutes, scrape the frozen lemon mixture off the sides of the pan and into the center; repeat scraping every 30 minutes, until you have an icy, slushy mixture.

4. Arrange the frozen lemon halves onto each of six small plates. Spoon some of the granita onto each and serve immediately.

chapter nine

From the Cookie Jar
Wholesome and Homemade

No matter what our age, we are all cookie monsters. The fragrance of freshly baked cookies cooling on a rack on the counter is the stuff of happy thoughts, compared with ripping into an inferior package of rock-hard store-bought cookies—many made with artificial ingredients, preservatives, and trans fats. Here we've again incorporated wholesome ingredients, often making use of white whole-wheat flour, which you can purchase from King Arthur Flour or your supermarket.

Cookie baking is a wonderful activity to do with your children. If your experience with making cookies doesn't go beyond cutting slices of premade cookie dough bars, we have provided essential baking tips.

Chocolate Chip Flying Saucers

Chocolate Snaps

Chocolate Sandwich Cookies

Mom-Mom's One-Pot Brownies

Ultimate Oatmeal Cookies

Chocolate-Raisin Oatmeal Cookies

Wheat Biscuit Shortbread

Chocolate-Dipped Shortbread

Peanut Butter Blondies

Chocolate Chip Peanut Butter Bars

Simply Splendid Sugar Cookies

Sugar Cookie Cutouts

Yin-Yang Black and White Cookies

Mini-Whoopee Pies

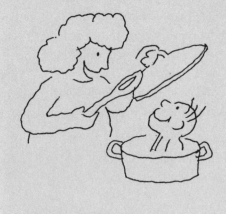

Chocolate Chip Flying Saucers

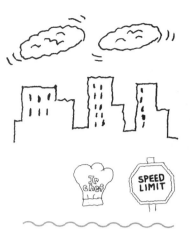

These flat, chewy, half whole-wheat cookies are for the chocolate chip purist: no nuts, no frills—pure bliss. They will fly out of the kitchen mysteriously. Use a 1-ounce (2-tablespoon-capacity) ice-cream scoop for easy measuring.

2 sticks unsalted butter, at room temperature

1 cup granulated sugar

1 cup (packed) dark brown sugar

2 large eggs

1 teaspoon vanilla extract

¾ teaspoon fine salt

½ teaspoon baking soda

1 cup unbleached all-purpose flour

⅔ cup white whole-wheat flour

1 cup semisweet chocolate chips

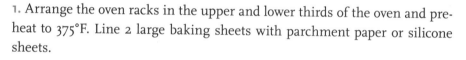

PREP: 15 minutes plus cooling
BAKING: 28 minutes
SPEED LIMIT: 43 mpr

Makes about twenty 4-inch cookies

PER COOKIE:
243 calories, 13g fat (8g saturated), 32g carbohydrates, 1g fiber, 3g protein

1. Arrange the oven racks in the upper and lower thirds of the oven and preheat to 375°F. Line 2 large baking sheets with parchment paper or silicone sheets.

2. In the bowl of an electric mixer, cream the butter and sugars, beating at medium-high speed until fluffy, about 5 minutes. Add the eggs, vanilla, salt, and baking soda and beat at medium speed just until the eggs are incorporated, 1 to 2 minutes. Add the flours and mix at low speed just until blended, scraping down the bowl as necessary. Stir in the chocolate chips.

3. Drop 6 heaping tablespoons of dough on each cookie sheet, spacing the tablespoons of dough evenly apart. Bake for 7 minutes, switch and rotate the pans, and bake 5 to 7 minutes more, until the cookies are evenly golden. Let the cookies cool on the pans for a minute or two and then transfer with a spatula to racks to cool completely. Repeat with the remaining dough.

Chocolate Snaps

These crisp chocolate cookies are satisfying and great for dunking in milk (or coffee, Mom and Dad)! You can grind them for serving over ice cream, or to make them into sandwiches (see below).

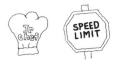

PREP: 20 minutes plus chilling
BAKING: 20 minutes
SPEED LIMIT: 40 mpr

Makes about 3 dozen cookies

PER COOKIE:
70 calories, 4g fat (1.5g saturated), 12g carbohydrates, 0g fiber, 1g protein

1 stick unsalted butter, softened
1 cup sugar
1 large egg
$\frac{1}{2}$ teaspoon baking soda
$\frac{1}{4}$ teaspoon fine salt
$\frac{1}{2}$ cup unsweetened cocoa powder (preferably Droste brand)
1 cup unbleached all-purpose flour
$\frac{1}{2}$ cup whole-wheat flour
About 1 cup confectioners' sugar, for decorating

1. Cream the butter and sugar in the bowl of an electric mixer, beating at high speed until fluffy, about 5 minutes. Add the egg, baking soda, and salt and mix until blended. Add the cocoa powder and mix at low speed until incorporated. Add the flours and mix at low speed until blended.

2. Divide the dough in half, form into 2 disks, and wrap in plastic or waxed paper. Chill until firm, at least 1 hour or up to 2 days.

3. Take 1 piece of dough out of the refrigerator. Arrange the racks in the upper and lower thirds of the oven and preheat the oven to 350°F. Take out 2 large cookie sheets and line with parchment paper or silicone sheets.

4. Lightly flour a work surface and then roll out the dough $\frac{1}{4}$ to $\frac{1}{8}$ inch thick. Cut out the cookies with a 3- to 4-inch round cookie cutter. Transfer the cookies with a metal spatula to the baking sheets and then chill for 10 minutes. Bake the cookies for about 10 minutes, until somewhat firm to the touch. (Do not overbake or the cookies will be bitter.) Let cool on the pans for 2 minutes and then transfer with a metal spatula to racks and let cool completely. Repeat with the remaining dough.

5. To decorate, lay a lacy doily on top of the cookies and dust with confectioners' sugar.

Chocolate Sandwich Cookies: Fill pairs of our crisp chocolate cookies with our Old-Fashioned Vanilla Frosting (page 249); much tastier than those famous chocolate-vanilla sandwich cookies!

Mom-Mom's One-Pot Brownies

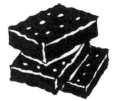

These brownies, from Tracey's mom, are fast to make and not overly sugary, and since you're mixing the batter in one pot, it's an easy cleanup.

2 sticks unsalted butter
4 ounces unsweetened chocolate
1¾ cups granulated sugar
4 large eggs
1 cup unbleached all-purpose flour
2 teaspoons vanilla extract
½ teaspoon fine salt
¾ cup chopped walnuts or pecans (optional)

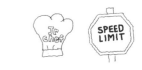

PREP: 10 minutes plus cooling
BAKING: 30 minutes
SPEED LIMIT: 40 mpr

Makes 2 dozen small bar cookies

PER BROWNIE
(WITH NUTS):
180 calories, 12g fat
(7g saturated),
16g carbohydrates,
1g fiber, 3g protein

1. Preheat the oven to 350°F. Lightly butter a 13- by 9-inch metal baking pan.

2. Combine the butter and chocolate in a medium saucepan. Cook over medium heat, stirring, until melted and smooth, about 5 minutes. Remove from the heat and whisk in the sugar. Whisk in the eggs, one at a time, and then whisk in the flour, vanilla, and salt. If you're using nuts, add them now, and mix to incorporate.

3. Scrape the batter into the prepared pan, being sure to spread into the corners. Bake for 25 to 30 minutes, until soft but springy to the touch in the center. Let cool completely in the pan on a rack and then cut into bars.

Four-year-old Miles A., from San Diego, California:
"Good, Mama, can I have another one?"
His sister, three-year-old Betsy A.:
"Great, Mama, can I have another one?"

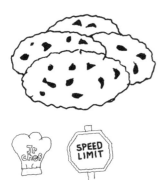

Ultimate Oatmeal Cookies

Our friend Susan Jaslove, a longtime cooking and nutrition teacher, puts chocolate-covered raisins in her oatmeal cookies. We think she would agree that these are the best plain oatmeal cookies, but you can add whatever mix-ins you like. The cookies are even better the next day.

PREP: 15 minutes
BAKING: 30 minutes
SPEED LIMIT: 45 mpr

Makes about 3 dozen cookies

PER COOKIE
(WITH PECANS):
140 calories, 8g fat
(3.5g saturated),
16g carbohydrates,
1g fiber, 2g protein

2 sticks (½ pound) unsalted butter
1 cup (packed) dark brown sugar
½ cup granulated sugar
2 large eggs
¾ teaspoon fine salt
½ teaspoon baking soda
½ tablespoon vanilla extract
¾ cup unbleached all-purpose flour
¾ cup white whole-wheat flour
2½ cups old-fashioned rolled oats
1 cup pecans, coarsely chopped (optional)

1. Arrange oven racks in the upper and lower thirds of the oven and preheat the oven to 350°F. Line 2 large cookie sheets with parchment paper.

2. In the bowl of an electric mixer, cream the butter and sugars until fluffy, 5 to 6 minutes. Add the eggs and beat until incorporated, scraping the bowl as necessary. Add the salt, baking soda, and vanilla and mix at medium speed until blended. Add the flours and mix at low speed until smooth. Stir in the oats and nuts, if using, and mix until incorporated.

3. Drop generous tablespoons of dough 2 inches apart on the prepared sheets. Bake in the upper and lower thirds of the oven for about 15 minutes, switching the sheets halfway through, until the cookies are nearly set and golden brown. Let cool on the sheets for 1 minute, and then transfer the cookies with a metal spatula to a rack to cool completely.

Chocolate-Raisin Oatmeal Cookies: Add 1½ cups of chocolate-covered raisins (or raisins, chopped dried fruit, or semisweet chocolate chips or chunks) to the cookie dough.

Bobby S., a big kid who goes to James Madison University in Harrisonburg, Virginia, says that these are his favorite cookies of all time.

Wheat Biscuit Shortbread

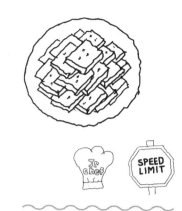

This buttery shortbread is a treat for all ages. Kids can help stir the dough with a wooden spoon.

> 2 sticks unsalted butter, at room temperature
> 2/3 cup granulated sugar
> 2 teaspoons vanilla extract
> 1/2 teaspoon fine salt
> 1 1/4 cups unbleached all-purpose flour
> 1 cup white whole-wheat flour

PREP: 10 minutes plus chilling and cooling
BAKING: 17 minutes

Makes about 3 dozen cookies

PER COOKIE:
81 calories, 5g fat (3g saturated), 8g carbohydrates, .5g fiber, 1g protein

1. Arrange the racks in the upper and lower thirds of the oven and preheat the oven to 325°F. Line 2 large cookie sheets with parchment paper or silicone sheets.

2. In a large bowl, combine the butter, sugar, vanilla, and salt at medium-low speed just until smooth. Add the flours and mix until just blended. Divide the dough in half and then shape, without overhandling, into 2 disks.

3. On a lightly floured surface, roll 1 piece of dough out into a 13-inch 1/4-inch-thick square. Using a ruler and a fluted pastry wheel or a large knife, trim the edges and cut into 2- by 1-inch rectangles. Transfer the cookies to the baking sheets, spacing 1 1/2 inches apart. Reroll the scraps and repeat with the remaining dough. Mark each cookie several times by poking with the tines of a fork and then chill the pans in the refrigerator for 10 minutes. Bake the cookies for about 17 minutes, until golden and nearly firm in the center. Let cool for 5 minutes on the baking sheets and transfer to racks to cool completely.

Chocolate-Dipped Shortbread: Finely chop 8 ounces semisweet chocolate. Place half of the chocolate in a heatproof bowl set over a saucepan with 1 inch of simmering water and stir until the chocolate is melted and smooth. Add the remaining chocolate to the bowl; remove the bowl from the pot and place on a folded towel. Stir occasionally until the chocolate is smooth. Scrape the chocolate into a small bowl. Line a baking sheet with clean parchment or waxed paper. Dip the cookies halfway into the chocolate, let the excess drip off, and then place on the paper-lined sheet; let stand until set and dry, at least 1 hour.

Peanut Butter Blondies

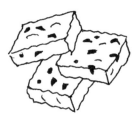

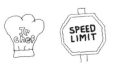

PREP: 10 minutes plus cooling
BAKING: 30 minutes
SPEED LIMIT: 40 mpr

Makes 25 bar cookies

PER COOKIE:
117 calories, 6.5g fat
(3g saturated),
13g carbohydrates,
1g fiber, 2g protein

Peanut butter lovers rejoice! These subtle bars are full of protein and nutty flavor. If your peanut butter is unsalted, add an extra ¼ teaspoon salt to the dough.

> 1 stick unsalted butter, softened
> ½ cup (packed) light brown sugar
> ½ cup granulated sugar
> 1 large egg
> ½ cup unsweetened natural peanut butter
> ½ teaspoon baking soda
> ½ teaspoon fine salt
> ¾ cup white whole-wheat flour
> ¾ cup unbleached all-purpose flour

1. Preheat the oven to 325°F. Lightly butter an 8-inch square metal baking pan.

2. Cream the butter and sugars in the bowl of an electric mixer at high speed until fluffy, about 5 minutes. Add the egg and beat at medium speed until incorporated. Add the peanut butter, baking soda, and salt and mix at low speed until blended. Add the flours and mix until incorporated.

3. Transfer the dough to the prepared pan, pressing evenly with a rubber spatula. Bake for about 30 minutes, until golden and puffed. Let cool completely before cutting into 25 squares.

Cooks' Note

❖ For easy cutting and quicker cooling, line the baking pan with foil: Tear off a 14-inch-long sheet of foil. Invert the pan and mold the foil over the outside. Remove the foil, invert the pan, and fit the foil inside, carefully pressing into the corners. Lightly butter the foil and proceed with the recipe. After baking, let the cookies cool in the pan on a rack for 5 minutes, grasp the foil, and transfer the blondies in the foil directly to the rack to cool.

"Those peanut butter blondies are so awesome!" exclaims Mikey S., a college-age kid from Jackson Hole, Wyoming.

Chocolate Chip Peanut Butter Bars: Mix ½ cup mini-chocolate chips into the finished dough and bake as directed.

Simply Splendid Sugar Cookies

King Arthur's white whole-wheat flour is a must for these crispy, buttery sweets. Use festive sprinkles on them if baking for the holidays.

> 2 sticks (½ pound) unsalted butter, at room temperature
> 1½ cups confectioners' sugar
> 2 teaspoons vanilla extract
> ½ teaspoon baking soda
> ½ teaspoon fine salt
> 1 large egg
> 1⅓ cups white whole-wheat flour
> 1⅓ cups unbleached all-purpose flour
> Coarse white sugar sprinkles, or turbinado (raw) sugar

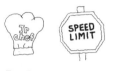

PREP: 10 minutes plus cooling
BAKING: 24 minutes
SPEED LIMIT: 34 mpr

Makes about 40 cookies

PER COOKIE:
90 calories, 5g fat
(3g saturated),
10g carbohydrates,
.5g fiber, 1g protein

1. Arrange the racks in the upper and lower thirds of the oven and preheat the oven to 375°F. Line 2 large cookie sheets with parchment paper. Place some sugar sprinkles in a small bowl.

2. Cream the butter and confectioners' sugar in the bowl of an electric mixer until fluffy, about 5 minutes. Add the vanilla, baking soda, and salt and beat at medium speed until incorporated. Add the egg and beat until incorporated. Add the flours and mix at low speed just until blended.

3. Scoop up enough dough to form into a 1-inch ball, rolling between the palms until smooth. Roll the dough ball in the sugar sprinkles to coat and place on the prepared cookie sheet. Repeat, arranging a dozen coated dough balls evenly spaced on each sheet and then, using a drinking glass, press on the dough balls to flatten to about ¼ inch thick.

4. Bake the cookies for about 12 minutes, switching and rotating the pans halfway through, until the cookies are golden and somewhat firm to the touch. Transfer the cookies with a metal spatula to racks and let cool completely. Repeat with the remaining dough.

Cooks' Note

❖ You can use chocolate sprinkles (from King Arthur) for coating the cookies before baking. Indiatree.com offers colored sugar sprinkles that are dyed with vegetable juices—the pink, orange, and yellow are particularly pretty.

Sugar Cookie Cutouts: Divide the dough in half, wrap in waxed paper, and chill for at least 1 hour. Lightly flour a work surface and then roll out 1 piece of dough to a ¼-inch thickness. Cut out the cookies with cookie cutters. Transfer the cookies with a metal spatula to baking sheets and chill for 10 minutes. Bake the cookies for about 15 minutes, let cool on the baking sheets for 5 minutes, and transfer to racks.

"I like plain cookies and I love these plain cookies!"
sings John-John C., sixteen years old,
of Middletown, New Jersey.

Yin-Yang Black and White Cookies

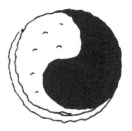

We think these cakelike cookies have excellent karma; eating them will ensure that you have a great day. You can make the cookies ahead: If you wrap them well and unfrosted, they can be frozen for up to a month. Ice them the day you want to serve them. (We have included instructions for both 5-inch cookies and 2½-inch cookies.)

Cookie Batter

- 1 stick plus 2 tablespoons unsalted butter, at room temperature
- ¾ cup plus 2 tablespoons granulated sugar
- 2 large eggs, at room temperature
- 2 teaspoons vanilla extract
- ½ teaspoon fine salt
- ½ teaspoon baking soda
- 1¼ cups unbleached all-purpose flour
- ½ cup plain low-fat yogurt or reduced-fat sour cream
- ½ cup white whole-wheat flour, such as King Arthur

White Frosting

- 1½ cups confectioners' sugar
- 3 pinches of salt
- 2 tablespoons hot water
- 1 tablespoon honey

Black Frosting

- ¾ cup confectioners' sugar
- ¼ cup unsweetened cocoa powder, preferably dark cocoa or Dutch process
- Pinch of salt
- 2½ tablespoons hot water
- 2 tablespoons honey

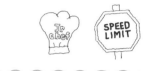

PREP (INCLUDES FROSTING):
15 minutes
BAKING: Small: 14 minutes;
large: 16 minutes
SPEED LIMIT: 30 mpr

Makes 1 to 2 dozen frosted cakelike cookies

PER 1 LARGE COOKIE OR
2 SMALL COOKIES:
155 calories, 6g fat
(3g saturated),
26g carbohydrates,
.5g fiber, 2g protein

1. Make the cookie bases: Arrange the racks in the upper and lower thirds of the oven and preheat the oven to 350°F. Line 2 large baking sheets with parchment paper or silicone sheets.

2. Cream the butter and sugar in the bowl of an electric mixer at high speed until fluffy, about 5 minutes. Add the eggs, one at a time, beating well until blended. Add the vanilla, salt, and baking soda and mix at low speed. Add the all-purpose flour and mix at low until almost blended. Mix in the yogurt and the whole-wheat flour until incorporated.

3. For large cookies: Use a ¼-cup-capacity ice-cream scoop (regular-size scoop) with a release lever to drop the batter in 6 mounds on each baking sheet (or 2 heaping tablespoons for each cookie); top off the mounds with any extra batter. Bake for 11 minutes and quickly switch and rotate the pans and bake for 4 to 5 minutes more, until golden and springy to the touch. For 2½-inch cookies: Drop the batter in 12 mounds, 1 heaping tablespoon each, on both baking sheets; top off the mounds with any remaining batter. Bake for 7 minutes and quickly switch and rotate the pan and bake for about 7 minutes more. Transfer the baking sheets to racks and let the cookies cool completely.

4. Meanwhile, make the frostings. For the white frosting: Combine the confectioners' sugar and salt in a small bowl. Add the water and honey and stir with a fork until smooth. For the black frosting: Combine the confectioners' sugar, cocoa, and salt in a small bowl and stir with a fork to mix. Add the water and honey and stir until smooth. (The icings should be thick enough to spread; if they are at all runny, add more confectioners' sugar, a little at a time, to thicken to the desired consistency.)

5. Spreading a generous tablespoon of white frosting on one half of the flat side of each large cookie (use ½ tablespoon of frosting for each side of the smaller cookies). Then on the other half of each cookie, spread the black frosting. Let dry for at least 15 minutes to set before serving.

Mini-Whoopee Pies

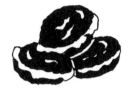

These wee sandwich cakes, also known as Moon Pies, got their start in Pennsylvania Dutch country. They are known as whoopee pies because children exclaim "Whoopee!" when the cakes are ready. Whole Foods sells Tiny Trapeze brand marshmallow cream, made with "no junkie stuff," as the container states.

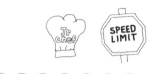

CAKE

1¼ cups unbleached all-purpose flour
¾ cup whole-wheat flour
½ cup unsweetened cocoa, such as Droste
½ teaspoon baking soda
½ teaspoon fine salt
1 stick unsalted butter, at room temperature
1 cup granulated sugar
1 large egg
1 cup milk

FILLING

1 stick unsalted butter, softened
1⅔ cups confectioners' sugar
½ teaspoon vanilla extract
2 cups marshmallow cream

PREP: 20 minutes, plus cooling
BAKING: 14 minutes
SPEED LIMIT: 34 mpr

Makes 3 dozen small sandwich cakes

PER SANDWICH:
146 calories, 6.5g fat (3g saturated),
24g carbohydrates,
.5g fiber, 1.5g protein

1. Arrange the oven racks in the upper and lower thirds of the oven and pre-heat the oven to 425°F. Line 2 large baking sheets with parchment paper.

2. Make the cakes: Whisk together the flours, cocoa, baking soda, and salt in a medium bowl.

3. Cream the butter and sugar in the bowl of an electric mixer at high speed until fluffy, about 4 minutes. Add the egg and milk and beat at medium speed until incorporated. At low speed, add the flour mixture in 2 batches, alternating with the milk, mixing until just blended.

4. Using a half-tablespoon measure, drop 18 generous teaspoons of batter onto each sheet, leaving about 2 inches between cakes. Bake the 2 sheets at the same time, 5 to 7 minutes, until springy to the touch. Let cool on the sheets for 5 minutes, and transfer to racks to cool completely. Change the parchment and repeat using the remaining batter (72 cakes in total).

5. Make the filling: Beat the butter and confectioners' sugar at low speed until blended and then beat at high speed until fluffy, about 5 minutes. Add the vanilla and marshmallow cream and mix at low speed until blended, about 1 minute.

6. Match the pairs of cakes with the same shapes and spread the bottom side of 1 cake with filling and sandwich together with the other cake. (Store the finished whoopee pies in a covered plastic container and chill for up to 3 days.)

"I call them cow pies, because they are brown and white like the cows near my house," says eight-year-old Maddison M., of Traverse City, Michigan. "They're delicious. They feel squishy in my mouth!"

cookie tips

Here are a few steps to ensure your cookie doesn't crumble when you bake it. For more baking tips, check out our dessert chapter.

The Big Chill: Chilling cutout cookies before baking helps them keep their shape during baking.

On a Roll: If rolling out dough, chill it sufficiently and use just enough flour to prevent sticking when rolling out. Try to roll dough evenly for consistent texture. Brush off any excess flour when finished rolling.

Sugar and Spice: When making cookies, be sure your spices are fresh—if older than six months old, throw them out and buy new ones. Also, have on hand a variety of sanding sugar and other sprinkles to decorate cookies.

Dunk It Right: If dipping cookies in chocolate, begin with a bar of high-quality chocolate and chop it fine. Melt half of the chocolate in a double boiler over simmering water; add the remaining chocolate, remove from the heat, and stir until smooth. Don't stir the chocolate more than necessary, and, for best results, dip the cookies into the chocolate as soon as the chocolate is ready.

It's a Wrap: The best way to keep cookies fresh is in a tin. Keep different varieties in separate tins to keep the flavors pure and the cookies crisp or soft. Place sheets of waxed paper in between layers of delicate cookies for extra protection. For gifts, choose sturdier cookies, such as shortbread, oatmeal, blondies, or sugar cookies, and wrap them carefully with waxed paper.

chapter ten

An Introduction to Food Sensitivities

Gluten-Casein-Soy-Free Recipes

Parenthood—it's a whole new world. No matter what you expect, whether it's your first or your fifth child, sometimes things run smoothly, almost carefree, but sometimes they don't.

There are children who will try foods without a thought, almost with haste—those who can immediately appreciate the sight and smell of steamed spring asparagus or pungent roasted wild Alaskan salmon. On the flip side are the skeptics, the ones who look at you with disbelief at the mere suggestion that they dip their forks into what they think could be akin to a bucket of bats, or green beans laced with poison. The wheel of life spins, and we do the best we can with either type of child. It is, after all, one of our duties, besides caring for them nutritionally, to expose our kids to the pleasures of food.

But food preferences and foods that disagree with our genetic makeup are two different matters. As adults we know when we aren't feeling quite "right," but a child may be too young to express this. When something doesn't look right with our child—and the change may seem sudden—it can be alarming, particularly when a legitimate cause is not apparent. An energetic, happy child may become lethargic, irritable, even hostile and aggressive—or appear flushed, feverish. Perhaps his abdomen is bloated. He might exhibit behavior indicating (or complain about) a tummyache, a headache, or even joint pain. Sometimes you'll see dark circles under your daughter's eyes and think these are from a lack of sleep. However, all of these signs can be indicative of food sensitivity.

We are not talking about food allergies but food sensitivities. The two are very different: Allergies and sensitivities are mediated by different elements of the immune system. Allergies, usually more dramatic, can cause hives, vomiting, swelling, trouble breathing, shock, or even death—for example, a severe peanut allergy. Sensitivities are usually subtle—in the intensity of their appearance and in the time they take to develop. Changes in behavior, for instance, can take so long to develop that you may not notice the change until it has become quite significant.

The fairly rapid increase in food sensitivity over the past thirty years is thought to be due to a dysfunction of the immune system, perhaps secondary to environmental influences. It has happened too quickly to be attributed to genetic changes in our body constitution. Regardless of the reason for their presence, food sensitivities have become quite mainstream: There are camps with meal plans for kids on special diets and numerous magazines, newsletters, and websites dedicated to food sensitivities and related chronic illnesses, such as celiac disease. So help and, more important, support is definitely out there (see the list of helpful contacts in the "Experts File" chapter).

The concept of food sensitivity has not enjoyed the support of traditional medicine. For necessary advice, support, and diagnostic testing, we often must access other parents, support networks, and nontraditional or alternative physicians who have expertise in this area. As an example, one mom we know was sure that her son, at age three, was sensitive to cow's milk. She asked his doctor if he would test his food allergies. The doctor indicated that the insurance company would be "mad at him" for doing that kind of testing, and that she should just give the boy soy milk. It was obvious to her that this particular physician wasn't versed at all in the intricacies of food sensitivity. When she did have an appropriate test done, it showed that her son was sensitive to dairy, wheat, beans, and legumes, but, interestingly, much more sensitive to soy than anything else. Metametrix Clinical Laboratory processes food allergy and sensitivity tests (www.metametrix.com). You can also contact them or the Autism Research Institute (www.autism.com and click on DAN—Defeat Autism Now) for a list of practitioners.

Changing a child's diet when food sensitivities are present can literally change the life of that child and his family. Don't underestimate the power of food! We personally know of several cases of children who were diagnosed within the autistic spectrum, but after following a gluten-free, casein-free diet were considered cured within six months. In the early nineties it was unheard of to put an autistic child on a gluten-free, dairy-free diet. Within ten years it has become much more commonplace. However, these sensitivities are not only operative in just those with severe behavioral disorders such as autism; a very significant percentage of "typical" children are affected as well. (Recent studies have shown a link between food additives and hyperactivity.)

Adjusting to a special diet is something the whole family deals with, but it is easier than you might think. Some individuals need to completely adhere to a special diet, and if they are young and have other developmental problems, they may not completely comprehend how important it is. It may mean that certain foods such as cookies and other snacks will be banned from the home. This may lead to some other unhappy campers, but know that the effect of the proper diet on a child cannot be underrated.

A special diet is not cause for heartbreak—for many it is an answer from heaven. Many have seen their child literally bloom when an offending food is removed from her diet. Also, a child with food sensitivities can actually be malnourished because he doesn't absorb nutrients properly. Often these children are very picky eaters, who will test you endlessly. By using some of the recipes that follow and others, you can master the art of patience and learn that a limited, proper diet can be a blessing.

∼ TIPS AND INGREDIENTS ∼

The following information pertains to a diet that is gluten-free, casein-free, and soy-free. Removing gluten, especially in baking, is the most difficult adjustment for a home baker.

Milk

Soy is a common substitute for cow's milk, but if your child is sensitive to soy, it's logical to try rice milk. Be sure the rice milk is gluten-free—many brands contain problematic barley malt (as do many wheat-free cereals). Another option is potato flake milk. A young child will drink these substitutes, and even if an older child refuses to drink any of them, you can use them in cooking.

Butter, Oil, and Shortening

Many vegetable oils, margarines, and shortenings contain soy, and children with sensitivities are often allergic to soy. Safflower oil is rich in monounsaturated fat and light in flavor. For mixing a cake batter, when a creamed butter and sugar mixture is desired, there are some shortening products made of palm oil. Again, know your own child's sensitivities. Ghee is readily available; this is a Middle Eastern product, which is essentially clarified butter with the milk solids removed, so it's safe for those with casein sensitivities. (Make sure the brand you buy is labeled casein-free.) It can be used in place of butter for frying.

Flours

More supermarkets are selling specialty flours, especially rice flour, but there is a greater assortment at the health food store. Be sure to check out the expiration dates on the products you buy, and stock up your freezer when there are sales.

Grains that are safe:

❖ arrowroot, amaranth, buckwheat, corn, millet, potato, quinoa, rice, sorghum, tapioca

Grains to avoid:

❖ wheat, durum, semolina, kamut, spelt, rye, barley

An Oat and Corn Controversy

It is questionable as to whether oats contain gluten. Studies indicate that they probably do not, but they are grown so close to wheat that they may be cross-contaminated from the beginning. Technically are they gluten-free? You have to use your own judgment. Unfortunately in these days of mega lawsuits, many packaged-good companies have changed their labels. For instance, a particular brand of cornflakes would be gluten-free—they are processed on clean equipment—but because the same company makes other products, some of them with wheat, they don't claim that the cereal is gluten-free even though corn doesn't have gluten. They don't even label it as wheat-free.

Gums

The gluten in wheat flour is what gives baked goods their elasticity. Gluten is what makes bread crusty, cakes springy, and bagels chewy. Gluten-free baked goods can be crumbly and dense. To contend with this problem we add xanthan gum or you can add guar gum to your batter. These gums are available at the health food store.

Eggs

Egg whites are a problem for some, but there are a number of egg substitutes in powder form available at the health food store. Often when we use eggs in baking, the whites are whipped separately for improved volume and texture.

Other Leaveners

Look for gluten-free aluminum-free baking powder. Baking soda is not a problem.

Sweeteners

For the sensitive, artificial sweeteners are not advised. Avoid products with high fructose corn syrup, and in your own recipes use honey, preferably locally produced, pure maple syrup, and sugar, preferably organic and unbleached.

Cheese

This popular ingredient is a tough one for some to give up. When cow's milk cheese is a no-no, there is goat cheese, but those who must be casein-free have to avoid that, too.

There are cheeses made of tofu (soy), which are a great option for many. We have found that there are some rice-based cheese products, but they were developed for vegans and usually contain gluten or casein. So, again, be careful and read labels.

Nuts

Tree nuts include the walnut, almond, hazelnut, cashew, pistachio, and Brazil nut. Some people may be sensitive or allergic to certain or all tree nuts. We like to add nuts to baking for texture and nutritional value. The peanut is a legume, so if your daughter has a problem with peanuts it doesn't mean she can't eat tree nuts. Some children do well substituting cashew butter for peanut butter, but again, comprehensive testing is the best way to avoid problems.

Chocolate

Look for organic unsweetened chocolate and bittersweet chocolate that is dairy-free, although keep in mind that the two types are not interchangeable in your baking. (Semisweet and milk chocolate contain milk solids.)

Flavorings

Your health food store will carry gluten-free vanilla and other extract substitutes.

Label Conscious

Read the labels on processed packaged goods, especially lunch meats, pasta, sauces, and salad dressings—even gluten-free products may have other ingredients that are undesirable for you specifically. Avoid products containing modified food starch or modified starch; artificial colors and flavorings; anything with the word *malt* attached to it (these are usually made from barley); caramel coloring; and brown rice syrup (often made from barley). Hydrolyzed plant protein and hydrolyzed vegetable protein contain casein. Those with soy sensitivities should be on the lookout for unspecified types of vegetable oil; these are typically soybean oils. Soy lecithin, which is an emulsifying agent, is permitted because the allergens have been removed during processing.

Storage Wraps and Containers

When you make a batch of rolls or muffins, individually wrap and freeze them. Waxed paper and cellophane bags are best for those who are sensitive in general. Try www.nycake .com for a selection of cellophane bags.

Opening Up the Lunch Box Question

It is hard to believe that some lunch boxes are toxic, and yet some are. Those in question are made of soft vinyl, which is popular because of its insulating qualities. According to the Center for Environmental Health (800-652-0827; www.cehca.org), lead was found on the surface of some vinyl lunch boxes and on the inside surface, where the food is stored. Some boxes have painted designs on them, which also were found to contain lead. You can purchase a simple, inexpensive kit at the hardware store to test your lunch box. (Remember to swab inside and out.) To be on the safe side, when buying a new lunch box, avoid soft vinyl. Look for eco-friendly brands made of cloth or buy an old-fashioned metal box, which never goes out of style. (For more information, go to www.reusablebags.com, www.seventhgeneration.com, and www.simplepureclean.com.)

~ ESPECIALLY DELICIOUS GLUTEN-FREE/ CASEIN-FREE RECIPES ~

The recipes that follow are designed for a diet free of gluten, casein, and soy. Some are simple, but a number of them contain a lot of ingredients. This is due to the nature of baking wheat-free. (We have often added xanthan gum to a combination of flours to help with the texture of the baked goods.) To help with your busy life: Premix batches of dry ingredients for specific recipes, label, and store in the freezer. You will note that we have abbreviated GF for gluten-free and CF for casein-free.

Brown Rice Sandwich Rolls

Gluten-Free Flapjacks

Gluten-Free Waffles

GF Blueberry-Corn Muffins

Thanksgiving Muffins

GF Nutty Carrot Cake Cookies

Flourless Chocolate Cake

GF-CF Marble Cake with
Fudgy Frosting

Meringues for Margie

Peppermint Meringues

Shaved Chocolate Meringues

Tropical Fruit Coconut Macaroons

Chocolate-Covered Strawberries

Brown Rice Sandwich Rolls

The inspiration for these moist and tender rolls, which are better than anything you can buy, and great for sandwiches and toasting, came from Tracey's friend Karen Antone, a mom who is the salt of the earth. There are a lot of ingredients, but once you have measured them out and combined them, mixing and making these rolls is easy. The dough resembles thick cookie dough, which is too moist for kneading and is best portioned out with an ice-cream scoop that has a release lever. You can use all brown rice flour or a mixture of brown and white rice flours.

1 cup warm water (105°F to 115°F)
1 teaspoon sugar
One ¼-ounce packet active dry yeast
½ cup GF vanilla-flavored rice milk, at room temperature
¼ cup honey
¼ cup olive oil, preferably extra-virgin
1 tablespoon cider vinegar
3 large eggs, at room temperature
1 cup brown rice flour
1 cup white rice flour
½ cup sorghum flour, buckwheat flour, or quinoa flour
   (see Cooks' Notes)
½ cup tapioca flour
⅓ cup potato flour, plus more for forming rolls
⅓ cup ground flaxseed (optional)
1 tablespoon xanthan gum
2 teaspoons GF baking powder
1½ teaspoons fine salt
1 teaspoon baking soda

PREP: 20 minutes plus resting and cooling
BAKING: 20 minutes

Makes 1 dozen 3- to 4-inch rolls

PER ROLL:
273 calories, 8g fat (1g saturated), 46g carbohydrates, 3g fiber, 5.5g protein

1. Place the warm water in a glass measuring cup; stir in the sugar. Sprinkle the yeast on top, stir to mix, and let stand.

2. Meanwhile, combine the rice milk, honey, oil, vinegar, and eggs in a medium bowl and beat with a fork or a whisk to blend.

3. Combine the brown rice flour, white rice flour, sorghum flour, tapioca flour, potato flour, flaxseeds, if using, xanthan gum, baking powder, salt, and baking soda in the bowl of a standing electric mixer with the paddle attachment. Mix at low speed until the dry ingredients are well blended. Make

a well in the center of the dry mixture and then pour in the yeast mixture and the eggs mixture. Mix at low speed until well blended, scraping down the bowl as necessary. Cover the bowl with a kitchen towel and let the dough rest for 20 minutes to mature the flavors.

4. Line a large baking sheet with parchment paper. Using a ⅓-cup-capacity ice-cream scoop, scoop out 12 scoops of dough, spacing the mounds evenly on the sheet. Place another half-scoop on top of each mound and, working with floured hands (using more potato flour), lightly shape each mound into a smooth ball. Return to the parchment and shape into a patty (like an English muffin) ¾ inch high. Cover with a towel and let rest while you preheat the oven to 350°F.

5. Bake the rolls in the center of the oven for about 20 minutes, until golden on top, golden brown underneath, and hollow sounding when you tap on top with your finger. Let cool for at least 15 minutes before serving.

Cooks' Notes

❖ Sorghum, buckwheat, and quinoa flours all have specific flavors they lend to the rolls. Any of them is a good choice because they add protein and fiber, but because they are intense, we only suggest a small amount; you can also substitute rice flour for any of them in this recipe. Brown rice flour is also more nutritious than white rice flour.

❖ The addition of tapioca and potato flours and xanthan gum adds chewy texture to the rolls and should not be substituted.

Phillip A., twelve, of Leonardo, New Jersey, loves these rolls with a hamburger or sliced turkey for lunch at school.

Gluten-Free Flapjacks

Pancakes are a treat for breakfast or dinner and are easy enough to make on a weekday morning. Serve with a side of fresh fruit or several strips of nitrate-free bacon. You can double this recipe as needed and can freeze any extra cakes (see Cooks' Note).

½ cup GF vanilla-flavored rice milk
1 large egg
1 tablespoon safflower oil
1½ tablespoons sugar
1 teaspoon GF baking powder
½ teaspoon baking soda
Pinch of salt
¾ cup brown rice flour
¼ cup corn flour
¼ cup tapioca starch
Pure maple syrup, warmed, for serving

PREP: 5 minutes
COOKING: 12 minutes
SPEED LIMIT: 17 mpr

Makes 1 dozen 3- to 4-inch pancakes to serve 4

PER TWO 3½-INCH PANCAKES (4 SERVINGS): 256 calories, 6g fat (1g saturated), 50g carbohydrates, 2g fiber, 4g protein

1. Combine the milk, egg, and oil in a medium bowl, whisking until smooth. Whisk in the sugar, baking powder, baking soda, and salt. Add the rice flour, corn flour, and tapioca starch and stir with the whisk just until smooth.

2. Heat a well-seasoned or nonstick large skillet or griddle over medium heat. Spoon 2 tablespoons batter for each 3½-inch pancake. Cook until bubbles appear on the surface, 1 to 2 minutes. Flip with a spatula and cook until springy to the touch and golden, about 1 minute. Serve with warmed maple syrup.

Cooks' Note

❧ To freeze any extra pancakes, let cool completely and then wrap in pairs in cellophane bags, separated with sheets of waxed paper. To reheat frozen pancakes, unwrap and toast in a toaster oven at medium or place in a single layer on a plate and microwave for about 45 seconds at medium (50%) power or until hot. Serve immediately.

Gluten-Free Waffles: Ladle about ½ cup of batter onto a hot waffle iron and cook according to the manufacturer's instructions.

GF Blueberry-Corn Muffins

Although some prepared gluten-free muffins are available at the health food store and some supermarkets, they tend to be pricey and may contain ingredients unsuitable for your child. These muffins are easy and satisfying—moist and tender, with an ample amount of fruit and a touch of cinnamon. Tracey's son gobbles them up. Serve warm for breakfast, split and spread with nut butter and all-fruit jam for lunch, or as an after-school pick-me-up.

PREP: 10 minutes plus cooling
BAKING: 18 minutes
SPEED LIMIT: 28 mpr

Makes 1 dozen regular-sized muffins

PER MUFFIN:
188 calories, 11g fat (1g saturated), 22g carbohydrates, 1g fiber, 2.5g protein

2 large eggs, separated
$\frac{1}{4}$ cup plus 1 tablespoon sugar
$\frac{1}{2}$ cup safflower oil
2 teaspoons GF baking powder
$\frac{1}{2}$ teaspoon baking soda
$\frac{1}{4}$ teaspoon xanthan gum
$\frac{1}{4}$ teaspoon fine salt
1 $\frac{1}{3}$ cups brown rice flour
1 cup GF vanilla-flavored rice milk
$\frac{2}{3}$ cup corn flour
1 cup organic blueberries, rinsed and patted dry
$\frac{1}{4}$ teaspoon cinnamon

1. Place the oven rack in the upper third of the oven and preheat the oven to 400°F. Lightly oil a 1 muffin pan with 1 dozen $\frac{1}{2}$-cup-capacity muffin cups and set aside.

2. Combine the 2 yolks and $\frac{1}{4}$ cup sugar in the bowl of an electric mixer and beat at high speed until fluffy and pale, about 3 minutes. Gradually drizzle in the oil while beating at medium speed. Add the baking powder, baking soda, xanthan gum, and salt and mix at low speed until incorporated. Add the rice flour and milk and mix at low speed until smooth. Add the corn flour and mix until blended.

3. In a clean, dry mixing bowl, beat the egg whites until stiff. Fold one-third of the whites into the batter lightly and then fold in the remaining whites. Fold in the berries.

4. Spoon the batter into the prepared pan, filling about three-quarters full. Mix the remaining tablespoon of sugar with the cinnamon, sprinkle on top of the muffins, and bake for about 18 minutes, until lightly golden and springy to the touch. Let the muffins cool in the pan on a rack for about 15 minutes;

cut around the edge of each muffin with a small knife and remove from the pan. Let cool completely before serving or freezing.

Cooks' Notes

❖ The muffins freeze nicely: Wrap individually in cellophane and store in the freezer; thaw overnight in the fridge and rewarm or split and toast before serving.

❖ Use the muffins as a sandwich base: Split muffins horizontally and spread with nut butter and your child's favorite jam.

Thanksgiving Muffins: Omit the blueberries and add ⅔ cup finely chopped homemade turkey, ⅓ cup chopped pecans, and ¼ cup dried cranberries or dark currants to the batter.

GF Nutty Carrot Cake Cookies

Can't decide between cookies and cake? Here is the dessert for you. We love the homespun look and texture of these large cookies. They make a great after-school treat for the whole troop.

PREP: 10 minutes
plus cooling
BAKING: 15 minutes
SPEED LIMIT: 25 mpr

Makes about 14 cookies

PER COOKIE:
161 calories, 8g fat
(1g saturated),
21g carbohydrates,
1g fiber, 2g protein

⅓ cup packed light brown sugar
⅓ cup granulated sugar
2 large eggs, at room temperature
¼ cup safflower oil
1 teaspoon gluten-free vanilla flavoring
¼ teaspoon xanthan gum
¼ teaspoon baking soda
¼ teaspoon cinnamon
1¼ cups brown rice flour
2 medium carrots, peeled and coarsely grated (about ½ cup packed)
½ cup pecans, chopped
Confectioners' sugar, for dusting

1. Arrange the racks in the upper and lower thirds of the oven and preheat the oven to 350°F. Line 2 large baking sheets with parchment paper.

2. Combine the brown sugar, granulated sugar, and eggs in the bowl of an electric mixer and beat at high speed until thick and fluffy, about 2 minutes. With the machine running, still at high speed, gradually drizzle in the oil, beating until incorporated. Add the vanilla, xanthan gum, baking soda, and cinnamon and mix at low speed until blended. Mix in the flour at low speed and add the carrots and pecans and mix at low speed until incorporated.

3. Spoon the batter in heaping tablespoons onto the baking sheets, spooning 7 mounds on each sheet, spacing the cookies 3 inches apart. Bake for about 15 minutes, switching and rotating the pans after 12 minutes, until lightly golden and springy to the touch. Transfer the sheets to racks and let the cookies cool completely.

4. Just before serving, lightly dust the cookies with confectioners' sugar.

Cooks' Note

❖ You can individually wrap the cookies in small cellophane bags and freeze. Just pop a frozen cookie into your child's lunch bag and it will come to room temperature and be perfect by midday!

Flourless Chocolate Cake

The pure chocolate of this shallow rich cake goes a long way. It will be pleasing to anyone, and the cake is simple to mix and bake. Dress it up with a dusting of cocoa powder. In summer, you can decorate the platter, around the circumference of the cake, with black-eyed Susans. Tracey often makes this cake for her son's birthday and serves coconut sorbet alongside.

8 ounces dairy-free bittersweet chocolate, preferably organic, finely chopped

1 cup ghee (clarified butter), solid coconut oil, or vegetable shortening (see Cooks' Notes)

1½ cups sugar

6 large eggs

1 cup unsweetened cocoa powder, preferably Dutch-process

2 teaspoons GF vanilla flavoring

PREP: 10 minutes plus cooling
BAKING: 50 to 60 minutes

Makes 1 shallow, dense 9-inch cake to serve about 10

PER SERVING (BASED ON 10 PORTIONS):
480 calories, 41g fat (13g saturated),
40g carbohydrates,
4g fiber, 7g protein

1. Place a rack in the lower third of the oven and preheat the oven to 350°F. Lightly oil a 9- by 2-inch springform pan, line with parchment paper, and oil the paper.

2. Combine the chocolate and ghee in a stainless-steel medium bowl and place on top of a saucepan with 1 inch of simmering water. Whisk occasionally until melted and smooth, and then remove from the heat. Add the sugar and whisk until incorporated. Crack the eggs into a separate bowl and add to the chocolate mixture one at a time, quickly whisking after each addition. Add the cocoa and vanilla and stir with the whisk until smooth.

3. Scrape the batter into the prepared pan and smooth the top. Bake for 50 to 60 minutes, until the top has a thin crust and moist crumbs appear when a cake tester is inserted into the center of the cake. Let cool completely in the pan on a rack and then remove the side of the pan, invert the cake onto a platter, and peel off the paper. Garnish as desired.

Cooks' Notes

❖ Ghee is butter that has been clarified, thus all of the milk solids have been removed. Look for jars marked casein-free in the ethnic section of the supermarket, at Indian markets, and health food stores. Refrigerate any leftover opened ghee.

❖ Adding the eggs quickly helps cool the chocolate mixture. However, it is preferable to add them one at a time for easier blending.

"I want cake"—simple words from Tracey's son Darren after blowing out the candles.

GF-CF Marble Cake with Fudgy Frosting

Birthday parties are really something to celebrate with this moist and tender cake! It has the texture of a typical marble cake—light and springy with delicious chocolate. It is best served the day it is baked.

PREP: 25 minutes plus cooling
BAKING: 50 minutes

Makes 16 servings

PER SERVING:
358 calories, 12g fat
(5g saturated),
62g carbohydrates,
1g fiber, 3.5g protein

CAKE

    3 ounces casein-free bittersweet chocolate, chopped
    4 large eggs, separated, plus 1 egg white at room temperature
    ¾ cup plus ½ cup granulated sugar
    ½ cup safflower oil
    2 teaspoons GF baking powder
    1 teaspoon xanthan gum
    ½ teaspoon baking soda
    ½ teaspoon fine salt
    1½ cups white rice flour
    ¾ cup tapioca flour
    1 cup GF vanilla-flavored rice milk

FROSTING

    3 ounces unsweetened chocolate, chopped
    ½ cup nonhydrogenated all-vegetable shortening (such as Spectrum Organic)
    One 1-pound box confectioners' sugar (4 cups)
    2 teaspoons GF vanilla flavoring
    ¼ teaspoon fine salt
    1 to 2 tablespoons rice milk

1. Make the cake: Arrange an oven rack in the lower third of the oven and preheat the oven to 350°F. Lightly oil a 13- by 9-inch baking pan, line with parchment paper, and oil the paper.

2. Place the bittersweet chocolate in a microwavable small bowl. Microwave at medium (50%) power for 1½ minutes; stir and then repeat heating and stirring until smooth. Reserve while you prepare the batter.

3. Combine the egg yolks and ¾ cup of the sugar in a mixing bowl and beat with an electric mixer at high speed until fluffy and pale in color, about 3 minutes. Gradually drizzle in the oil, mixing at medium speed until incor-

porated. Add the baking powder, xanthan gum, baking soda, and salt and mix at low speed until blended. Add the rice flour, tapioca flour, and milk and mix at low speed until smooth.

4. Place the egg whites in a clean, dry bowl and beat with clean beaters at high speed until soft peaks form when the beaters are lifted. Mixing at medium speed, sprinkle in the remaining $\frac{1}{2}$ cup sugar, 1 tablespoon at a time. Once all of the sugar has been added, mix at high speed until the mixture is thick and glossy. Fold one-third of the whites into the batter to lighten and then add the remaining whites, folding until no streaks of white remain.

5. Scrape two-thirds of the vanilla batter into the prepared pan. Add the cooled chocolate to the remaining batter and fold just until incorporated. Spoon blobs of chocolate batter on top of the batter in the pan, spacing evenly around the pan, and then swirl the batters with the rubber spatula to make a marble pattern. (The batter will rise substantially.)

6. Bake for about 50 minutes, until a cake tester inserted into the center comes out clean. Let cool for 15 minutes. Cut around the sides of the cake with a small sharp knife, turn the cake out onto a rack, peel off the paper, and let cool completely.

7. Prepare the frosting and ice the cake: Place the unsweetened chocolate in a small microwavable bowl. Microwave at medium (50%) power for $1\frac{1}{2}$ minutes; stir and then repeat heating and stirring just until smooth.

8. Place the shortening in a mixing bowl and beat with an electric mixer at high speed until fluffy. Add the confectioners' sugar a little at a time, mixing at low speed until incorporated. Gradually drizzle in the melted chocolate, add the vanilla and salt, and mix at medium speed until smooth. Add 1 to 2 tablespoons of the rice milk and beat until the desired consistency is reached. Invert the cake onto a serving platter and spread the frosting on the top and sides of the cake.

"Yummmmmmyyyy," says seven-year-old Daniel K., of Middletown, New Jersey.

Meringues for Margie

These cookies were named for Tracey's auntie Marge, who spent several years in Paris as a young girl. (At that time, she ate meringues—her favorite thing—every day for at least four years!) Tracey's son, Darren, loves them in a variety of flavors (see the variations). They are an easy homemade treat and keep well in a tin.

PREP: 15 minutes
BAKING: 1 hour

Makes about 2 dozen cookies

PER COOKIE:
*17 calories, 0g fat,
5g carbohydrates,
0g fiber, .5g protein*

*2 egg whites, at room temperature
Pinch of salt
Pinch of cream of tartar
¾ cup superfine sugar
1 teaspoon GF vanilla flavoring*

1. Arrange the racks in the upper and lower thirds of the oven and preheat the oven to 350°F. Line 2 large cookie sheets with parchment paper.

2. Place the egg whites in the bowl of an electric mixer and beat at medium speed until foamy, about 2 minutes. Add the salt and cream of tartar, beat again at medium, and gradually add the sugar, slowly sprinkling in 1 tablespoon at a time. Once the sugar is added, continue beating until the mixture is stiff. Add the vanilla and fold until barely incorporated.

3. Drop the batter by heaping teaspoons onto the prepared cookie sheets, spacing them 1½ inches apart. Place in the hot oven, shut the door, and turn off the oven. Do not open the oven for at least 1 hour.

Cooks' Notes

❖ Egg whites are easier to separate when they are cold.

❖ Be sure when separating the whites from the egg yolks that absolutely no yolk gets mixed in with the whites, or the whites will not whip up to full volume.

❖ When beating egg whites it is important to use bowls and beaters that are dry and grease-free.

❖ Store meringues in a cookie tin at room temperature to maintain their crispness.

Peppermint Meringues: Gently fold 1 cup of crushed red-and-white peppermint hard candies into the stiff sweetened egg whites.

Shaved Chocolate Meringues: Gently fold a finely chopped 4-ounce bar of dairy-free bittersweet chocolate into the stiff sweetened egg whites.

Tropical Fruit Coconut Macaroons

You can substitute your favorite dried fruit in these chewy bonbons, which are best served slightly crispy on the day they are made. Tracey made something similar to these for a Christmas issue of *Nick Jr.* magazine.

3 tablespoons filtered water
⅔ cup sugar
1 tablespoon light corn syrup
¼ teaspoon fine salt
2 cups unsweetened shredded coconut
4 pieces dried mango, finely chopped (⅓ cup)
2 slices dried pineapple, finely diced (about ½ cup)
2 slices dried papaya, finely diced (¼ cup)
2 large egg whites
½ teaspoon GF vanilla flavoring

PREP: 15 minutes
BAKING: 12 minutes
SPEED LIMIT: 27 mpr

Makes about 2 dozen

PER MACAROON:
61 calories, 2g fat
(2g saturated),
11g carbohydrates,
1g fiber, 1g protein

1. Arrange the racks in the upper and lower thirds of the oven and preheat the oven to 400°F. Line 2 large cookie sheets with parchment paper.

2. Combine the water, sugar, corn syrup, and salt in a small saucepan and bring to a boil. Remove from the heat and pour into a heatproof large bowl. Stir in the coconut, mango, pineapple, and papaya until well mixed. In a small bowl, beat the egg whites and vanilla together with a fork until frothy and then stir into the coconut mixture.

3. Drop heaping tablespoons of dough onto the cookie sheets, spacing the mounds about 1½ inches apart. Bake for 10 to 12 minutes, until golden. Let cool completely on the baking sheets on a rack.

Cooks' Note

❖ Store macaroons in a tin or covered plastic container at room temperature for up to 3 days.

Chocolate-Covered Strawberries

Do you remember the first time you ate a chocolate strawberry? Well, we both do. The key to success is to melt half of the chocolate so it is smooth and warm and then add the remaining chocolate and stir until smooth. The chocolate is guaranteed to set. It's a trick we learned from our favorite *chocolatier*, Jacques Torres.

PREP: 10 minutes plus standing

Makes 20 strawberries

PER STRAWBERRY:
45 calories, 3g fat
(1.5g saturated),
7g carbohydrates,
1g fiber, 1g protein

20 ripe large strawberries, at room temperature
6 ounces dairy-free organic bittersweet chocolate, finely chopped
$\frac{1}{4}$ teaspoon safflower oil

1. Rinse the berries, leaving the stem leaves intact, and gently pat dry. Line a large baking sheet with parchment and set aside.

2. Place half of the chocolate in a small metal bowl over a small saucepan with 1 inch of simmering water. Stir the chocolate until completely melted and warm. Remove the bowl from the saucepan; immediately add the remaining chocolate and let stand for 3 minutes. Add the oil and stir until smooth.

3. Dip the strawberries one by one in the chocolate: Hold a berry by the leaves and dunk, covering about five-sixths of the fruit with chocolate. Lift up over the bowl, let the excess chocolate drip off, and transfer the berry to the prepared baking sheet. Repeat with the remaining berries and chocolate.

4. Let stand until set, about 30 minutes. Serve at room temperature.

Cooks' Note

❖ Use room-temperature berries for dipping; chilled fruit will cool the melted chocolate too quickly and blooming (discoloration of the chocolate) may occur.

store-bought gluten-free mixes we like

Here are some gluten-free products and manufacturers we use. Because this is a rapidly changing food industry, there are new products popping up all the time. Read the labels on all products—even if you have used them before. Many items that are gluten-free contain dairy ingredients. For more recommendations, go to www.realfoodforhealthykids.com.

Van's Wheat Free Waffles
Cherrybrook Kitchens cake mixes
Frozen Muffins by George
Bob's Red Mill Gluten-Free flours
Arrowhead Mills flours, mixes, and cereals
Spectrum Naturals products
Hain Gluten-Free Baking Powder
Erewhon cereals
Barbara's Gluten-Free cereals
Pamela's cookies
Health Valley cereals and snacks
Gluten-Free Pantry products
Bearitos chips and snacks
Ener G products
Quinoa Corp. flour and pastas
Pacific Rice Milk products
Rapunzel Bittersweet Chocolate
Planet Harmony Organic Fruit Candies
Mary's Gone Crackers

chapter eleven

First Foods
Great Recipes for Six to Thirty-Six Months Old

t's an exciting day when baby supplements the breast or bottle with solid food. The first time he or she tastes real food, it is a startling experience for the baby and a hilarious one for the parents, as the food comes careening out of the little one's mouth, since the concept of swallowing food is a learned one.

After the first weeks of baby cereal (usually barley, rice, and oat varieties), he moves on to real food. The question then becomes what, how much, and at what time. Our best advice is to follow your pediatrician's recommendations as to timing, schedules, and amounts. If you buy factory-processed baby food, be sure to buy organic. (One recommended brand is Earth's Best; for others, see "Store-Bought Baby Foods We Like," on page 337). However, even with the best brands, you're still giving your baby processed products that have sat on shelves for who knows how long. But while making the food yourself seems too big a task for exhausted, stressed parents, it's actually easy and much more inexpensive to make your own. All it requires on your part is a small amount of planning. Here are recipes, from A to Z, for purees and suggestions for finger foods, as well as information on storing issues, food allergies, milk, and when to introduce foods.

~ SOUND BITES ~

As hard as it is to believe, it will never be easier to get your kids to eat broccoli puree or spinach pie than at this age, so this is the time to truly feed them well. Hopefully, they will end up liking many of the things you first feed them; plus, you will have given them a healthy start. Amazingly, a lot of parents don't take advantage of this time: A study of infants and toddlers published in 2005 and financed by Gerber found that most children up to the age of two did not have anywhere near the recommended daily fruit and vegetable intake. In fact, one-third of toddlers did not eat any fruit on a given day and about a fifth had no vegetables. And the most common "vegetable"? French fries.

While there is no definitive evidence that a lack of healthy produce at the beginning of one's life will have long-lasting irreparable effects—although deficiencies of calcium and iron can occur as the result of an unhealthy diet—it can make it more difficult for kids to like fresh, wholesome foods as they grow.

When a baby or a toddler (and even older) tries a new food, it can take up to twelve times before her palate gets used to the dish. Many parents give up after a few times, so it's important to introduce a food—and, once no allergic reaction occurs within the subsequent two to three days—to continue to serve it up. If after more than a dozen times baby still refuses kale, try peas. Just keep experimenting, but then do try to reintroduce the food he doesn't like later on.

As to the important issue of organics: As *Consumer Reports* magazine concluded in 2005, "Because children's developing bodies are especially vulnerable to the toxins found in nonorganic baby food, it pays to buy organic food for baby as often as possible. Children may be at risk of higher exposure to the toxins found in nonorganic food because baby food is often made up of condensed fruits or vegetables, potentially concentrating pesticide residues." The same applies to making your own. *Consumer Reports* recommends always buying organic for these items: meat, poultry, eggs, dairy, apples, bell peppers, celery, cherries, imported grapes, nectarines, peaches, pears, potatoes, raspberries, spinach, and strawberries. When organic is not available, make sure to wash produce extremely well, even things you peel, such as melon, oranges, and bananas.

~ GOT MILK? ~

When baby turns one, he or she can be switched from breast or formula to whole milk (baby cannot digest the protein in cow's milk before then) and should not be given low-fat milk until at least the age of two, unless a pediatrician has given the go-ahead. Toddlers need about 2 cups of whole milk daily divided throughout the day.

Soy milk is a popular alternative to cow's milk, but the decision to give that instead should be discussed with your pediatrician first. (Soy milk does not contain all of the vitamins cow's milk does.)

Finally, a few words on the condition of lactose intolerance: The inability to digest lactose, the predominant sugar found in milk, is not uncommon in toddlers and could vanish suddenly, when a child is older. If your child experiences stomach discomfort or actual diarrhea after drinking milk, consult your pediatrician. The doctor may have you cease or limit dairy products, switch to soy or rice milk, or have your child take a lactase liquid or tablet. For more information, log on to the website for the National Digestive Diseases Information Clearinghouse (see the "Experts File" chapter).

~ FOOD GLORIOUS FOOD ~

Once your pediatrician has given the go-ahead for solids—usually when baby reaches about six months—you can introduce your little loved one to the wonderful world of food. Generally, bland cereal mixed with breast milk or formula is the only solid for a couple of weeks (see our homemade baby cereal recipe, D Is for Delicious Baby Cereal). Your doctor will no doubt advise to always start the meal, whether breakfast, lunch, or dinner, with breast milk or formula, followed by cereal (usually barley, then rice, then oatmeal), followed by a veggie or fruit puree. One note: Just as you wouldn't give a ten-year-old a cupcake before her green beans, do not start baby with something sweet followed by savory. Always give savory items first and if baby is still hungry, a fruit puree is the follow-up.

The First Solids: Six to Twelve Months

These are foods that baby can try. With the exception of the banana and avocados, all should be cooked (baked, boiled, or steamed) through.

Dairy: breast milk or formula
Grains: barley, rice, oats
Fruits: apples, apricots, avocados, bananas, nectarines, peaches, pears, plums, prunes, pumpkin
Protein/Meat: chicken, turkey, tofu purees
Vegetables: acorn/butternut squash, green beans, peas, yellow squash, sweet potatoes, zucchini, potatoes

The I-Can-Feed-Myself Months: Twelve to Twenty-Four Months

All of the above foods plus:

Dairy: whole milk plain yogurt, cream cheese, cottage cheese, pasteurized unaged cheeses, ice cream
Grains: Cheerios, multigrain no-salt crackers, graham crackers without honey, pasta, bagels
Fruits: blueberries, cantaloupe, kiwi, mangos, papaya
Protein/Meat: egg yolks, lean beef or pork, lentils
Vegetables: asparagus, broccoli, cauliflower, eggplant, spinach

The Not-So-Terrible Twos: Twenty-Four Months to Thirty-Six Months

All of the above foods plus:

Dairy: low-fat milk, if desirable, any type of cheese as long as it's pasteurized
Grains: any, preferably whole or multigrain
Fruits: berries, pitted cherries, oranges, lemon, grapes cut into quarters or halves
Protein/Meat: whole eggs, mild white fish (no tuna or other high-mercury fish), cut-up nuts
Vegetables: beets, corn, cucumbers

A Is for Applesauce

B Is for Butternut Squash

C Is for Carrots

D Is for Delicious Baby Cereal

E Is for Eggs

F Is for Fruit Purees

G Is for Gobble-Gobble Turkey

H Is for Honeydew Ice

I Is for Instant Banana Snack

J Is for Jellied Fruit

K Is for Kiwi

L Is for Lentils

M Is for Mango Mixer

N Is for Nummy Pasta and Cheese

O Is for Oats and Groats

P Is for Petit Peas

Q Is for Quick Dinner

R Is for Rich Rice Pudding

S Is for Spinach

T Is for Tofu

U Is for Ultimate Juice

V Is for Veggie Mash

W Is for Whole-wheat Teething Biscuits

X Is for Xcellent Meat and Taters

Y Is for Yams

Z Is for Zucchini

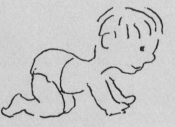

A Is for Applesauce

This applesauce was a big hit with Tanya's twins when they were first eating solids. You can make it in big batches because it freezes well (and when baby is about 9 months, you can make this blend chunkier). These three varieties are particularly complementary, but any organic apple works, except for the undelicious Red Delicious. You can always add things to applesauce such as banana puree, baby cereal, or mashed mango.

1 Granny Smith apple, peeled, cored, and sliced
1 Golden Delicious apple, peeled, cored, and sliced
1 Fuji apple, peeled, cored, and sliced
1 cup water
Pinch of cinnamon (optional)

In a large saucepan, cook the apple slices with the water over medium heat until tender, about 12 minutes. Add the cinnamon, if using, and stir. With a handheld immersion blender, blender, or food processor, puree the apples and add some or all of the cooking liquid until the desired consistency is created.

PREP: 5 minutes
COOKING: 12 minutes
SPEED LIMIT: 17 mpr

Makes 2 cups (4 to 8 servings)

B Is for Butternut Squash

At the Steel household, butternut squash is made almost every week and turned into soups and mashes. Here is a simple mash-up that your baby will undoubtedly love. It needs no adornment and is packed with vitamins. We use the cooking water to make it smoother but you can also use breast milk or formula.

Pinch of cinnamon (optional)
1 medium to large butternut squash, halved lengthwise and deseeded
1 cup water

PREP: 2 minutes
COOKING: 45 minutes
SPEED LIMIT: 47 mpr

Makes 6 servings

1. Preheat the oven to 400°F. Sprinkle the cinnamon, if using, on each squash half and then place flesh down on an aluminum foil–lined baking sheet. Add the water. Bake until the flesh is very soft when pierced with a fork, about 45 minutes.

2. Remove the flesh from the skin with a spoon. Using either a handheld immersion blender, a blender, or a food processor, puree the squash and then add cooking liquid (or breast milk/formula) for the desired consistency. Serve at room temperature.

C Is for Carrots

Loaded with vitamins and an inherent sweetness, organic carrots are a great starter food for baby.

2 carrots, peeled and sliced into ½-inch-thick rounds
Breast milk or formula

In a large saucepan of boiling water, cook the carrots until tender, about 12 minutes. Drain, then using a food processor or a handheld immersion blender, puree the carrots and add a tablespoon or two of the breast milk/formula until the desired consistency is reached.

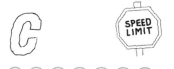

PREP: 1 minute
COOKING: 12 minutes
SPEED LIMIT: 13 mpr

Makes 1 to 2 servings

D Is for Delicious Baby Cereal

Here is a good basic cereal. As baby gets a little older, you can add a few things to the cereal such as a tablespoon of banana puree. You can make this ahead and refrigerate it for a day or two—at most—or simply have the rice, barley, or oatmeal ground and ready to go.

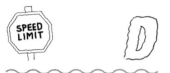

PREP: 1 minute
COOKING: 3 minutes
SPEED LIMIT: 4 mpr

Makes 1 serving

*¼ cup brown or long-grain white rice or oatmeal (not instant
    or quick-cook variety)*
⅓ cup filtered water
Breast milk or formula

In a food processor, grind the brown rice or oatmeal until it is a fine powdery substance (babies over 7 months can have unground). Transfer to a medium saucepan, add the water, and cook on medium heat until thick and cooked through, about 3 minutes. Let cool and add a tablespoon or two of breast milk or formula until the desired consistency is reached. Serve lukewarm or at room temperature.

E Is for Eggs

Eggs are a great way for baby to get protein. However, until baby has reached one, she should only have the yolk, not the white. The key is to buy organic eggs and make sure that you cook them thoroughly to guard against salmonella. Once baby is older, go to the breakfast chapter for omelets, poached eggs, and other egg ideas. To start baby off on eggs, here is a foolproof way to make hard-cooked eggs.

2 organic eggs
1 tablespoon breast milk or formula

Fill a small saucepan with cold water, leaving 2 inches of room at the top. Place the eggs in the cold water to cover and bring to a boil. Remove from the heat, cover with a lid, and let stand for 10 minutes. Drain, cover with iced water to cool, and transfer to a small bowl and store in the fridge. (Don't peel until ready to use, and discard after 2 days.) Peel gently, cut in half, and remove the yolk. Smash with a fork and add the breast milk or formula until the desired consistency is reached.

PREP: 12 minutes
SPEED LIMIT: 12 mpr

Makes 2 servings

F Is for Fruit Purees

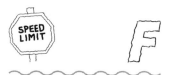

PREP: 2 minutes
COOKING: 25 minutes
SPEED LIMIT: 27 mpr

Makes 1 serving

Fruit makes a great puree and a thirst-quenching smoothie, and is just plain fun to pick up and eat for toddlers. You can serve fruit raw, but the flavor intensifies if you bake it. This recipe applies to any firm fruit, such as apples and pears, and stone fruit, such as peaches, pears, plums, and apricots. This can be frozen, although nutrients will be lost.

Pinch of cinnamon (optional)
1 piece ripe hard fruit, such as an apricot, apple, or pear (if using
*   plums, use 2), halved and pitted or cored*
¼ cup filtered water

1. Preheat the oven to 400°F. Sprinkle a pinch of cinnamon, if using, on each apricot half and place flesh down on a glass baking dish. Pour in the water and bake for 20 to 25 minutes, until the flesh is very soft when pierced with a fork.

2. Remove the skin from the flesh with a knife. Using a handheld immersion blender, a blender, or a food processor, puree the fruit and add some or all of the pan juices until the desired consistency is reached. If the fruit is too tart for baby, you can add a ¼ teaspoon of sugar. Serve at room temperature.

G Is for Gobble-Gobble Turkey

Turkey is a tom-terrific way to introduce baby to meaty puree. We've added some yam/sweet potato puree to the mix so he can enjoy a plateful of Thanksgiving any day of the year. If you want to speed this recipe up, you can use 1 cup cooked turkey breast cut into 1-inch pieces and ½ cup Y Is for Yams puree blended together.

½ yam or sweet potato, peeled, trimmed, and cut into ⅓-inch slices
1 cup raw ground turkey or ground chicken

1. In a saucepan of boiling lightly salted water over medium heat, cook the yam until tender, about 5 minutes. Reserve ½ cup of the yam cooking water and then drain.

2. Meanwhile, place the turkey in the saucepan and cook, stirring and adding a tablespoon or two of the yam liquid, until no pink remains, about 4 minutes. Transfer the turkey and yam to a blender or a food processor and puree until smooth, adding the reserved cooking water to achieve the desired consistency.

PREP: 2 minutes
COOKING: 10 minutes
SPEED LIMIT: 12 mpr

Makes 2 to 4 servings

H Is for Honeydew Ice

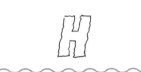

PREP: 5 minutes
FREEZING: 2 hours

**Makes about 8 ice pops or
3 ice-cube trays**

If it's a hot summer's day, nothing will be more refreshing to your little one than some lightly sweet honeydew ice. If you have a toddler who can hold an ice pop, you can pour the mixture into plastic cups or molds, put a wooden stick in, and make your own ice pop. This recipe was inspired by one that ran in *Gourmet* magazine several years back and became a favorite in the Steel household.

One small (2-pound) honeydew melon (or watermelon or cantaloupe)
3 tablespoons sugar
¼ cup filtered water

1. Halve, quarter, and seed the melon. Using a knife, cut the slice away from the peel and cut each slice into 1-inch pieces.

2. Combine the sugar and water in a small saucepan and cook over medium heat, stirring, until dissolved, about 1 minute. Let cool. Place half of the melon in a blender, pour in the sugar syrup, and blend until smooth. Add the remaining melon and blend again. Pour into an ice-cube tray or ice-pop mold and let freeze, about 2 hours.

I Is for Instant Banana Snack

To make this a more substantial meal, mix in ¼ cup cooked baby cereal.

2 ripe bananas
¼ cup breast milk or formula

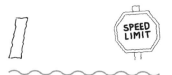

Using an immersion blender, a blender, or a food processor, puree the bananas with the milk until the desired consistency is created.

Cooks' Note

❖ Bananas are loaded with potassium and make a great dessert, but if baby suffers from constipation, you need to limit banana intake.

PREP: 1 minute
COOKING: 1 minute
SPEED LIMIT: 2 mpr

Makes 2 servings

J Is for Jellied Fruit

Instead of making gelatin mixes with artificial coloring and lots of sugar, you can whip up an easy gelatin with fresh fruit.

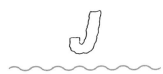

PREP: 1 hour including chilling

Makes 4 servings

One 2-pound wedge seedless watermelon, cut up, at room temperature
One ¼-ounce packet unflavored gelatin
2 tablespoons granulated sugar
1 tablespoon fresh lemon juice

1. Force the watermelon through a juicer or puree in a food processor; strain through a fine sieve. (You should have about 2 cups of juice.)

2. Place ¼ cup of the watermelon juice in a heatproof bowl. Sprinkle the gelatin on top and let stand to soften for 5 minutes, then microwave for 30 seconds to melt the gelatin. Stir in the sugar and lemon juice and then stir the gelatin mixture into the remaining watermelon juice. Spoon the mixture into four 6-ounce custard cups or ramekins, wrap, and chill until set, about 30 minutes. Cut into small squares to serve baby.

K Is for Kiwi

Kiwi is loaded with vitamin C but can be hard for toddlers to pick up, as it's so slippery—here's an easy way for them to eat kiwi.

1/4 cup Cheerios or three 2-inch plain graham cracker squares
1 slightly soft ripe kiwi

In a food processor, pulse the Cheerios or graham crackers until fine. Place into a plastic sealable bag. Peel the kiwi and cut into small cubes, about 1/4 inch each. Add to the plastic bag, shake repeatedly until the kiwi is coated with the crumbs, and serve.

PREP: 2 minutes
SPEED LIMIT: 2 mpr

Makes 1 serving

Cooks' Note

❖ Avoid graham crackers with honey or added sugar coating.

L Is for Lentils

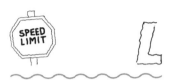

COOKING: 45 minutes

Makes 6 to 8 servings

Legumes, of which lentils are one variety, are a great source of protein and fiber. This takes a bit of time to prepare but will keep baby happy and full. Legumes can sometimes make baby gassy, so watch the first time he or she eats this to see if that results. You can add tofu or cheese to the lentils.

2 cups dried green lentils
½ teaspoon kosher salt
¼ cup breast milk or formula (optional)
¼ cup shredded mozzarella cheese (optional)

Rinse the lentils twice and discard any debris. Cook in a large pot of boiling salted water until the lentils are very soft, about 45 minutes. Drain, return to the pot, and add milk or formula, if using, as desired for a creamy consistency, or stir in the cheese, if using. Serve warm or at room temperature.

M Is for Mango Mixer

Mango is a fruit that baby will love eating any which way. It is rich in vitamins A, B, and C, but when the baby is under a year, it can be hard to digest. If baby does have problems digesting it raw, steam or boil it and let cool before blending. This drink is better suited for a toddler, as it's thick and needs to be drunk out of a sippy cup or with a straw.

> 1 ripe mango, peeled and cut into cubes (see page 229 for cutting tips)
> ½ cup plain whole milk yogurt
> 1 tablespoon wheat germ
> Breast milk, formula, or whole milk (optional)

Using a handheld immersion blender, a blender, or a food processor, puree the mango, yogurt, and wheat germ until smooth. If it seems too thick for your baby, thin it with breast milk, formula, or milk, if using, until the desired consistency is created.

PREP: 2 minutes
COOK: 1 minutes
SPEED LIMIT: 3 mpr

Makes 4 servings (12 ounces)

N Is for Nummy Pasta and Cheese

This is a simpler version of our Mega Mac 'n' Cheese for toddlers (page 171). We like to use fine, small whole-wheat macaroni, such as Da Vinci brand, which cooks fast and is nutritious. It also freezes well. See our Introduction for freezing tips.

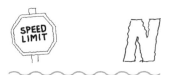

PREP: 5 minutes
COOKING: 10 minutes
SPEED LIMIT: 15 mpr

Makes 5 cups (about 10 servings)

1⅓ cups (6 ounces uncooked) small whole-wheat elbow macaroni, such as Da Vinci brand
1 tablespoon unsalted butter
1 tablespoon unbleached all-purpose flour
1 tablespoon cornstarch
1 cup whole milk, formula, or breast milk
1 cup mild Cheddar cheese, coarsely shredded

1. Bring a large saucepan of water to a boil; add the macaroni and cook, stirring often, until nicely tender, about 5 minutes. Drain in a colander and rinse with cool water until cool. Reserve.

2. Melt the butter in the same pasta pot over medium heat. Stir in the flour and cook, stirring, for 1 minute. Whisk the cornstarch into the milk and add to the pot, whisking, until the mixture is thick. Bring to a boil, reduce the heat, and simmer, whisking, for 1 minute longer. Add the pasta and cheese and stir until melted.

O Is for Oats and Groats

Oatmeal is a nutritious way to start the day off for baby, but it also makes a great gloppy filling snack for any time.

> 1/4 cup rolled or old-fashioned oats or baby oatmeal cereal
> 1/3 cup breast milk, formula, or milk
> 1/3 ripe banana, mashed with a fork

Pulse the whole oats in a food processor until fine. Combine the oatmeal, milk, and banana in a small saucepan. Bring the mixture to a boil, reduce the heat, and simmer, stirring often until tender, about 3 minutes. Add more milk as desired to thin the mixture.

PREP: 1 minute
COOKING: 3 minutes
SPEED LIMIT: 4 mpr

Makes 1 serving

P Is for Petit Peas

Baby peas are one of the best foods for toddlers; they love picking them up and feeding themselves.

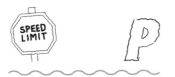

PREP: 2 minutes
COOKING: 5 minutes
SPEED LIMIT: 7 mpr

*Makes 1 cup (2 to
4 servings)*

1 cup frozen petit peas
½ teaspoon olive oil or ¼ tablespoon unsalted butter (optional)

Bring 1 cup of salted water to a boil in a small saucepan. Add the peas, reduce the heat, and simmer until soft, about 5 minutes. Drain and then toss with oil or butter, if using, and serve as is, or mash or puree to the desired consistency.

Q Is for Quick Dinner

When your toddler is hungry, she needs some protein and carbohydrates. An omelet can be whipped up in a flash and you can add anything to it. Try some finely diced boiled ham (about a half slice) or a tablespoon or two of thawed frozen peas or finely chopped cooked spinach. After a baby is one, whole eggs are fine, but before then, simply use the yolk.

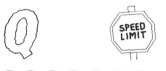

PREP: 1 minute
COOKING: 2 minutes
SPEED LIMIT: 3 mpr

Makes 1 serving

1 large egg, preferably cage-free or organic
1½ teaspoons cold water
1 teaspoon extra-virgin olive oil or unsalted butter
1 tablespoon shredded cheese, such as Cheddar, Swiss, or Monterey Jack

1. Combine the egg and water in a small bowl; beat with a fork until well blended.

2. Heat the oil in a small well-seasoned skillet over medium-high heat. Pour in the egg and cook, scrambling constantly with a fork, a silicone spatula, or a wooden spatula until the egg is almost cooked through, about 1 minute. Remove from the heat.

3. Spread the egg in an even layer and sprinkle the cheese on top. Place the pan over very low heat and let stand for 1 minute to set. Fold over in half and transfer to a plate and let stand for a minute to melt the cheese. Let cool before serving.

R Is for Rich Rice Pudding

This pudding has more protein than a basic rice pudding. Because of the whole milk and eggs, it is suitable for children only over one year old.

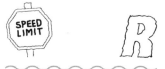

PREP: 5 minutes
COOKING: 30 minutes
SPEED LIMIT: 35 mpr

Makes 6 servings

2 cups Perfect Rice (page 196)
1½ cups whole milk, plus more if desired
2 tablespoons sugar
2 large eggs, beaten

1. Combine the rice, milk, and sugar in a heavy small saucepan, cover, and bring to a boil over medium heat. Reduce the heat to low and simmer gently for 15 minutes.

2. Beat the eggs with a fork in a heatproof medium bowl. Add half of the hot rice mixture and mix well to blend. Transfer that mixture back to the saucepan and stir over low heat until steaming hot but not boiling. Transfer the pudding to a food processor and process for 1 minute. (The mixture will still have texture.) Scrape the pudding into a clean bowl and chill for 30 minutes, stirring occasionally, before serving. Cover any remaining pudding after it has cooled.

S Is for Spinach

This puree can be made heartier with ground cooked brown rice. For those under one, use formula or breast milk to make this creamy.

½ pound organic baby spinach leaves, well rinsed
½ tablespoon unsalted butter
1 teaspoon unbleached all-purpose flour
¼ cup milk, formula, or breast milk

1. Bring ½ inch of water to boil in a medium skillet. Add the spinach leaves and stir until wilted, 1 to 2 minutes. Drain in a colander. Rinse with cold running water until cool. Squeeze the spinach in batches by hand or through a fine-mesh sieve to remove as much liquid as possible.

2. Melt the butter in the same pan over medium heat, add the flour, and stir for 1 minute. Whisk in the milk and bring to a boil.

3. Transfer the spinach mixture to a food processor. Puree until smooth and then let cool before serving.

PREP: 10 minutes
COOKING: 10 minutes
SPEED LIMIT: 20 mpr

Makes 4 servings

T Is for Tofu

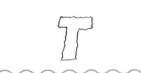

Tofu is packed with protein and isoflavones and is a great partner for many foods. You can cut some firm tofu into small cubes and combine with cut-up pear or roll tofu cubes in crushed graham cracker crumbs. For babies over one, you can whip silken tofu in a blender with a little bit of yogurt or cream cheese and some strawberries and/or banana to make a smoothie.

When buying tofu, look for the type (firm, soft, and silken) that is right for the dishes you are making. Purchase tofu in sealed tubs with a freshness date stamped on the container, not bulk tofu that is stored in a large container of water at the market.

U Is for Ultimate Juice

Breast milk or formula is the drink of choice until baby is one, and water is a great next choice, but for variety, homemade juice can be an option for toddlers and older kids. Make sure to use only organic fruit, and if you don't have a juicer, think about investing in one. You can use a blender or a food processor, but it's important then to strain the juice.

> 1 small apple, preferably McIntosh, peeled, cored, and quartered
> 1 small navel orange or blood orange, peeled, sectioned,
>   and pitted
> 1 medium carrot, peeled and cut into chunks

Process the apple, orange, and carrot in a juicer to extract the juice, or place in a blender or a food processor with $1/4$ cup of water and blend until smooth; strain through a fine-mesh sieve.

PREP: 2 minutes
COOKING: 1 minute
SPEED LIMIT: 3 mpr

Makes 1 to 2 servings
($3/4$ cup)

V Is for Veggie Mash

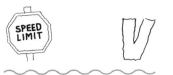

PREP: 5 minutes
ROASTING: 20 minutes
SPEED LIMIT: 25 mpr

Makes 2 to 4 servings

You can roast just about any vegetable for this mash (check out our other Monster Mashes in our dinner chapter). If you don't have time to roast the veggies, you can steam or boil them until tender.

> 1 parsnip, peeled, trimmed, and cut into 1/3-inch slices
> 1 carrot, peeled, trimmed, and cut into 1/3-inch slices
> 1 small yam or sweet potato, peeled, trimmed, and cut into
>   1/3-inch slices
> Extra-virgin olive oil, for drizzling
> 1/4 cup formula, breast milk, or milk

1. Preheat the oven to 450°F and line a large shallow baking sheet with foil. Peel the parsnip, carrot, and yam, cut into 1/3-inch-thick slices, and transfer to the prepared baking sheet. Drizzle the oil on top, toss well, and spread the vegetables out on the pan.

2. Bake for 15 to 20 minutes, until the vegetables are tender and golden brown on the edges. Let cool slightly and transfer to a bowl, add the milk, and mash to the desired consistency.

W Is for Whole-Wheat Teething Biscuits

Many teething biscuits crumble and break too easily. These are a little sturdier and safer for baby to eat.

¼ cup milk or formula
1 large egg yolk
1½ tablespoons vegetable oil
1 teaspoon pure vanilla extract
1 cup whole-wheat flour
1 tablespoon rolled oats
1 tablespoon wheat germ
Pinch of cinnamon
1 teaspoon sugar
1 tablespoon nonfat dry milk

PREP: 10 minutes
BAKING: 15 minutes
SPEED LIMIT: 25 mpr

Makes 10 biscuits

1. Preheat the oven to 350°F. Lightly grease a large cookie sheet. Combine the milk, yolk, oil, and vanilla in a medium bowl and whisk to blend. Add the flour, oats, wheat germ, cinnamon, sugar, and dry milk and stir together to make a stiff dough.

2. On a lightly floured work surface, roll out the dough to a ¼-inch-thick rectangle, and using a cookie cutter or glass with a 3-inch rim, cut into cookies. Transfer to the prepared sheet, spacing 2 inches apart. Bake for 15 minutes, or until golden and firm.

X Is for Xcellent Meat and Taters

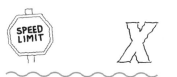

PREP: 1 minute
COOKING: 2 minutes
SPEED LIMIT: 3 mpr

Makes 2 to 4 servings

Take advantage of your leftovers for baby's dinner! You can use any cooked meat in this recipe.

½ cup finely diced or chopped cooked meat or poultry
¼ cup thawed frozen peas
¼ cup cooked mashed potatoes, rice, or pasta
¼ cup breast milk, formula, or milk

In a small saucepan, combine all of the ingredients and cook, stirring, over medium heat until thoroughly hot. Using a handheld immersion blender, a blender, or a food processor, puree the mixture, adding a little more breast milk or formula as necessary, until the desired consistency is reached. Serve at room temperature.

Y Is for Yams

You can use yam or sweet potato in this dish. Both are rich in vitamins A and C. If you are pressed for time, you can boil or steam the veggie.

Pinch of cinnamon (optional)
1 medium yam or sweet potato, scrubbed and halved, ends trimmed
½ cup filtered water

1. Preheat the oven to 400°F. Sprinkle the cinnamon, if using, on the yam halves and put cut side down on a glass baking dish. Pour in the water and bake until the potato is soft, about 30 minutes.

2. Scoop out the flesh from the skin. Using a handheld immersion blender, a blender, or a food processor, puree the yam and cooking liquid (or breast milk or formula) until the consistency you desire is created. Serve at room temperature.

PREP: 3 minutes
COOKING: 30 minutes
SPEED LIMIT: 33 mpr

Makes 2 servings

Z Is for Zucchini

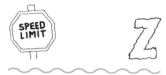

PREP: 2 minutes
COOKING: 10 minutes
SPEED LIMIT: 12 mpr

Makes 2 servings

Toddlers can eat raw sticks of zucchini and will love dipping them into a yogurt-based sauce, such as Rockin' Ranch Dressing (page 219). This mild zucchini mash is a great first vegetable for baby.

1 medium zucchini, peeled and sliced into ½-inch-thick slices
1 teaspoon olive oil (optional)

Bring 1 inch of water to a boil in a medium saucepan. Insert a steamer and fill with the zucchini. Cover with a lid and cook until the zucchini is tender, about 8 minutes. Using a handheld immersion blender, a blender, or a food processor, puree the zucchini and add the oil, if using, or a little bit of the cooking liquid (or breast milk or formula) until the consistency you desire is created. Serve at room temperature.

~ TIPS FOR MAKING FIRST FOODS ~

❖ Generally, salt, sugar, and pepper are unnecessary to add to baby's food. Let the flavor come from the food itself.

❖ Freezing breast milk destroys its nutritious qualities. Do not freeze breast milk or food you make with it.

❖ Allow frozen food to thaw overnight in the refrigerator, and then warm gently in a saucepan.

❖ If you do microwave food, make sure to use a microwave-safe glass container. Microwave at brief intervals (about 30 seconds) and stir often while heating.

❖ Let toddlers feed themselves by offering them foods such as cooked sweet potato pieces or banana slices in ice-cube trays or muffin baking tins.

~ STORING HOMEMADE BABY FOOD ~

Refrigerating: In general, use fresh homemade baby food within seventy-two hours, keeping it chilled in the refrigerator.

To Warm: Heat food gently in a small saucepan over medium-low heat, stirring, until warm. Test the heat by spooning a little of the warm mixture onto your wrist.

To Freeze: Spoon a freshly made fruit or vegetable puree into a glass container with a lid or into an ice-cube tray and cover with plastic. Freeze until firm and then release the cubes from the tray and transfer to a freezer bag. Mark the bag with a label indicating the contents and date. Use frozen puree within two weeks of freezing to maintain the nutritional content.

To Defrost: Thaw puree overnight in the refrigerator or place in a bowl on top of a saucepan over an inch of simmering water, cover, and let "steam" over a hot water bath to quickly thaw. Do not leave out on the counter overnight to thaw, as bacteria can grow.

~ CHOKING HAZARDS ~

Here is a partial list of foods that should not be served whole to children until they are at least two years old:

Hot dogs
Raisins
Popcorn
Grapes
Nuts
Seeds

food allergies

These foods have been known to cause allergic reactions in little ones, so introduce these foods one at a time and then watch for any reactions, including hives, rashes, difficulty breathing, and vomiting, for forty-eight hours after ingesting. Generally, these foods can be introduced between twelve and twenty-four months, but consult your pediatrician first and read our food allergy section in the Introduction.

Peanuts and peanut butter
Soy products, including vegetable oil
Cow's milk and other dairy products containing casein
Tree nuts, such as walnuts and pecans
Fish and shellfish
Egg whites
Honey
Strawberries
Chocolate
Wheat

~ BABY TEETHING? ~

Hand her a frozen mini-bagel or frozen banana to gnaw on. It will chill her gums a little, provide a snack, and take her mind off the pain.

~ FINGER FOOD TIPS ~

* When baby has more than just gums for mashing up food and shows an interest in putting things in his mouth—usually by about ten months—talk to your pediatrician about starting him on finger foods.
* Never leave baby unattended when she is eating, and make sure she is sitting upright.
* Begin with foods you already know he likes, cutting tender pieces into small dice instead of mashing.
* For foods that are slippery, such as small tofu cubes and diced fruit, place in a resealable plastic bag, add crushed cracker or graham cracker crumbs, and shake to coat for easy handling.

~ FINGER FOODS FOR TODDLERS ~

Just about anything that is small (pea-sized) and healthful can be given to toddlers. They love to feed themselves but can cram too much food in at once, so never leave them alone when they are chowing down. Here is a small sampling of finger food ideas:

Whole-wheat pasta shapes, such as wheels or rotelle, cut up
Cut-up raw, steamed, or roasted vegetables, such as carrots, zucchini, and broccoli
Thawed frozen shelled edamame (soybeans)
Toasted whole-wheat soldiers (toast cut into thin sticks)
Cut-up pasteurized organic cheeses
Cut-up fruit
Small chunks of tofu
Mini-meatballs, quartered
Diced dried fruit, such as apricots or pears
Diced pieces of ham, cooked turkey, or chicken

~ STORE-BOUGHT BABY FOODS WE LIKE ~

Here are a few baby food companies making high-quality products. For more suggestions, log on to www.realfoodforhealthykids.com.

Evie's Organic Edibles
Homemade Baby
Garden of Eating line
Happy Baby (FreshDirect)

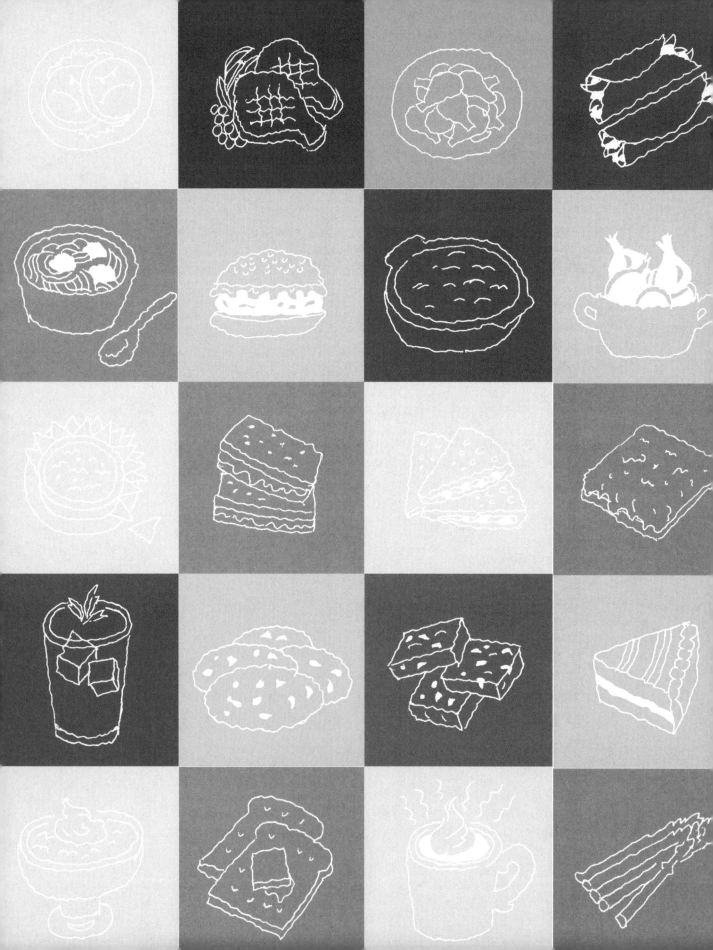

chapter twelve

The Experts File

Want to learn more about health and nutrition? Find a Community Sponsored Agriculture unit near you? Get books on creating birthday parties? Here are some great resources we found that will help guide you in your quest to raise healthy, happy children. For more sources, books, websites, and other information, log on to www.realfoodforhealthykids.com. (Please note: Some website URLs might have changed since publication.)

~ NUTRITION GUIDES AND COOKBOOKS ~

A Parent's Guide to Childhood Obesity: A Road Map to Good Health by the American Academy of Pediatrics

Guide to Your Children's Nutrition by the American Academy of Pediatrics

Jane Brody's Nutrition Book: A Lifetime Guide to Good Eating for Better Health and Weight Control

Eat, Drink, and Be Healthy: The Harvard Medical School Guide to Healthy Eating

The American Dietetic Association's Complete Food and Nutrition Guide

Great Parties for Kids: Fabulous and Creative Ideas for Children Aged 0–10 by Charlotte Packer and Rose Hammick

The Kids Pick-A-Party Book by Penny Warner

The Surprising Power of Family Meals: How Eating Together Makes Us Smarter, Stronger, Healthier and Happier by Miriam Weinstein

~ WEBSITES AND NEWSLETTERS ~

For more helpful websites and newsletters, go to our website, realfoodforhealthykids.com.

American Dietetic Association (www.eatright.org)
American Academy of Pediatrics (www.aap.org)
The National Institutes of Health's Medline Plus (www.nlm.nih.gov/medlineplus/nutrition.html)
The Mayo Clinic (www.mayoclinic.com/health/food-and-nutrition/NU99999)
The United States Department of Agriculture (www.mypyramid.gov)
Tufts Health and Nutrition Letter (www.healthletter.tufts.edu)
Nutrition for Kids (www.nutritionforkids.com/)
Eat Smart, Grow Strong (www.eatsmartgrowstrong.org)
Kids Health (www.kidshealth.org)
The Eat Well Guide (www.eatwellguide.org)
Home Food Safety (www.homefoodsafety.org)
NutritionData (www.nutritiondata.com)

Autism Organizations

Autism Speaks is a support group for families and a link to many other sites (www.autismspeaks.org).
Autism Research Institute can help you find an MD to help test your child for food sensitivities (www.autism.com).
Halo (Helping Autism through Learning and Outreach) Clinic offers teaching methods for nonverbal children (www.halo-soma.org).

~ KIDS COOKING CLASSES—VIRTUAL AND ACTUAL ~

Check out *Shaw Guides to Cooking Schools* (www.shawguides.com) and these individual schools and sites:

Little Chefs (www.littlechefs.com)
Culinary Institute of America (www.ciachef.edu/enthusiasts/programs/hp-kids.asp)
Kids Cooking Company (www.kidscookingcompany.com)
Les Petites Gourmettes (www.lespetitesgourmettes.com)
Chefs2Be (www.chefs2be.com)

~ FARMER'S MARKET SOURCES ~

Great sites for information on farmers' markets:

Local Harvest (www.localharvest.org)
The United States Department of Agriculture (www.ams.usda.gov/
    farmersmarkets)

For community-supported farms:

Sustainable Agriculture Research and Education (www.sare.org)
National Sustainable Agriculture Information Service (www.attra.ncat.org)
Biodynamic Farming and Gardening Association (www.biodynamics.com/
    csa.html)
The New Farm (newfarm.org/farmlocator)

~ MAIL-ORDER FOODS ~

Companies that deliver high-quality foods include:

Whole Foods (www.wholefoods.com)
FreshDirect (www.freshdirect.com)
Wegman's (www.wegmans.com)
Shaw's (www.shaws.com)
Peapod (www.peapod.com)
Pioneer Organics (www.pioneerorganics.com)
Niman Ranch (www.nimanranch.com)

~ FOOD SENSITIVITY INFORMATION ~

There are a lot of resources out there but probably the best clearinghouses are these:

Food Allergy Initiative (www.foodallergyinitiative.org)
The National Digestive Diseases Information Clearinghouse (digestive.niddk
    .nih.gov)
Peanut Allergy Home Page (www.peanutallergy.com)
Celiac.com: A Celiac and Gluten-Free Resource (www.celiac.com)

chapter thirteen

The Last Course
Critics and More

Here you will find a list of our esteemed food critics who faithfully tasted these recipes and gave their very considered opinions, plus some seasonal weekly meal planners.

~ REAL FOOD FOR HEALTHY KIDS FOOD ~ CRITICS PANEL

These kids across America spent time critically judging our recipes. Their opinions—and great quotes—are greatly appreciated!

Adam M., Cornish, Maine

Aidan C., Bronx, New York

Alexander C., Princeton, New Jersey

Alfred M., Royal Palm Beach, Florida

Allaire M., Port Chester, New York

Andrea S., Cornish, Maine

Andrew M., Rye, New York

Betsy A., San Diego, California

Blaine G., Cornish, Maine

Bobby S., Harrisonburg, Virginia

Brendan D., Rye, New York

Brenna M., Port Chester, New York

Brian L., Rye, New York

Brian S., Boca Raton, Florida

Brittany R., Porter, Maine

Caroline C., Weston, Connecticut

Catherine D., Rye, New York

Ceri D., Valencia, California

Christina H., Atlanta, Georgia

Clayton Z., Port Chester, New York

Cole H., New York, New York

Connor D., Bronx, New York

Connor G., Oxford, Mississippi

Darren F., Middletown, New Jersey

Elijah S., Booneville, Indiana
Emma S., Rye, New York
Emory Z., Port Chester, New York
Fiona G., New York, New York
Gabriel B., Oxford, Mississippi
Gabriel C., Bronx, New York
Greg M., Rye, New York
Hayley K., Rhinebeck, New York
Isabel G., New York, New York
Isabelle M., Matawan, New Jersey
Jack B., Rye, New York
Jackson F., Brooklyn, New York
Jacob E., Westport, Connecticut
Jacob S., Booneville, Indiana
John-John C., Middletown, New Jersey
Julia B., Rye, New York
Kaylen M., Port Chester, New York
Kelly M., Middletown, New Jersey
Kelsey S., Rye, New York
Kevin M., Rye, New York
Kobey W., Porter, Maine
Lila E., Westport, Connecticut
Lua L., Amagansett, New York
Lucas M., Rye, New York
Macey M., New York, New York
Maddison M., Traverse City, Michigan
Maeve D., Valencia, California
Margot F., Middletown, New Jersey

Mark L., Rye, New York
Martin C., Bronx, New York
Max D., Tavernier, Florida
Max M., Bethel, Connecticut
Megan L., LaGrange, Kentucky
Mia H., New York, New York
Mikey S., Jackson Hole, Wyoming
Miles A., San Diego, California
Nathan S., San Diego, California
Owen C., Bronx, New York
Owen F., Brooklyn, New York
Pablo L., Brooklyn, New York
Patrick N., Kezar Falls, Maine
Paul-Michael M., Royal Palm
    Beach, Florida
Phillip A., Leonardo, New Jersey
Rosey M., Studio City, California
Ruby S., Amagansett, New York
Sanger S., Port Chester, New York
Sara H., Rye, New York
Sarah C., Rye Brook, New York
Stephen M., Rye, New York
Taven M., Traverse City, Michigan
Tehmina P., Brooklyn, New York
William S., Port Chester, New York
Wyatt Z., Port Chester, New York
Zane S., Amagansett, New York
Zuzu F., Brooklyn, New York

∼ SEASONAL WEEKLY MEAL PLANNERS ∼

Use these menu ideas to assist you in planning meals for your family. Serve portions that are appropriate for your children's specific needs and make use of leftovers when you can.

Autumn

Sunday

Breakfast: Brioche French Toast (page 48) with sliced pears
Lunch: Harvest Tomato Tart (page 184)

Snack: Chunky Guacamole (page 104) with whole-grain tortilla chips
Dinner: Slow-Roasted Pork Shoulder (page 147), Rainbow Slaw (page 205),
    A Is for Applesauce (page 307)
Dessert: Big Peach and Blackberry Cobbler (page 259)

Monday

Breakfast: Hole-y Eggs! (page 29)
Lunch: Edamame Succotash Salad (page 82)
Snack: Celery stuffed with cottage cheese
Dinner: Mexican Tomatoes Rellenos (page 148), mixed salad with Mexican
    Adobo Dressing (page 217)
Dessert: Pan-grilled fresh pineapple slices

Tuesday

Breakfast: Good Day Pear Crisp (page 36)
Lunch: Choppy-Choppy Salad (page 84) with cold roast pork
Snack: Mini-antipasto
Dinner: Lazy Lasagna (page 161), green salad with ABC Vinaigrette
    (page 215)
Dessert: Fresh berries with cinnamon whipped cream

Wednesday

Breakfast: Broccoli 'n' Cheese Breakfast Burrito (page 32)
Lunch: California-Style Tuna Salad Rolls (page 78)
Snack: Celery stuffed with natural peanut butter
Dinner: Easy-Bake Scampi (page 129), steamed broccoli
Dessert: Baked apples

Thursday

Breakfast: Carrot Cake Oatmeal (page 33)
Lunch: Bento Box Chef's Salad (page 73)
Snack: Tree House Trail Mix (page 100)
Dinner: Sultan's Chicken-Couscous Bake (page 160), Squish Squash (page 208)
Dessert: Sautéed fresh plums with vanilla low-fat yogurt

Friday

Breakfast: Scrambled eggs, The Great Pumpkin Toddy (page 236)
Lunch: Classic Tabbouleh (page 81), sliced turkey
Snack: Ba-Ba Banana Bread (page 52)
Dinner: Pop's Spinach Pie (page 182)
Dessert: The Great Pumpkin Toddy (page 236), Easy-Does-It Applesauce Cake (page 258)

Saturday

Breakfast: Best Eggs on Earth (page 39)
Lunch: Mellow Yellow Split Pea Soup (page 167), whole-grain toast
Snack: Veggies and Homemade Onion Dip (page 105)
Dinner: Spaghetti and Meatballs (page 169), Hail Caesar, Jr. (page 119)
Dessert: Vanilla Angel Food Cake (page 257)

Winter

Sunday

Breakfast: Green Eggs-in-Ham Quiche Cups (page 40)
Lunch: Vegetable Grilled Cheese Quesadillas (page 87)
Snack: Golden Garlic Hummus (page 108) with baby carrots and baked pita chips
Dinner: Perfectly Punctual Prime Rib (page 136), Special Occasion Biscuits (page 64), Blasted Winter Vegetables (page 199)
Dessert: Lively Lemon Granita (page 268)

Monday

Breakfast: Sunshine Parfait (page 37)
Lunch: Country Ham Gems (page 80)
Snack: Chewy Granola Bars (page 99)
Dinner: Roast Beef Hash (page 137), Zucchini-Parmesan Pancakes (page 200)
Dessert: Sliced bananas with frozen yogurt and wheat germ

Tuesday

Breakfast: Strongman's Oatmeal (page 34), sliced mango
Lunch: Turkey Pinwheels (page 79)
Snack: Happy Apple Toddy (page 236)

Dinner: Crabby Cakes (page 128), Creamed Spinach (page 198)
Dessert: Blueberry Cheesecake Smoothie (page 228)

Wednesday

Breakfast: Tomorrow's French Toast (page 35)
Lunch: Roast Beef Siberians (page 77)
Snack: stoned wheat crackers, Homemade Onion Dip (page 305)
Dinner: Thai Green-Curry Chicken (page 120), Perfect Rice (page 196)
Dessert: Low-fat vanilla yogurt with fresh orange segments and cinnamon

Thursday

Breakfast: Apple-Maple Oatmeal (page 33)
Lunch: Bacon Banana-Rama (page 74)
Snack: Cottage cheese with carrots, celery, and breadsticks
Dinner: Super Steak Fajitas (page 126), green salad
Dessert: Sliced apple and low-fat vanilla yogurt

Friday

Breakfast: Potato and cottage cheese omelet
Lunch: Choppy-Choppy Salad (page 84), Blue on Blue Dressing (page 218),
    sesame bread sticks
Snack: Tree House Trail Mix (page 100)
Dinner: Easy-Bake Scampi (page 129), Harvest Ratatouille (page 201)
Dessert: Vanilla Angel Food Cake (page 257)

Saturday

Breakfast: Perfect Poached Eggs (page 43) in a cup with toasted soldiers
Lunch: Popeye's Panini Presto (page 89)
Snack: Zucchini Tempura (page 102), Horseradish Dunk (page 103)
Dinner: Nan's Shepherd's Pie (page 158), green salad
Dessert: Flourless Chocolate Cake (page 295), whipped cream

Spring

Sunday

Breakfast: Protein Power Pancakes (page 47)
Lunch: Chickpea Pita Pockets (page 94)

Snack: Homemade Onion Dip (page 105) with baked potato chips and fresh vegetables
Dinner: Good-as-Gold Roast Chicken (page 149), Tater-Brocky (page 207)
Dessert: Chocolate-Covered Strawberries (page 300)

Monday

Breakfast: Spinach and Bean Taco (page 31)
Lunch: Hail Caesar, Jr. (page 119) with cold chicken
Snack: Tree House Trail Mix (page 100)
Dinner: Chicken Enchilada Casserole (page 140), Hasty Hash Browns (page 193)
Dessert: Cheddar cheese and sliced apple

Tuesday

Breakfast: Carrot Cake Oatmeal (page 33)
Lunch: Peanut Butter Berry-wich (page 74)
Snack: Low-fat yogurt, Extreme Granola (page 50)
Dinner: Chicken Salad Melt (page 90), green salad with ABC Vinaigrette (page 215)
Dessert: Semisweet chocolate

Wednesday

Breakfast: Bursting Berry Muffins (page 53)
Lunch: Crunchy Asian Chicken Salad (page 75)
Snack: Strawberry Cheesecake Smoothie (page 228)
Dinner: Mexican-Style Pan-Roasted Pork with Pineapple (page 123), Totem Poles (page 202)
Dessert: Mango sorbet

Thursday

Breakfast: Sunshine Parfait (page 37)
Lunch: Bento Box Chef's Salad (page 73)
Snack: Kamikaze Eggs (page 109)
Dinner: Super Steak Fajitas (page 126)
Dessert: Ricotta cheese with fresh strawberries

Friday

Breakfast: Cold cereal with sliced banana
Lunch: Egg Salad Double-Decker Sandwiches (page 76), celery sticks
Snack: Lovey's Parmesan Treats (page 101)
Dinner: Grilled Wild Salmon (page 143), Turkish Green Beans (page 203)
Dessert: Lemon Sour Cream Cake (page 254)

Saturday

Breakfast: Blue Ribbon Pancakes (page 46), pan-fried ham
Lunch: Sumo Salmon Cakes with Salad (page 144)
Snack: Golden Garlic Hummus (page 108), whole grain crackers
Dinner: Grilled Pint-Sized Pizzas (page 133), Boardwalk Fresh Lemonade (page 225)
Dessert: Dreamy Creamy Cheesecake (page 265)

Summer

Sunday

Breakfast: Best Eggs on Earth (page 39)
Lunch: Middle Eastern Veggie Burgers (page 95) with Sesame Sauce (page 95)
Snack: Lovey's Parmesan Treats (page 101)
Dinner: Juicy Flank Steak (page 141), Hasty Hash Browns (page 193), steamed
   broccoli
Dessert: Brown Mouse (page 264)

Monday

Breakfast: Huevos Rancheros (page 88)
Lunch: Classic Tabbouleh (page 81)
Snack: Sliced cantaloupe with cottage cheese
Dinner: My Hero! (page 142),
   Super-Mash! (page 206)
Dessert: Watermelon Gell-ee (page 267)

Tuesday

Breakfast: Strongman's Oatmeal (page 34), carrot juice
Lunch: Turkey Pinwheels (page 79)
Snack: Fresh cherries

Dinner: Penne Primavera (page 181), Choppy-Choppy Salad (page 84),
   Blue on Blue Dressing (page 218)
Dessert: Lively Lemon Granita (page 268)

Wednesday

Breakfast: Cheese Omelet (page 42), small green salad
Lunch: Peanut Butter Berry-wich (page 74)
Snack: Sliced watermelon
Dinner: Crispy Jamaican Pork with Pan-Fried Bananas (page 122), sautéed spinach,
   corn on the cob
Dessert: Low-fat yogurt with Extreme Granola (page 50)

Thursday

Breakfast: Toaster Oven Use-Yer-Bean Taco (page 31)
Lunch: Roast Beef Siberians (page 77)
Dinner: Middle Eastern Couscous with Tofu and Vegetables (page 189)
Dessert: Mango Lassi (page 229)

Friday

Breakfast: Hole-y Eggs! (page 29)
Lunch: California-Style Tuna Salad Rolls (page 78)
Snack: Sliced apple and peanut butter
Dinner: Not-Your-Basic Turkey Burger (page 121), Grilled Spudniks (page 197)
Dessert: Sliced plums with yogurt and Extreme Granola (page 50)

Saturday

Breakfast: Belgian Waffles (page 45) with mixed berries
Lunch: Grilled Vegetable Cheese Quesadillas (page 87), cucumber slices, grape
   tomatoes
Snack: Island-Style Smoothie (page 227)
Dinner: Peachy Keen Chicken (page 115), Creamed Spinach (page 198),
   Berry Delicious Iced Tea (page 226)
Dessert: Cheery Cherry Plank (page 260), whipped cream

index